The Vascular System: Health and Preservation of Vessel

The Vascular System: Health and Preservation of Vessel

Jayce Spencer

FOSTER ACADEMICS
www.fosteracademics.com

www.fosteracademics.com

FOSTER ACADEMICS

Cataloging-in-publication Data

The vascular system : health and preservation of vessel / Jayce Spencer.
p. cm.
Includes bibliographical references and index.
ISBN 978-1-64646-586-6
1. Cardiovascular system--Diseases. 2. Cardiovascular system. 3. Blood-vessels--Physiology.
4. Cardiovascular system--Physiology. I. Spencer, Jayce.
RC669 .V37 2023
616.1--dc23

Foster Academics,
118-35 Queens Blvd., Suite 400,
Forest Hills, NY 11375, USA

ISBN 978-1-64646-586-6 (Hardback)

Contents

Preface

Every book is a source of knowledge and this one is no exception. The idea that led to the conceptualization of this book was the fact that the world is advancing rapidly; which makes it crucial to document the progress in every field. I am aware that a lot of data is already available, yet, there is a lot more to learn. Hence, I accepted the responsibility of editing this book and contributing my knowledge to the community.

Blood vessels are tubular structures through which the body fluids i.e., blood and lymph circulate. There are three main types of vessels, namely, arteries, veins and capillaries. Most of the patient care management plans usually require that the medical staff is able to access the vessels of the patient's body in addition to preserving the vessels. In administering medicines and vital fluids to patients, vascular access is a standard technique. Vascular access procedure requires that a flexible and sterile plastic tube (called catheter) is inserted into the blood vessel of a patient for drawing blood from the body or to inject medication into the body. There are many complications associated with administering medicines or essential fluids through this procedure like phlebitis (inflammation of the vein), deep vein thrombosis (DVT), and infections leading to discomfort to the patients. To protect the veins, and minimize damage and consequences, it is critical that vessel health should be assessed for each patient. This book elucidates the concepts around future developments with respect to vascular health and preservation. With its detailed analyses and data, it will prove immensely beneficial to professionals and students involved in this area of medicine at various levels.

While editing this book, I had multiple visions for it. Then I finally narrowed down to make every chapter a sole standing text explaining a particular topic, so that they can be used independently. However, the umbrella subject sinews them into a common theme. This makes the book a unique platform of knowledge.

I would like to give the major credit of this book to the experts from every corner of the world, who took the time to share their expertise with us. Also, I owe the completion of this book to the never-ending support of my family, who supported me throughout the project.

Editor

Part I

VHP: An Overview

1

Vessel Health and Preservation Model

Nancy L. Moureau

Abstract

More than 90% of patients admitted to acute care receive intravenous access for the delivery of treatment. The concepts of vessel preservation and risk reduction incorporate the topics that apply to all aspects of vascular access insertion and management for patient intravenous (IV) medical treatment. By following a specific clinical pathway of care that adheres to evidence-based practice, the outcomes are optimized, veins are preserved, and the treatment plan completed while minimizing delays and complications. VHP promotes patient-focused practices that reduce morbidity of untoward effects associated with intravenous devices.

Keywords

Vessel health · Vessel health and preservation
Quadrants of care · Vascular access assessment and selection · Vein assessment
Insertion · Care and management
Vascular access evaluation

N. L. Moureau (✉)
PICC Excellence, Inc., Hartwell, GA, USA

Menzies Health Institute, Alliance for Vascular Access Teaching and Research (AVATAR) Group, Griffith University, Brisbane, QLD, Australia
e-mail: nancy@piccexcellence.com

1.1 Introduction to Vessel Health and Preservation

Vessel health and preservation (VHP) is a model applied to vascular access and the administration of IV medications and treatment that structures evidence-based practices within four quadrants of medical care: assessment/selection, insertion, management, and evaluation of vascular access devices. The model incorporates evidence-based practices, guidelines, and recommendations from many countries to guide practice from patient admission through completion of treatment. Application of the VHP is designed to ensure a higher level of safety for the patient, reduce risk with device selection, limit negative consequences of insertion using specially trained clinicians, promote complication-free device longevity through proper care and maintenance practices, and complete the process by evaluating and removing devices as soon as treatment is completed. From the first quadrant to the last, evidence guides practice as implemented in education to clinicians providing care.

The aim of the VHP model and pathway is to improve quality of care, reduce risks associated with vascular access devices (VADs), and increase patient satisfaction and efficiency in the use of healthcare resources. The model is represented in a pathway within quadrants of care that follow the patient treatment process. A clinical pathway is a step-wise process for management of patient care that promotes efficiency within a defined group of patients, those requiring vascular access devices, during a defined period such as the treatment process (De Bleser et al. 2006; Hanchett and Poole 2001). The content of a clinical pathway is based on scientific evidence, research, recommendations, and professional consensus. Clinical pathways improve patient outcomes by reducing variability, adding standardization, and reducing medical errors (Panella et al. 2003).

Assessment is represented in the first quadrant of the pathway with proactive site selection as the first stage of the VHP model (Fig. 1.1). Ensuring that each device is clinically indicated and the lowest risk necessary for the treatment and duration intended is vital to the patient safety (Chopra et al. 2015). Following patient and vein assessment, stage two is intravenous device selection and insertion by a qualified clinician.

Quadrant two includes the insertion stage where the final selection of the type of device, number of lumens, insertion procedure, and most qualified inserter are selected. Study and evaluation of intravenous device size, length, type, complications, insertion procedures with outcomes, and patient risk factors are all vital to this stage. It is within insertion that visualization technologies are employed to promote the highest degree of success.

Establishing and maintaining a route of access to the bloodstream is essential for patients in acute care. Quadrant three encompasses maintenance of the device, which is the longest stage in the life of the catheter. The last stage of the VHP model involves discontinuation of the treatment and removal of the device, followed by evaluation of patient outcomes and clinician competency. Education for clinicians inserting and managing the devices is an overarching theme of the entire model and is incorporated into all four quadrants of care.

Each of these stages forms an intentional process to guide selection, insertion, management, and discontinuation of the vascular access device (VAD). Often medical facilities are driven by default actions, based on crisis management when a VAD fails, opting to quickly select and replace with another similar device rather than thinking through the patient-specific process of selection. The concepts of vessel preservation and risk reduction incorporate the problems and subjects that apply to all aspects of vascular access insertion and management for patient IV medical treatment. VHP establishes a framework or pathway that follows each step of the patient

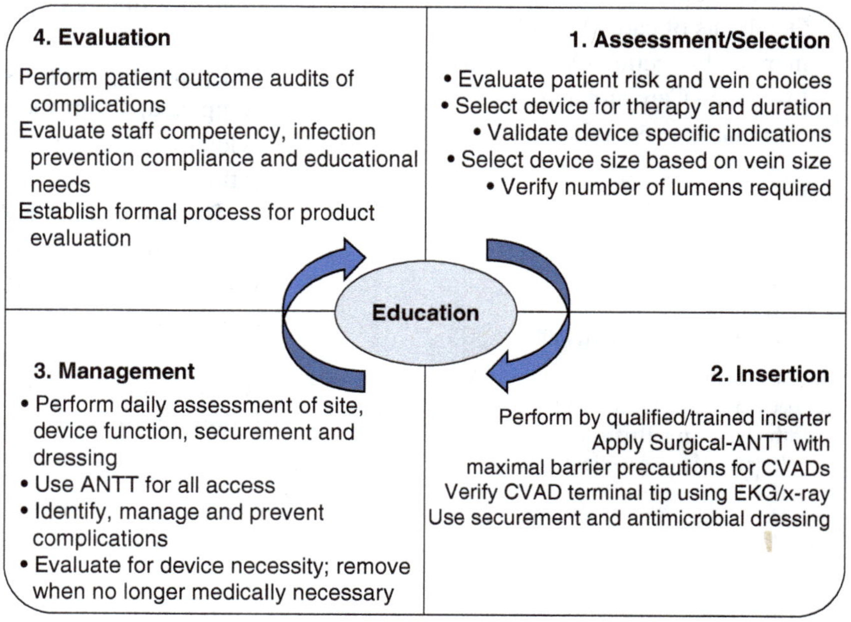

Fig. 1.1 Vessel health and preservation: Four quadrants of care (used with permission N. Moureau, PICC Excellence)

experience, intentionally guiding clinical care and improving and establishing a structure to reduce patient risk.

Comprehensive assessment and selection of the best vein and insertion location, performed by a highly skilled inserter using the most appropriate device, managed in a precise way, and removed at the right time is a process that requires commitment to education, policy development, and specialized clinicians. For facilities fortunate enough to have specialists or speciality teams performing insertion and assessment, the VHP process becomes intuitive. When bedside nurses, physicians, and others are responsible for single steps in the process, fragmentation results and the patient suffers (Castro-Sanchez et al. 2014; Moureau et al. 2012; Panella et al. 2003). The evidence suggests that reduction of fragmentation, by establishing a pathway and teaching a structured process to all stakeholders reduces complications with IV therapy, improves efficiency and diminishes cost (Gaddis et al. 2007; Gurzick and Kesten 2010; Hallam et al. 2016; Weston et al. 2017).

1.2 Four Quadrants of Care

1.2.1 Quadrant 1: Right Assessment, Vein, and Device Selection

Right assessment and selection of the best vein and location is the first stage of the vascular access cycle. This stage begins at the time of admission and continues as diagnosis is established. Most patients receive their first intravenous device hurriedly inserted in the emergency department; location and method of insertion are often not optimal. Once the patient has stabilized, consideration is given to the most appropriate vascular access device that will provide the administration of the prescribed therapy. Assessments of patient history, comorbidities, contraindications, available veins, diagnosis, and duration are factors that determine level of risk, the appropriate device, and most qualified inserter. Individuals with ultrasound training can apply these skills for assessment and selection of the right location and vein for device insertion.

1.2.2 Quadrant 2: Right Insertion and Training

Selection of the right device and the right inserter encompasses the second stage of the VHP process. Appropriate device selection and number of necessary lumens is a determination made according to lowest risk for patient insertion and potential for infection in conjunction with the needs of the therapy. Selection of the inserter and application of infection prevention principles are contributing factors for patient safety. Vascular access specialists and teams of specially trained clinicians function to aid in selection and insertion of the most appropriate device. Ensuring the insertion is performed by a trained and qualified clinician with ultrasound skills reduces insertion and post insertional complications.

1.2.3 Quadrant 3: Right Management

Management of vascular access devices represents the largest portion of time in the VHP cycle. Right management includes assessment of the insertion site, dressing, and device function prior to each infusion. Care and management using right infection prevention methods including Aseptic Non Touch Technique (ANTT) for device handling, disinfection of access site, pulsatile flushing the device before and after infusions, performing dressing changes consistent with policies, and evaluation of device necessity with prompt removal when the VAD is no longer needed are cornerstones to safe patient care. Incorporated into management are the right supplies and technology needed to ensure the right outcomes. Right management is a process that requires consistency established through commitment to education, policy development based on guidelines and research, and consistent evaluation of outcomes.

1.2.4 Quadrant 4: Right Evaluation

Improvement of care is impossible without an established process of evaluation. Right evaluation for VHP program application includes outcome measurement of complications, observation of policy performance, and plan to provide education for staff departments and units with negative outcomes or practice deficiencies. A multimodal quality program applies guidelines and recommendations ensuring that practices are consistent and that staff are well informed through education and outcome reporting. Integrated with a VHP program is the evaluation of products, supplies, and technology, both existing and consideration for new product trial testing. Each product should undergo periodic assessment to determine performance according to the facility needs and expected application.

VHP quadrants all work together to deliver the highest quality of patient care through evidence-based practice. Patients receiving medical care should be able to trust for vascular access that:

1. The VAD selected has the lowest risk for insertion location, device size not to exceed 33% of vein diameter, length, and number of lumen, and is the most appropriate to deliver the treatment. The aim for the patient is greater comfort with reduction of the risk of complications.
2. Standard-ANTT or Surgical-ANTT is used for insertion, device management, dressing care, and medication administration with hub disinfection.
3. The VAD is individualized to patient-specific condition and medical history and placed in a suitable anatomical position to optimize dressing adherence and securement to minimize movement and reduce risk of premature failure.
4. The number of IV attempts is limited and will be performed by well-trained, qualified inserters supervised for competency.
5. The VAD is assessed for complications, dressing adherence, and flushed with normal saline to evaluate device function at least daily in acute care and removed when device is no longer needed, and treatment is complete.
6. The VAD is monitored and maintained by trained, competency-assessed clinical staff who receive consistent education on best practices for management of intravenous devices. Evaluation and education are provided on a timely and consistent basis to all clinical staff in connection with routine care and with any negative outcomes (assumes monitoring and reporting of all outcomes).
7. Concentrate medical product usage on those with scientifically studied and published evidence of positive patient outcomes.

Through the delivery of these seven trust points, patients maintain confidence in the healthcare system, avoid unnecessary costs and interventions, and achieve greater satisfaction with their healthcare centers all consistent with VHP precepts.

Case Study

A 250-bed acute care hospital identified quality gaps with negative outcomes associated with peripheral and central venous catheters. In an effort to reduce complications and improve patient outcomes, they committed to adopt the VHP model and apply it to all levels of care. The first step in the process was to provide training for patient assessment, followed by infection prevention education for all clinicians inserting or managing VADs. In addition, the education was continued to improve the competence of inserters to use ultrasound when needed, to implement better Standard-ANTT and Surgical-ANTT procedures, and to select the most appropriate device for the patient and therapy. Implementation of the VHP stages began in one targeted unit instituting initial assessment of every patient admitted to the area. Patient and clinician satisfaction feedback was collected and evaluated to identify improvement needs. Each patient received a detailed vascular access daily assessment that included evaluation of right device and right time if the device was still necessary, insertion site, dressing adherence, patient response, and catheter function. The final stage of the VHP process of implementation was evaluation of the outcomes and compliance with the process. While this hospital achieved a moderate 82% compliance with initial assessment, right inserter, daily assessments, and discontinuation of unnecessary VADs, their results had a huge impact on patient satisfaction and staff appreciation. Efficiency had improved with insertion changing from an average of 2.2 attempts with PIVCs to 1.4 per patient, supply usage was down 54% with PIVCs changed only when clinically indicated, and even with the added staff time in VHP implementation, the savings continued to mount above $265,000 estimated annual cost reduction.

Summary of Key Points

1. Vessel health and preservation (VHP) is a model applied to vascular access and the administration of IV medications and treatment that structures evidence-based practices within four quadrants of medical care: assessment/selection, insertion, management, and evaluation of vascular access devices.
2. Comprehensive assessment and selection of the best vein and insertion site location, performed by a highly skilled inserter using the most appropriate device, managed in a precise way, and removed at the right time is a process that requires commitment to education, policy development, and specialized clinicians.
3. Assessments of patient history, comorbidities, contraindications, available veins, diagnosis, and duration are factors that determine level of risk, the appropriate device, and most qualified inserter.
4. Ensuring the insertion is performed by a trained and qualified clinician with ultrasound skills reduces insertion and post insertional complications.
5. Device management includes assessment of the insertion site, dressing, and device function prior to each infusion.
6. Improvement of care is impossible without an established process of evaluation.

References

Castro-Sanchez E, Charani E, Drumright LN, Sevdalis N, Shah N, Holmes AH. Fragmentation of care threatens patient safety in peripheral vascular catheter management in acute care—a qualitative study. PLoS One. 2014;9:e86167.

Chopra V, Flanders SA, Saint S, Woller SC, O'Grady NP, Safdar N, Trerotola SO, Saran R, Moureau N, Wiseman S, Pittiruti M. The Michigan Appropriateness Guide for Intravenous Catheters (MAGIC): results from a multispecialty panel using the RAND/UCLA appropriateness method. Ann Intern Med. 2015;163(6 Suppl):S1–40.

De Bleser L, Depreitere R, Waele KD, Vanhaecht K, Vlayen J, Sermeus W. Defining pathways. J Nurs Manag. 2006;14(7):553–63.

Gaddis GM, Greenwald P, Huckson S. Toward improved implementation of evidence-based clinical algorithms: clinical practice guidelines, clinical decision rules, and clinical pathways. Acad Emerg Med. 2007;14:1015–22.

Gurzick M, Kesten KS. The impact of clinical nurse specialists on clinical pathways in the application of evidence-based practice. J Prof Nurs. 2010;26:42–8.

Hallam C, Weston V, Denton A, Hill S, Bodenham A, Dunn H, Jackson T. Development of the UK Vessel Health and Preservation (VHP) framework: a multi-organisational collaborative. J Infect Prev. 2016;17:65–72.

Hanchett M, Poole SM. Infusion pathways: planning for success. J Vasc Access Devices. 2001;6(3):29–37.

Moureau N, Trick N, Nifong T, Perry C, Kelley C, Carrico R, Leavitt M, Gordon S, Wallace J, Harvill M, Biggar C, Doll M, Papke L, Benton L, Phelan D. Vessel health and preservation (Part 1): a new evidence-based approach to vascular access selection and management. J Vasc Access. 2012;13:351–6.

Panella M, Marchisio S, Di Stanislao F. Reducing clinical variations with clinical pathways: do pathways work? Int J Qual Health Care. 2003;15:509–21.

Weston V, Nightingale A, O'loughlin C, Ventura R. The implementation of the Vessel Health and Preservation framework. Br J Nurs. 2017;26:S18–22.

2

Right Location and Vein: Assessment and Selection

Evan Alexandrou

Abstract

Right assessment and selection of the best vein and location is the first stage of the vascular access cycle within quadrant 1 of VHP. This stage begins at the time of admission and continues as diagnosis is established and treatment initiated. Most patients receive their first intravenous device during the assessment in the emergency department, typically a PIVC is inserted in a hurried fashion, and location and method of insertion are often not optimal. Once the patient has stabilized, consideration can be given to the most appropriate vascular access device, one that will provide the administration of the prescribed therapy. Assessments of patient history, comorbidities, contraindications, available veins, diagnosis, and duration of therapy are factors that determine level of risk, the appropriate device, and most qualified inserter. Individuals with ultrasound training can apply their skills for assessment and selection of the right location and vein for device insertion.

Keywords

Assessment · Patient assessment
Vein assessment · Ultrasound assessment
Vein characteristics · RAPEVA · RACEVA

E. Alexandrou (✉)
School of Nursing and Midwifery, Western Sydney University, Penrith, NSW, Australia

Central Venous Access and Parenteral Nutrition Service—Liverpool Hospital, Liverpool, NSW, Australia

Menzies Health Research Institute—Alliance for Vascular Access Teaching and Research (AVATAR) Group, Griffith University, Brisbane, QLD, Australia

Faculty of Medicine, South West Sydney Clinical School, University of New South Wales Australia, Sydney, NSW, Australia
e-mail: e.alexandrou@westernsydney.edu.au

2.1 Introduction

Within the first 48 h of admission to an acute care facility, a patient receives a diagnosis, PIVC placement, and initiation of treatment (Santolucito 2001). Since most PIVCs fail within the first 48 h, the optimal window for patient vein assessment and device selection is within this time frame (Hallam et al. 2016; Jackson et al. 2013). A patient-centered approach is focused on the vascular assessment of the patient, recent and past history with access, critical or chronic nature of their illness, comorbidities that may affect the risk of infection or other complications, types of medications to be administered, duration of treatment, future needs, specific access needs, and risk assessment of all factors, followed by vein and device choice (Hallam et al. 2016; Jackson et al. 2013; Moureau 2017).

2.2 Patient and Vein Assessment

Gaining a patient history and clinical assessment assists in determining device selection. Clinical histories such as past surgery, comorbid conditions, hematological or oncological history, as well as past vascular access-related complications that include difficult venous access or thrombosis are important factors that influence device choice (Sou et al. 2017; Woller et al. 2016). Physical assessment of the patient should include neurological, cardiovascular, respiratory, and gastrointestinal assessment. The assessment of coagulation profile, electrolyte, and full blood count review informs the inserter of areas of potential risk (Lonsway 2010).

Assessment for either peripheral or central access is enhanced with the use of ultrasound (Moureau 2014; Sharp et al. 2015a, b). Determination of the need for central venous access device (CVAD) requires a risk benefit assessment to avoid unnecessary placement of these higher risk devices (Chopra et al. 2015). Risk ratios with CVADs are higher than with peripheral devices both with insertion and post insertion-related complications (Maki et al. 2006; Mcgee and Gould 2003; Sou et al. 2017). The goal with assessment and selection is to choose the lowest risk VAD, which will complete the prescribed treatment plan while minimizing both insertion and post insertion-related complications (Chopra et al. 2013, 2015). The vessel health and preservation model incorporates a planned vascular access assessment that evaluates the patient factors correlated with the treatment plan to select the most suitable device and inserter (Hallam et al. 2016; Hanchett and Poole 2001; Moureau et al. 2012; Rotter et al. 2010).

2.3 Vessel Assessment

Clinical evaluation of the blood vessels and the pathway determines anatomical placement and ultimately the most appropriate device. Evaluation through observation and palpation of vessels or visualization with ultrasound can facilitate successful insertion and longer dwell times (De La Torre-Montero et al. 2014). Vessels that are tortuous in nature, have bifurcations, or thrombosis make placement of the device difficult and should be avoided (Moureau 2014). Approaches developed by the Italian Group for Venous Access Devices (GAVeCeLT) that include the Rapid Assessment of the Central Veins (RaCeVA) and the Rapid Assessment of the Peripheral Veins (RaPeVA) are protocols that can be used to thoroughly evaluate vessels and surrounding structures (Pittiruti 2012).

Thorough ultrasound assessment for vein selection reduces insertion-related complications (Flood and Bodenham 2013; Pirotte 2008). When urgency of placement is not necessary, time taken with selection of a location for cannula insertion in a stable area, away from joints and movement, results in lower rates of failure (Marsh et al. 2017). Vein selection for PIVC placement must be balanced with consideration for speed versus longer dwell time and reduced complications. Placement of a device in the hand or antecubital fossa is initially easier in most respects due to identification of veins visually and through palpation; however, these devices become dislodged, are uncomfortable for patients, and often fail in less than 72 h (Alexandrou et al. 2018). Vein selection with CVAD is dictated by insertion risk related to site, vein size, depth, and surrounding structures that may impact risk of complications (i.e., nerves, lymphatic tissue, artery) (Moureau 2017).

2.4 Ultrasound Assessment of the Patient

Ultrasound for vascular access site selection is used to identify and map structures within the arm, chest, neck, and leg that may be most suitable for device insertion and treatment. Ultrasound is used widely for central venous access, PICCs, midlines, and in more recent times for PIVCs too. The patient safety benefits of using ultrasound are undisputed (Bodenham et al. 2016; Gorski et al. 2016; Lamperti et al. 2012; Loveday et al. 2014). Gorski et al., in INS Standards (2016), recommend using visualization technologies like infrared or ultrasound to increase insertion success for patients with difficult access.

With ultrasound imaging and the use of a conductive medium, such as gel, the probe or transducer transmits sound waves that are interpreted on a viewing screen. Scanning for peripheral veins and structures within the arms begins at the level of the forearm working toward the body. Optimal peripheral cannula site selection is one that allows ultrasound-guided needle access in a vein 2–4 mm in diameter or larger and 0.3–1.5 cm in depth (Witting et al. 2010).

It is essential to assess the veins with ultrasound prior to the procedure to select the vein with optimal characteristics including the size, depth, and pathway with minimal risk to arterial/nerve injury, check the vein for patency, ensure thrombosis is not present, and identify any anatomical variations. Ultrasound assessment is undertaken without using a tourniquet to assess the vein in its normal state. Assess the depth, patency, and respiratory collapse; for instance, a critically ill patient may present in a cardiovascular hyperdynamic state with the artery pounding and encroaching the vein, which may itself be collapsing with each respiratory cycle. Application of assessment methods, such as RACEVA and RAPEVA, covered later in this chapter, guides the inserter to select the best vein and identifies any venous abnormalities prior to insertion (Pittiruti and Scoppettuolo 2017).

Anatomy is not exact, and variations exist. For example, the basilic veins are only present in the text book or traditional form of anatomy in 66%, as discovered in a study by Anaya-Ayala et al. (2011), who mapped veins of 290 patients including 426 arms (221 right, 205 left arm). From the mapped veins, the authors identified that the basilic vein joins the axillary vein around the same area that the brachial veins do. In the remaining 34% of patients, either the basilic joins the paired brachial veins in the mid to lower arm or the basilic joins an unpaired brachial in the mid to lower section of the arm (Anaya-Ayala et al. 2011).

During scanning and vein selection, identify arteries and nerves based on anatomical knowledge for the area (e.g., median nerve for PICC, carotid artery for jugular CVAD, pleura for subclavian CVAD). As scanning of the patient continues, look for normal and abnormal features of the vessels: shape, size, path, patency, and flow (Moureau and King 2007).

- **Shape**: Observe for irregularities in lumen size and vessel wall thickness. These types of abnormalities are usually best visualized in the sagittal plane.
- **Size**: Measure basilic, brachial, and cephalic vein diameter in their native state without a tourniquet. Vein size determines suitability of desired catheter size and number of lumens (i.e., caliber of peripheral vein must at least equal diameter of midline or PICC in French size). Diameter may be measured in the transverse or sagittal plane. The occupation of more than one third of the diameter of a blood vessel with a catheter reduces blood flow within the region and increase thrombosis risk. Generally, the scale in Fig. 2.1 provides a guide for determining the most appropriate catheter for vein size (Sharp et al. 2015a, b, 2016).
- **Path:** Note any aberrancy along the course of the vessel (tortuosity), areas of dilation, or stenosis. Also observe for symmetry of the vessel wall looking for irregularities rather than the normal round vessel shape. Uniformity of the path and vein wall is viewed specifically in sagittal, longitudinal view providing a more detailed view of vein path or vein wall abnormalities.
- **Patency:** Compress veins. Look for echogenic material within non-compressible veins that may indicate thrombosis or other structures such as nerves or arteries (use pulse wave Doppler if indicated). Look for collaterals around areas of non-compressible or retracted veins.
- **Flow:** Observe arterial and venous flow. Flow in the arterial system pulsatile and rhythmical if the patient has normal heart function. Flow in the venous system is typically slower without pulsatility. It is important to note that the "red" and "blue" colors typically used do not demonstrate arterial or venous flow but rather movement toward and away from the probe.

CATHETER/VEIN SCALE
Chart for determining catheter size/length versus appropriate vein diameter and depth from ultrasound assessment
Peripheral vascular access devices PICC Excellence, Inc.

FRENCH SIZE	2	2.5	3	3.5	4	4.5	5	5.5	6	7	8
CATHETER GAUGE SIZE	24	22	20	19	18	17	16	15	14		12
CATHETER MEASUREMENT mm	0.55	0.75	0.9	1.06	1.27	1.47	1.65	1.8	2.1	2.3	2.7
INCHES	0.022	0.026	0.0355	0.042	0.05	0.058	0.065	0.072	0.083	0.092	0.105
VESSEL SIZE needed 1/3 vs 2/3 catheter to blood flow. French size is desired vein size	2mm	2.5mm	3mm	3.5mm	4mm	4.5mm	5mm	5.5mm	6mm	7mm	8mm

INS RECOMMENDATION for 2/3 catheter in vein

DEPTH using 45 degrees	0..25	0.5	.75	1.0	1.25	1.5
CATHETER LENGTH needed	1.2cm	2cm	3.2cm	4.25cm	5.25	6.4cm
DEPTH using 30 degrees	0.25	0.5	.75	1.0	1.25	1.5
CATHETER LENGTH needed	1.5cm	3cm	4.5cm	6cm	7.5cm	8cm

www.piccexcellence.com

Fig. 2.1 Catheter vein measurement scale (used with permission N. Moureau, PICC Excellence)

- **Pre-insertion Ultrasound Assessment of the Central and Peripheral Veins** (RACEVA & RAPEVA (Emoli et al. 2014; Pittiruti 2012; Pittiruti and Scoppettuolo 2017)): Pre-insertion scanning of the major blood vessels prior to catheter insertion and mapping pathway of the catheter improves success rates and minimize complications. The RACEVA protocol is a six-step assessment of the major central vessels and important associated structures.

2.5 Rapid Vein Assessment RAPEVA and RACEVA Protocols (Pittiruti and Scoppettuolo 2017)

Rapid assessment peripheral vein assessment (RAPEVA) and rapid assessment central vein assessment (RACEVA) are performed with ultrasound to determine the most appropriate location for catheter insertion. Scanning of the peripheral vasculature includes visualization by starting at the antecubital region of the arm, moving up medially, and toward the chest. More information on ultrasound scanning and the RAPEVA methods are found in the references (Pittiruti 2012).

2.5.1 RAPEVA Position 1

Position 1—This position identifies vessels of the antecubital fossa, sometimes visible without ultrasound. Probe position should begin at the lateral side of the arm at the cubital crease in transverse position. Assess the smaller cephalic vein for compressibility and thrombosis (Fig. 2.2).

2.5.2 RAPEVA Position 2

Position 2—Moving from lateral to medial along the antecubital fossa, visualize larger veins with position variation from person to person. Probe position should move to the medial side of the arm at cubital crease in transverse position. Assess the basilic vein in relation to the median cubital vein as well as brachial artery and median and ulnar nerve. Assess basilic vein for compressibility, thrombosis, diameter, and distance from the skin (Fig. 2.3).

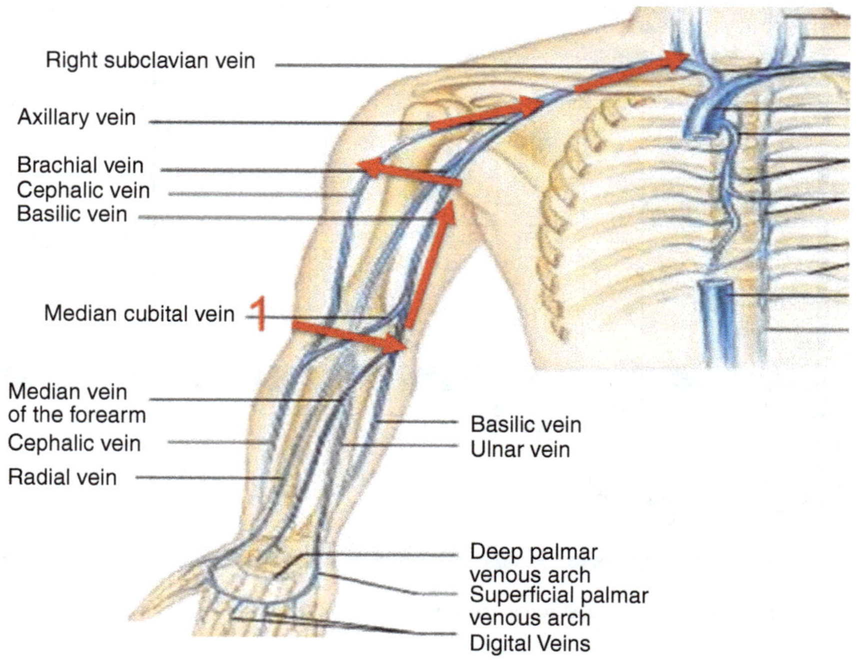

Fig. 2.2 RAPEVA Position 1: Antecubital cephalic vein assessment (used with permission Mauro Pittiruti)

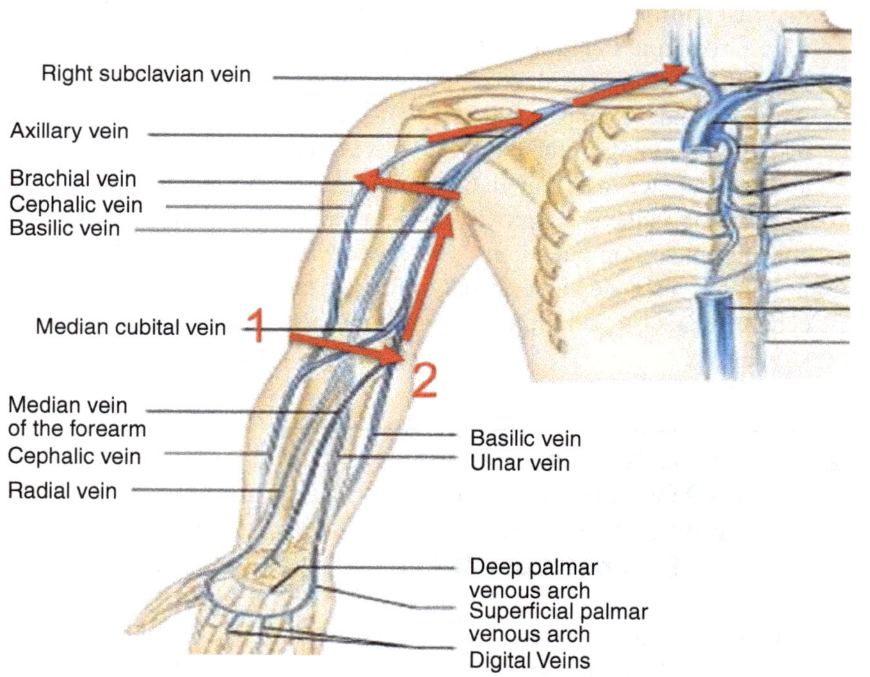

Fig. 2.3 RAPEVA Position 2: Antecubital basilic, brachial vein and nerve assessment (used with permission Mauro Pittiruti)

2.5.3 RAPEVA Position 3

Position 3—This position follows the basilic vein with the probe position on the medial side of arm in the bicipital humeral groove. Assess the basilic vein in relation to the ulnar nerve and brachial bundle with the brachial veins, artery, and median nerve. Assess basilic vein along the bicep groove for compressibility, thrombosis, diameter, and distance from the skin (Figs. 2.4, 2.5. This mid-upper arm position is a common location for PICC insertion stabilized by the surrounding bicep, brachialis, and coraco-brachialis muscle group.

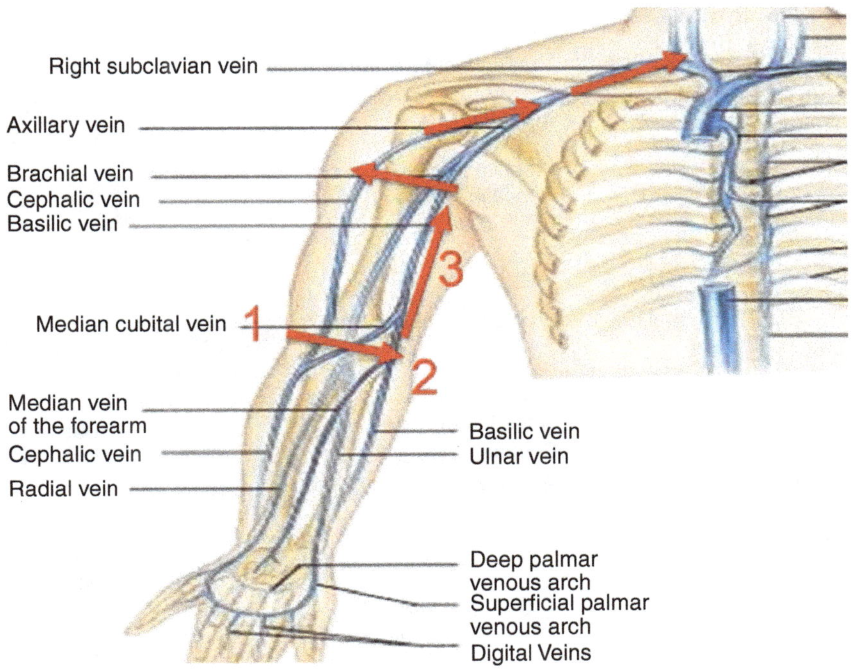

Fig. 2.4 RAPEVA Position 3: Medial position of arm for basilic vein, nerves, and brachial bundle (used with permission Mauro Pittiruti)

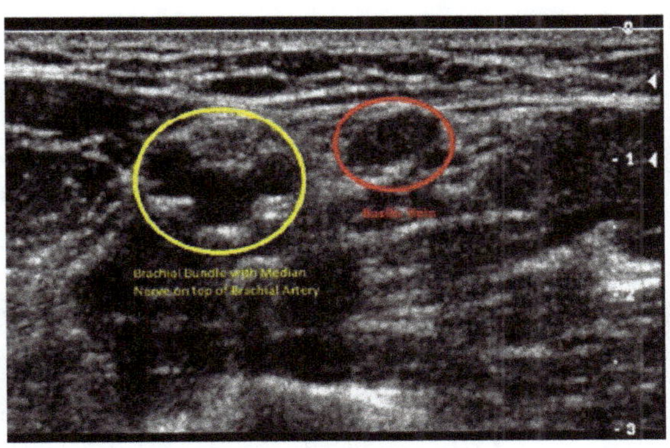

Fig. 2.5 Brachial bundle with median nerve and basilic vein (used with permission N. Moureau, PICC Excellence)

2.5.4 RAPEVA Position 4

Position 4—Probe position should be mid arm over bicep region. At this position the basilic vein is likely joined with the brachial veins but may vary in the exact location from person to person. Assess the brachial vein in relation to the brachial artery and median nerve. Brachial veins are paired veins, known as the venae comitantes situated on either side of the brachial artery with pulsations of the artery aiding in venous return. This bundle representing the brachial veins and artery includes the median nerve, one of the largest in the upper extremity. Assess brachial vein(s) for compressibility, thrombosis, diameter, distance from the skin, and optimal position to facilitate needle access while avoiding the artery and nerve (Fig. 2.6).

2.5.5 RAPEVA Position 5

Position 5—This position assesses the upper arm portion of the cephalic vein which can be difficult to locate. Probe position should be lateral side of the arm below the acromion in transverse mode. Assess the cephalic vein for compressibility and thrombosis (Fig. 2.7).

2.5.6 RAPEVA Position 6

Position 6—Following the cephalic vein from positions 5 to 6, identifies the intersection with the axillary vein. Probe position should be perpendicular and move to the pectoral groove in transverse mode, below the clavicle (lateral third of clavicle—as with Position 5 of RACEVA in the section that follows). This position assesses the axillary vein (AV) in short axis, axillary artery (AA) in short axis, and cephalic vein (CV) in long axis (Fig. 2.8).

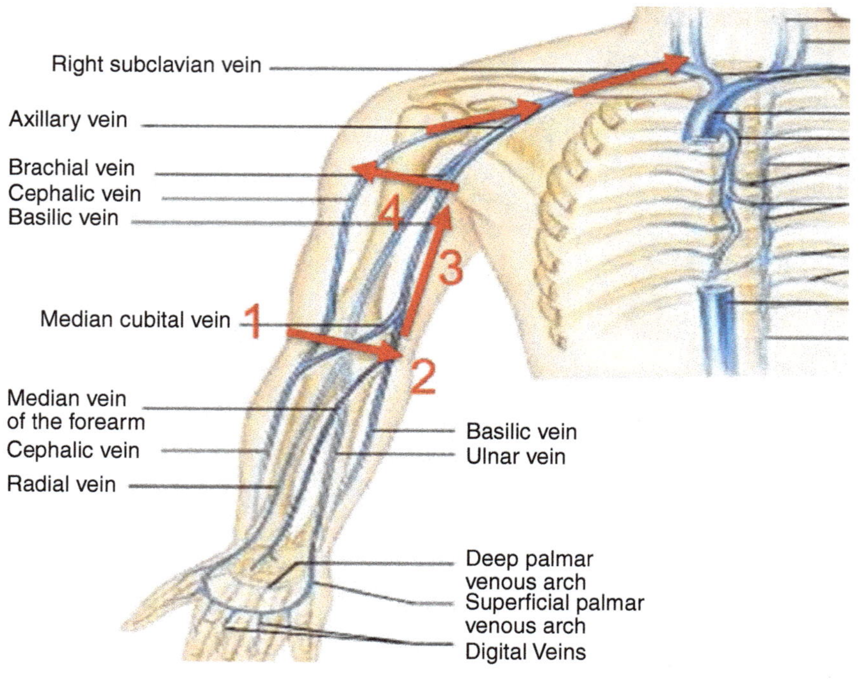

Fig. 2.6 RAPEVA Position 4: Brachial bundle assessment (used with permission Mauro Pittiruti)

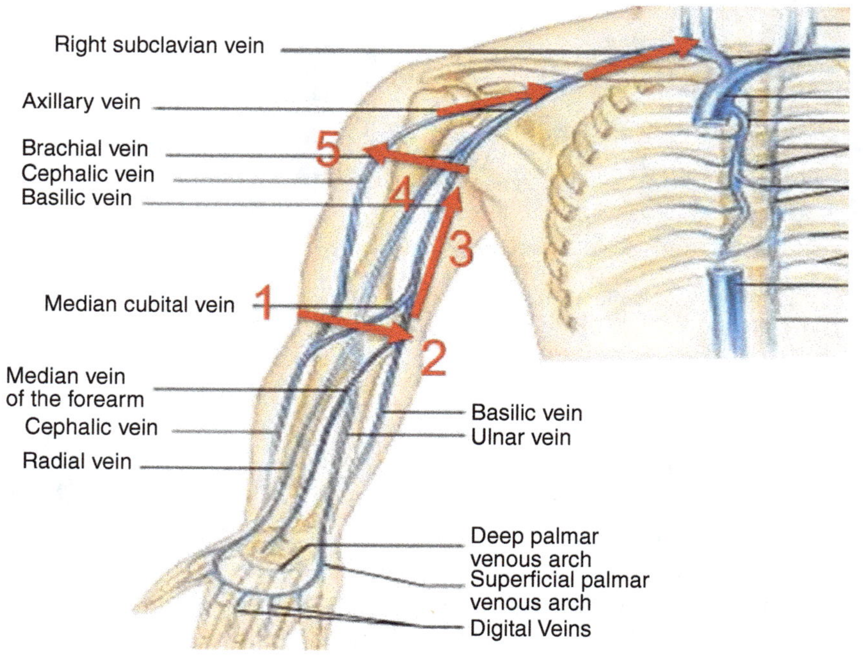

Fig. 2.7 RAPEVA Position 5: High cephalic vein assessment (used with permission Mauro Pittiruti)

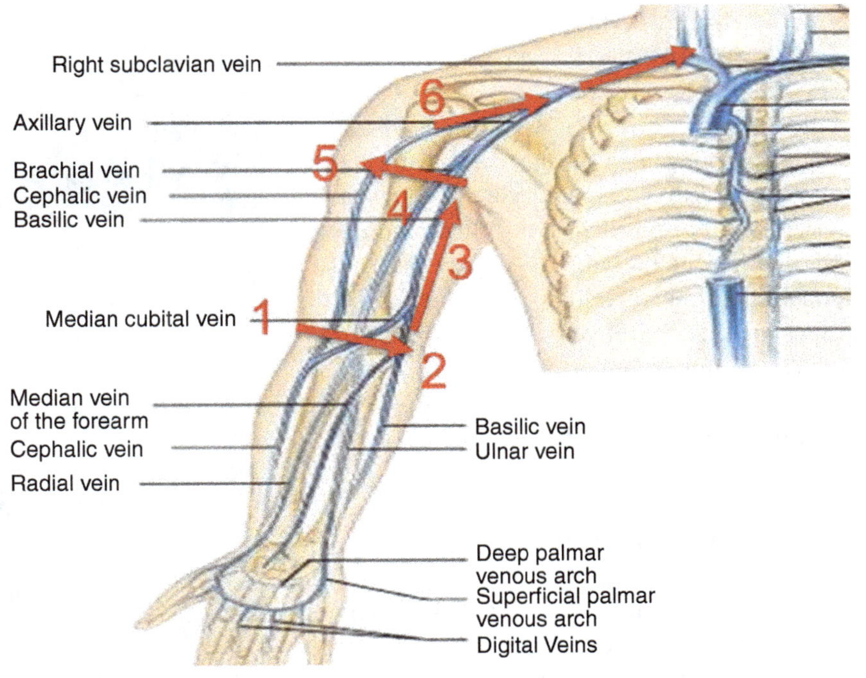

Fig. 2.8 RAPEVA Position 6: Axillary vein and artery assessment (used with permission Mauro Pittiruti)

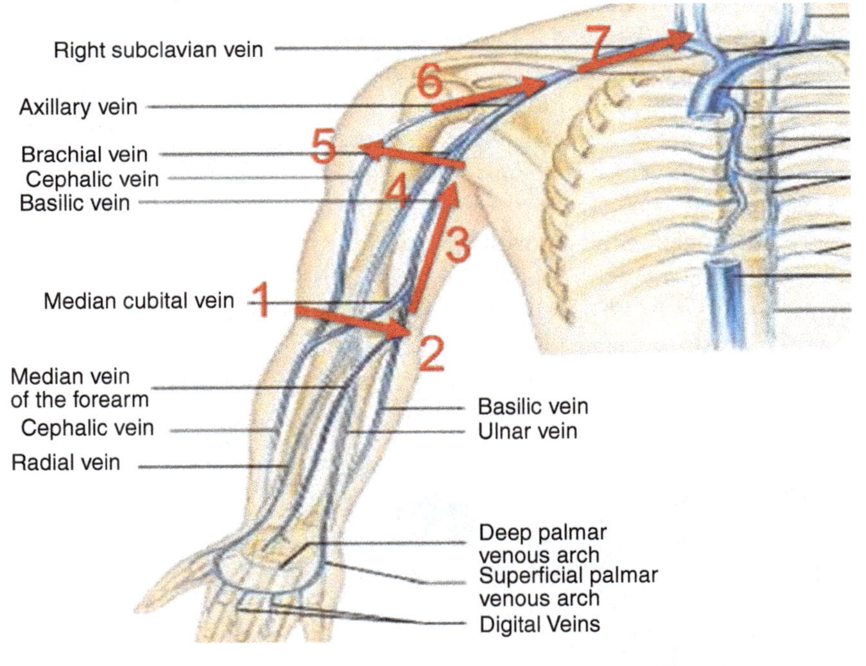

Fig. 2.9 RAPEVA Position 7: Subclavian and external jugular vein assessment (used with permission Mauro Pittiruti)

2.5.7 RAPEVA Position 7

Probe position is behind the clavicle (supraclavicular). This position assesses the subclavian vein (SV), external jugular vein (EJ) in long axis, and laterally the subclavian artery in short axis. Probe position moves to the lower neck in transverse plane to assess lower track of the IJV, subclavian artery in long axis as well as visualization of the distal IJV valve (Fig. 2.9).

2.6 RACEVA Rapid Central Vein Assessment

The RACEVA protocol uses ultrasound for thorough assessment of vascular structures in terms of size, patency and overal vialbility for catheterization. It also provides information on overall anatomy of the area do reduce inadvertant puncture of surrounding anatomic structures (Spencer and Pittiruti 2018). More information on ultrasound scanning and the RACEVA and RAPEVA methods are found in the references (Pittiruti 2012).

2.6.1 RACEVA Position 1

Position 1—Starting at the mid neck examining the internal jugular vessels and the carotid artery using a transverse view of the vessels. This position assesses the internal jugular vein (IJV) and carotid artery. Assess for compressibility, size, and shape (Figs. 2.10 and 2.11). Where possible and safe to do so for your patient, pressure should be applied to the veins to assess for compressibility and to check for patency and the presence of a thrombosis. The development of a thrombosis is a process, and in the early stages, the thrombus is still compressible (though the vessel is not likely to fully compress). At this stage it may also appear black and, like a normal vessel, only at the later stages does it start to take on a more solid form and then becomes more echogenic and the vein non-compressible. Any suspicion of a thrombus should be referred to the radiology and or vascular team for further investigation including Doppler ultrasound assessment.

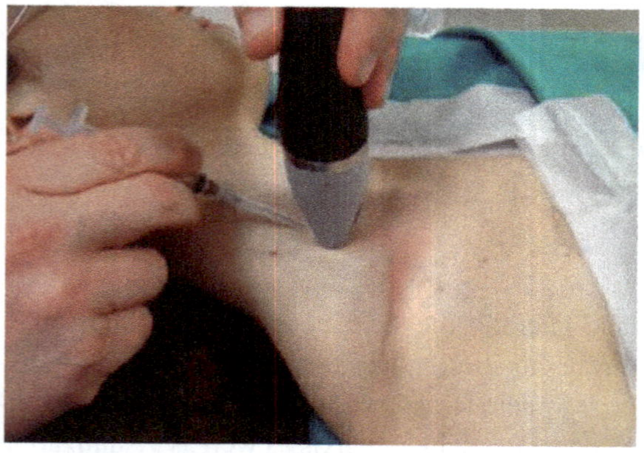

Fig. 2.10 RACEVA Position 1: Jugular vein assessment (used with permission Mauro Pittiruti)

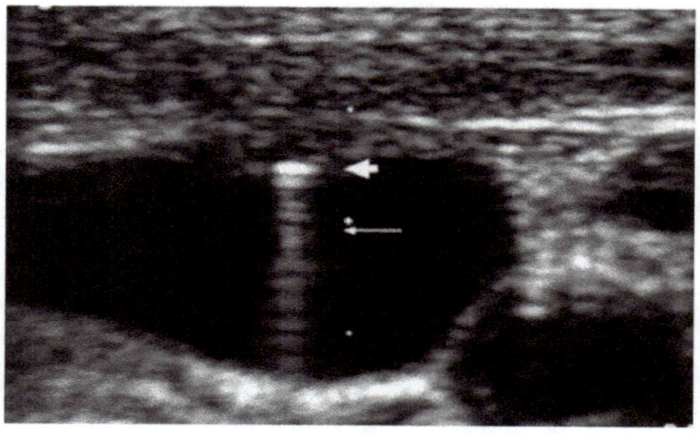

Fig. 2.11 RACEVA Position 2: Jugular assessment view with ultrasound (used with permission Mauro Pittiruti)

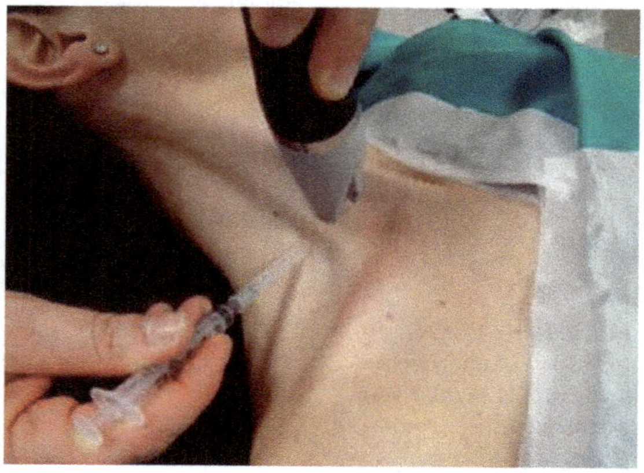

Fig. 2.12 RACEVA Position 2: Low IJV assessment and subclavian artery in in long axis (used with permission Mauro Pittiruti)

Position 2—Still in transverse position, transducer slides down to base of the neck, this allows view of the internal jugular and and carotid artery. The probe in transverse position at the base of the neck (supraclavicular) facilitates view of the lower track of the IJV, subclavian artery in long axis as well as the distal IJV valve. (Figs. 2.12 and 2.13).

2.6.2 RACEVA Position 3

Position 3—Transverse view, having followed the pathway of the internal jugular down to the

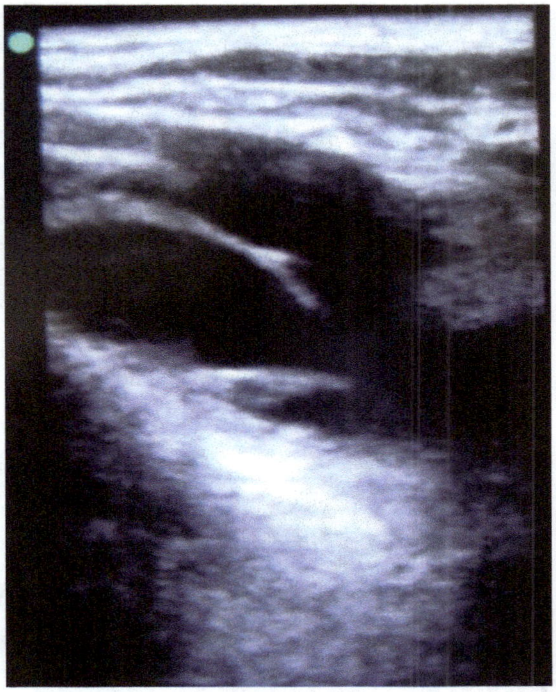

Fig. 2.13 View of the lower tract IJV with distal valve (used with permission Mauro Pittiruti)

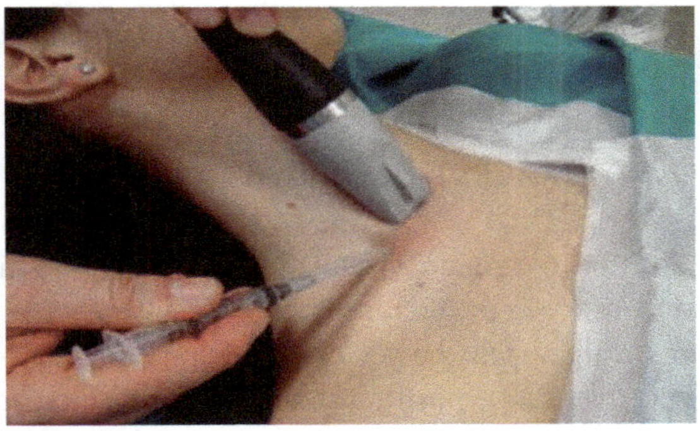

Fig. 2.14 RACEVA Position 3: Brachiocephalic vein (used with permission Mauro Pittiruti)

base of the neck now place the probe level with the sternal notch on the superior edge of the clavicle. Probe position should be above the clavicle to the side of the sternal notch in transverse plane. This position assesses the brachiocephalic vein. In order to view the brachiocephalic, angle the probe inferiorly toward the heart, and slight pressure may help achieve optimal visualization of the vessel. This is an ideal position for an "in-plane" puncture of the brachiocephalic vein (Figs. 2.14 and 2.15).

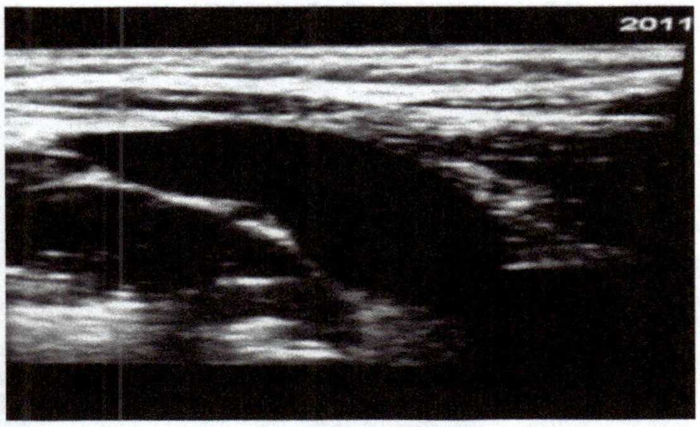

Fig. 2.15 Brachiocephalic vein assessment with ultrasound (used with permission Mauro Pittiruti)

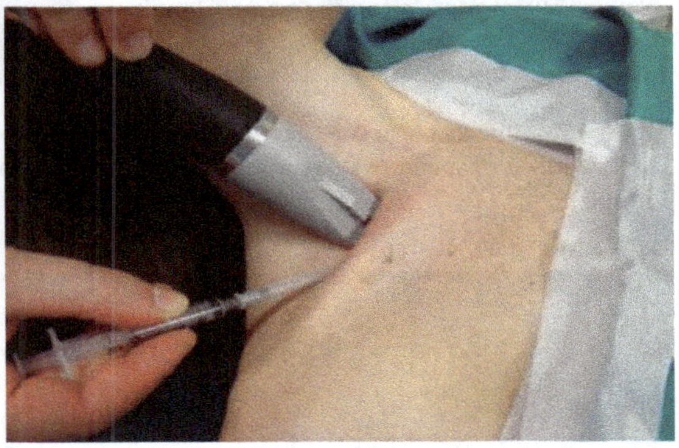

Fig. 2.16 RACEVA Position 4: Subclavian and external jugular vein assessment (used with permission Mauro Pittiruti)

2.6.3 RACEVA Position 4

Position 4—Probe position should be behind the clavicle (supraclavicular). This position assesses the subclavian vein (SV), external jugular vein (EJ) in long axis, and laterally the subclavian artery in short axis (Figs. 2.16 and 2.17). Sliding the probe slightly away from the sternal notch along the superior border of the clavicle and holding the probe in a similar angle used when examining the brachiocephalic allows view of the subclavian vein and artery, using both transverse and longitudinal views.

2.6.4 RACEVA Position 5

Position 5—Probe position should be perpendicular to the pectoral groove in short access,

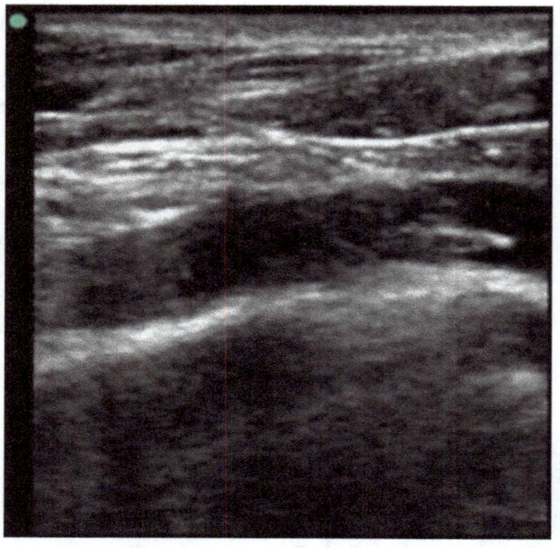

Fig. 2.17 Subclavian and external jugular vein assessment with ultrasound (used with permission Mauro Pittiruti)

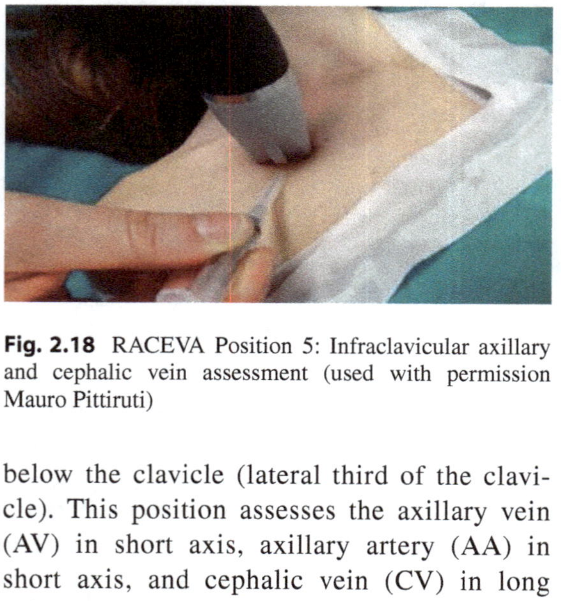

Fig. 2.18 RACEVA Position 5: Infraclavicular axillary and cephalic vein assessment (used with permission Mauro Pittiruti)

below the clavicle (lateral third of the clavicle). This position assesses the axillary vein (AV) in short axis, axillary artery (AA) in short axis, and cephalic vein (CV) in long axis. Ideal position for "out of plane": puncture of axillary vein (Figs. 2.18 and 2.19). Moving to the inferior border of the clavicle, visualize the axillary vein and artery in transverse view. A patient with increased respiratory demand may present with a vein that is opening and collapsing with the changes in intrathoracic pressure during the respiratory cycle. A patient with poor hydration status may also present with a collapsing vein as the venous pressure is low.

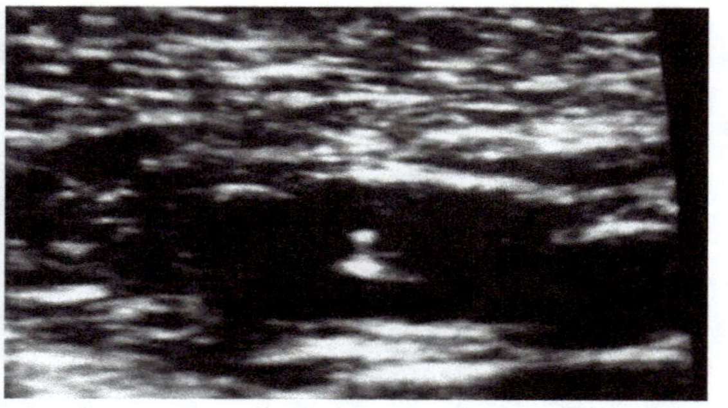

Fig. 2.19 Axillary and cephalic vein assessment with ultrasound (used with permission Mauro Pittiruti)

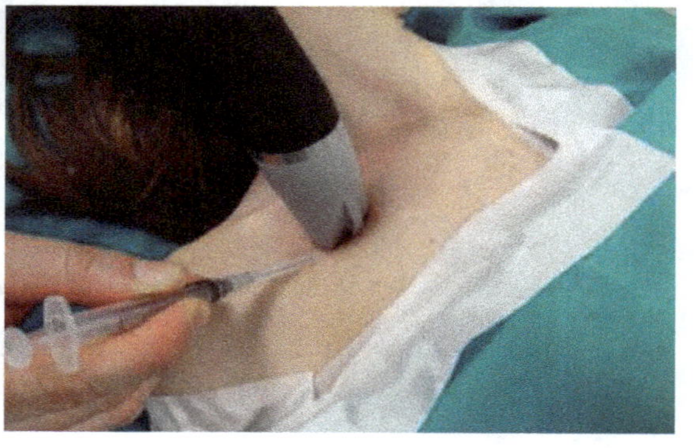

Fig. 2.20 RACEVA Position 6: Axillary vein assessment (used with permission Mauro Pittiruti)

2.6.5 RACEVA Position 6

Position 6—Again visualizing the axillary vein and artery in the deltopectoral or a subclavicular fossa area, view the vessels in a longitudinal perspective. Probe position should be perpendicular to the pectoral groove in long access, below the clavicle (lateral third of the clavicle).

This position assesses the AV in long axis, AA in long axis, and CV vein in long axis. Ideal position for "in-plane": puncture of the axillary vein (Figs. 2.20 and 2.21).

2.6.6 RACEVA Position 7

Position 7—Using the second intercostal space, the ultrasound is used to view the pleura and the lung tissue. The aim of identifying these structures is to identify the presence of a pneumothorax with the absence of sliding lung sign outlined

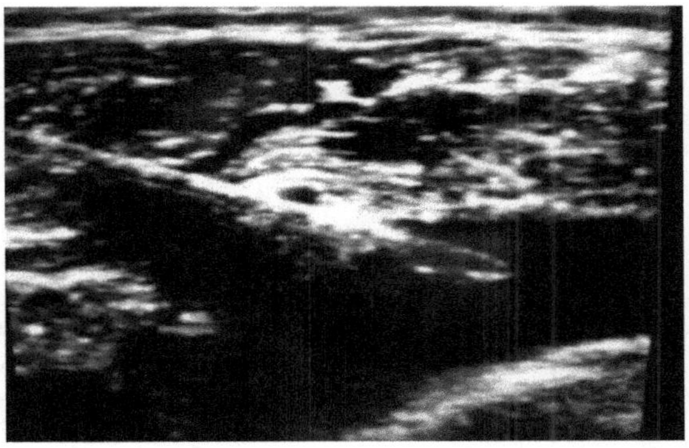

Fig. 2.21 Axillary vein in longitudinal view with ultrasound (used with permission Mauro Pittiruti)

in the next chapter with insertion. Sliding lung assessment should be performed pre- and post-CICC insertion, and although this will be covered in a separate section, it is important to note that ultrasound can be used as a reliable technique to assess lung movement and the presence or absence of a pneumothorax (Husain et al. 2012). As noted in the publication, there are several classic sonographic signs that include the "sliding lung" and "comet tail artifacts" that assess the normal function and integrity of the visceral and parietal pleura. Identify the horizontal, equally spaced hyperechogenic reflections of the pleura, and the conical-shaped shadows descending down the pleura deeper into the tissues known as comet tails indicate normal lung function for that lobe (Fig. 2.22).

2.6.7 RACEVA Position 8

More information on ultrasound scanning and the RACEVA and RAPEVA methods are found in the references (Pittiruti 2012; Pittiruti and Scoppettuolo 2017; Spencer and Pittiruti 2018).

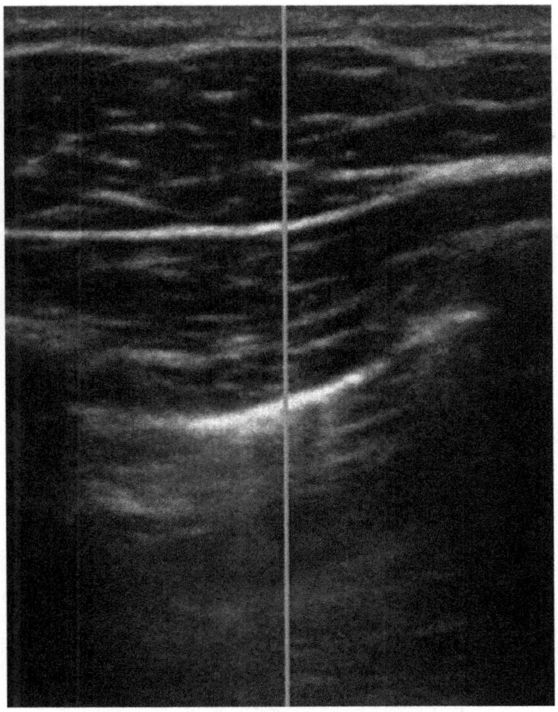

Fig. 2.22 Pleura with sliding lung comet sign (used with permission Mauro Pittiruti)

Case Study

A 45-year-old male entered the emergency room with elevated temperature, severe fatigue, weakness, shortness of breath, sleeping problems, some nausea, poor appetite, frequent small quantity urination, dry skin and poor turgor, and swelling to the legs and ankles with some muscle cramping. Laboratory blood work confirms a high creatinine level and a glomerular filtration rate (GFR) of 35 indicating moderate renal dysfunction. The issues noted with this patient include the need for dialysis, cautious fluid replacement for dehydration, and further testing to rule out sepsis. The emergency physician is trained in the RACEVA protocol and evaluates vein options, and configuration knowing the best choice for this patient is an internal jugular placement for the dialysis catheter. After numerous failed attempts at peripheral access, consideration was given to placement of a second axillary central catheter for fluids and antibiotic infusions. Prior to catheter placement, it was discovered that a tri-lumen dialysis catheter was available that included an extra lumen for the intravenous medications. The tri-lumen catheter was placed successfully in the right internal jugular vein under ultrasound guidance, the first infusion of antibiotics given, baseline central venous pressure and oxygen levels obtained, and the patient sent to dialysis for first treatment.

Summary of Key Points

1. The Vessel Health and Preservation process is designed to select the vein, location, and device that has lowest risk, preserves veins, and is most reliable for the treatment.
2. CVAD selection is optimal when individualized for the patient based on treatment plan, medication types, duration, and patient-specific factors.
3. Patients are the focus of VHP with individualized assessment, selection, and placement that reduces unnecessary trauma and VAD-related complications.
4. The use of visualization technology aids in assessment, vein selection, and insertion.

References

Anaya-Ayala JE, Younes HK, Kaiser CL, Syed O, Ismail N, Naoum JJ, et al. Prevalence of variant brachial-basilic vein anatomy and implications for vascular access planning. J Vasc Surg. 2011;53(3):720–4.

Alexandrou E, Ray-Barruel G, Carr PJ, Frost S, Inwood S, Higgins N, et al. Use of short peripheral intravenous catheters: characteristics, management, and outcomes worldwide. J Hosp Med. 2018;13 https://doi.org/10.12788/jhm.3039.

Bodenham A, Babu S, Bennett J, Binks R, Fee P, Fox B, Johnston A, Klein A, Langton J, Mclure H. Association of Anaesthetists of Great Britain and Ireland. Safe vascular access 2016. Anaesthesia. 2016;71:573–85.

Chopra V, O'Horo JC, Rogers MA, Maki DG, Safdar N. The risk of bloodstream infection associated with peripherally inserted central catheters compared with central venous catheters in adults: a systematic review and meta-analysis. Infect Control Hosp Epidemiol. 2013;34:908–18.

Chopra V, Flanders SA, Saint S, Woller SC, O'Grady NP, Safdar N, Trerotola SO, Saran R, Moureau N, Wiseman S, Pittiruti M, Akl EA, Lee AY, Courey A, Swaminathan L, Ledonne J, Becker C, Krein SL, Bernstein SJ, Michigan Appropriateness Guide for Intravenous Catheters Panel. The Michigan appropriateness guide for intravenous catheters (MAGIC): results from a multispecialty panel using the RAND/UCLA appropriateness method. Ann Intern Med. 2015;163:S1–40.

De La Torre-Montero J-C, Montealegre-Sanz M, Faraldo-Cabana A, Oliva-Pellicer B, Garcia-Real I, Fenwick M, Marcos CE, Rivas-Eguia B, Vila-Borrajo C, Valles-Andres J. Venous International Assessment, VIA scale, validated classification procedure for the peripheral venous system. J Vasc Access. 2014;15:45–50.

Emoli A, Cappuccio S, Marche B, Musaro A, Scoppettuolo G, Pittiruti M. [The ISP (Safe Insertion of PICCs) protocol: a bundle of 8 recommendations to minimize the complications related to the peripherally inserted central venous catheters (PICC)]. Assist Inferm Ric. 2014;33:82–9.

Flood S, Bodenham A. Central venous cannulation: ultrasound techniques. Anaesth Intensive Care. 2013;14:1–4.

Gorski L, Hadaway L, Hagle M, Mcgoldrick M, Orr M, Doellman D. Infusion therapy: standards of practice. J Infus Nurs. 2016;39(Suppl 1):S1–S159.

Hallam C, Weston V, Denton A, Hill S, Bodenham A, Dunn H, Jackson T. Development of the UK Vessel Health and Preservation (VHP) framework: a multi-organisational collaborative. J Infect Prev. 2016;17:65–72.

Hanchett M, Poole S. Infusion pathways: planning for success. J Vasc Access Devices. 2001;6:29–37.

Husain LF, Hagopian L, Wayman D, Baker WE, Carmody KA. Sonographic diagnosis of pneumothorax. J Emerg Trauma Shock. 2012;5:76.

Jackson T, Hallam C, Corner T, Hill S. Right line, right patient, right time: every choice matters. Br J Nurs. 2013;22(8):S24, S26–8.

Lamperti M, Bodenham AR, Pittiruti M, Blaivas M, Augoustides JG, Elbarbary M, Pirotte T, Karakitsos D, Ledonne J, Doniger S. International evidence-based recommendations on ultrasound-guided vascular access. Intensive Care Med. 2012;38:1105–17.

Lonsway RA. Patient assessment as related to fluid and electrolyte balance. In: Alexander M, Corrigan A, Gorski L, Hankins J, Perucca R, editors. Infusion nursing: an evidenced based approach. 3rd ed. St Louis: Saunders Elsevier; 2010.

Loveday H, Wilson J, Pratt R, Golsorkhi M, Tingle A, Bak A, Browne J, Prieto J, Wilcox M. EPIC3: national evidence-based guidelines for preventing healthcare-associated infections in NHS hospitals in England. J Hosp Infect. 2014;86:S1–70.

Maki DG, Kluger DM, Crnich CJ. The risk of bloodstream infection in adults with different intravascular devices: a systematic review of 200 published prospective studies. Mayo Clin Proc. 2006;81:1159–71.

Marsh N, Webster J, Larson E, Cooke M, Mihala G, Rickard C. Observational study of peripheral intravenous catheter outcomes in adult hospitalized patients: a multivariable analysis of peripheral intravenous catheter failure. J Hosp Med. 2017;13(2), 83-89.

Mcgee D, Gould M. Preventing complications of central venous catheterization. New Engl J Med. 2003;348:1123–33.

Moureau NL. Ultrasound anatomy of peripheral veins and ultrasound-guided venipuncture. In: Peripherally inserted central venous catheters. Milan: Springer; 2014.

Moureau NL. Vessel health and preservation: vascular access assessment, selection, insertion, management, evaluation and clinical education. Doctor of Philosophy by Publication (PhD) Thesis and Exegesis (PhD Doctorate), Griffith University; 2017.

Moureau N, King K. Advanced ultrasound assessment for venous access clinical education program and DVD. 2007.

Moureau N, Trick N, Nifong T, Perry C, Kelley C, Carrico R, Leavitt M, Gordon S, Wallace J, Harvill M, Biggar C, Doll M, Papke L, Benton L, Phelan D. Vessel health and preservation (Part 1): a new evidence-based approach to vascular access selection and management. J Vasc Access. 2012;13:351–6.

Pirotte T. Ultrasound-guided vascular access in adults and children: beyond the internal jugular vein puncture. Acta Anaesthesiol Belg. 2008;59:157–66.

Pittiruti M. RaCeVA: a guide for a rational choice of the most appropriate vein for central venous catheterization. Association for Vascular Access 26th Annual Scientific Meeting. San Antonio; 2012.

Pittiruti M, Scoppettuolo G. GAVeCeLT manual of PICC and midline—indications, insertion, management. Edra S.P.A.; 2017.

Rotter T, Kinsman L, James E, Machotta A, Gothe H, Willis J, Snow P, Kugler J. Clinical pathways: effects on professional practice, patient outcomes, length of stay and hospital costs. Cochrane Database Syst Rev. 2010;CD006632.

Santolucito J. A retrospective evaluation of the timeliness of physician-initiated PICC referrals: a continuous quality assurance/performance improvement study. J Vasc Access Devices. 2001;6:20–6.

Sharp R, Cummings M, Childs J, Fielder A, Mikocka-Walus A, Grech C, Esterman A. Measurement of vein diameter for peripherally inserted central catheter (PICC) insertion: an observational study. J Infus Nurs. 2015a;38:351–7.

Sharp R, Cummings M, Fielder A, Mikocka-Walus A, Grech C, Esterman A. The catheter to vein ratio and rates of symptomatic venous thromboembolism in patients with a peripherally inserted central catheter (PICC): a prospective cohort study. Int J Nurs Stud. 2015b;52:677–85.

Sharp R, Grech C, Fielder A, Mikocka-Walus A, Esterman A. Vein diameter for peripherally inserted catheter insertion: a scoping review. J Assoc Vasc Access. 2016;21:166–75.

Sou V, Mcmanus C, Mifflin N, Frost SA, Ale J, Alexandrou E. A clinical pathway for the management of difficult venous access. BMC Nurs. 2017;16:64.

Spencer TR, Pittiruti M. Rapid Central Vein Assessment (RaCeVA): a systematic, standardized approach for ultrasound assessment before central venous catheterization. J Vasc Access. 2018;1129729818804718.

Witting MD, Schenkel SM, Lawner BJ, Euerle BD. Effects of vein width and depth on ultrasound-guided peripheral intravenous success rates. J Emerg Med. 2010;39:70–5.

Woller SC, Stevens SM, Evans RS. The Michigan Appropriateness Guide for Intravenous Catheters (MAGIC) initiative: a summary and review of peripherally inserted central catheter and venous catheter appropriate use. J Hosp Med. 2016;11:306–10.

3

Selection of Vascular Access Device

Nancy L. Moureau and Evan Alexandrou

Abstract

Selection of the right vascular access device requires assessment using an algorithmic process, as represented in quadrants 1 and 2 of the VHP model, to provide the patient with a tailored device suited to patient-specific clinical conditions. The process of device selection includes a rational assessment of the patient's needs, vein anatomy and health and medical history as well as consideration of the characteristics of the prescribed therapy, in conjunction with proper knowledge of the proposed treatment. However, the first consideration must be whether the patient's therapy truly justifies administration via an indwelling VAD. This first step is often overlooked in acute healthcare settings, where more than 90% of therapies involve some form of IV administration. With developments in modern drugs, there may well be an oral administration alternative that is equally acceptable and, as such, is less risky to the patient. Perhaps the right VAD is no VAD at all!

Keywords

Selection · Catheter · Central venous Peripheral intravenous · Risk · Complications Infection · Vein anatomy · Vein size Infusion therapy

N. L. Moureau (✉)
PICC Excellence, Inc., Hartwell, GA, USA

Menzies Health Institute, Alliance for Vascular Access Teaching and Research (AVATAR) Group, Griffith University, Brisbane, QLD, Australia
e-mail: nancy@piccexcellence.com

E. Alexandrou
School of Nursing and Midwifery, Western Sydney University, Penrith, NSW, Australia

Central Venous Access and Parenteral Nutrition Service—Liverpool Hospital, Liverpool, NSW, Australia

Menzies Health Research Institute—Alliance for Vascular Access Teaching and Research (AVATAR) Group, Griffith University, Brisbane, QLD, Australia

Faculty of Medicine, South West Sydney Clinical School, University of New South Wales Australia, Sydney, NSW, Australia
e-mail: e.alexandrou@westernsydney.edu.au

3.1 Types of Vascular Access Devices

Vascular access devices are characterized as either peripheral or central, dependent on whether the distal end of the device terminates in the peripheral veins of the body or the larger central veins. Vascular access devices (Fig. 3.1) include:

- Peripheral cannula
- Extended dwell/ultrasound-guided cannula
- Midline catheters
- Central venous access devices

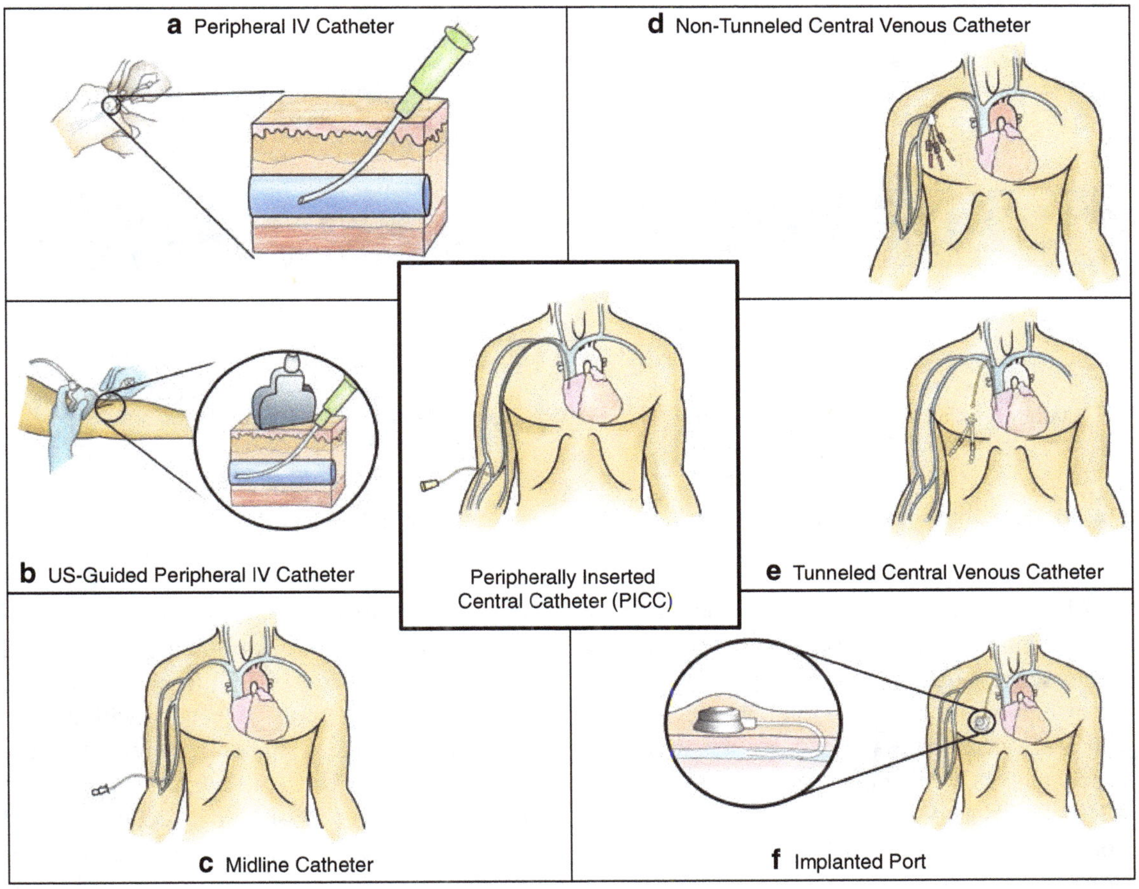

Fig. 3.1 Types of venous access devices (Chopra et al. 2015). *IV* intravenous, *US* ultrasonography. (**a**) Peripheral IV catheter. These devices are typically 3–6 cm, enter and terminate in the peripheral veins (*cross-section*), and are often placed in the upper extremity in veins of the hand. (**b**) US-guided peripheral IV catheter. Ultrasonography may be used to facilitate placement of peripheral intravenous catheters in arm veins that are difficult to palpate or visualize. "Long" peripheral IV catheters (typically ≥8 cm) that are specifically designed to reach deeper veins are also available for insertion under US guidance. (**c**) Midline catheter. These devices are 7.5–25 cm in length and are typically inserted in veins above the antecubital fossa. The catheter tip resides in the basilic or cephalic vein, terminating just short of the subclavian vein. These devices cannot accommodate irritant or vesicant infusions. (**d**) Nontunneled central venous catheter. Also referred to as "acute" or "short-term" central venous catheters, these are often inserted for durations of 7–14 days. They are typically 15–25 cm and are placed via direct puncture and cannulation of the internal jugular, subclavian, or femoral veins. (**e**) Tunneled central venous catheter. These differ from nontunneled catheters in that the insertion site on the skin and site of ultimate venipuncture are physically separated, often by several centimeters, reducing the risk for bacterial entry into the bloodstream and facilitating optimal location of the catheter for care of the exit site. Tunneled devices may be cuffed or noncuffed; the former devices have a polyethylene or silicone flange that anchors the catheter within the subcutaneous tissue and limits entry of bacteria along the extraluminal surface of the device. (**f**) Implanted port. Ports are implanted in the subcutaneous tissue of the chest and feature a reservoir for injection or aspiration (*inset*) and a catheter that communicates from the reservoir to a deep vein of the chest, thus providing central venous access. Ports are cosmetically more desirable than other types of central venous catheter and can remain in place for months or years. (**g**) Peripherally inserted central catheter. These long vascular access devices (>45 cm) are inserted into peripheral veins of the upper arm in adults and advanced so that the tip of the catheter resides in the lower portion of the superior vena cava or upper portion of the right atrium. They are similar to central venous catheters in that they provide access to the central circulation, but they do so without the insertion risks associated with direct puncture of deep veins in the neck, chest, or groin

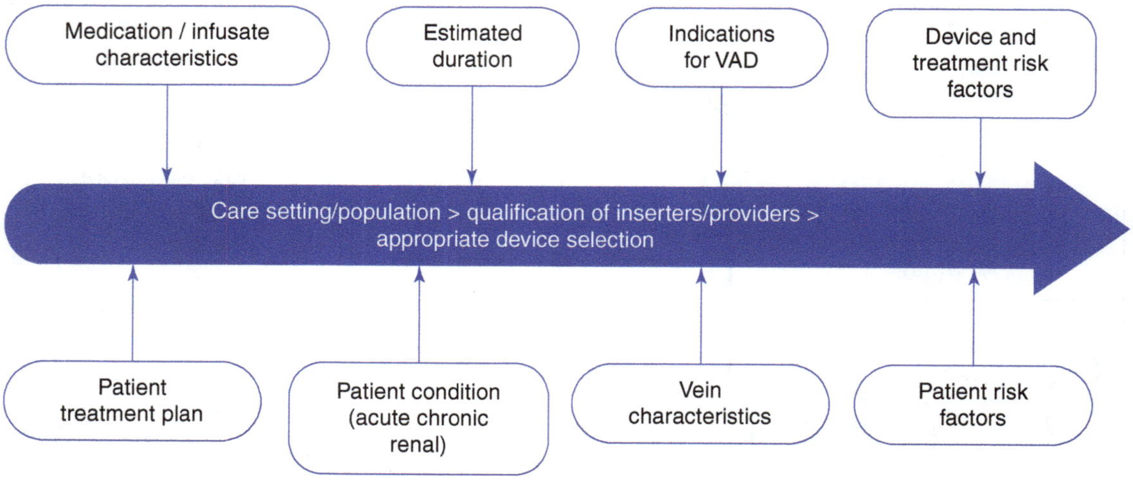

Fig. 3.2 Selection criteria for vascular access device (used with permission N. Moureau, PICC Excellence)

Although not considered a traditional form of VAD, administration of emergency drugs via the intraosseous route is gaining prominence in emergency care protocols where the insertion of a formal VAD cannot be successfully achieved in a timely manner. Whilst not central to discussion of VHP, the intraosseous (IO) route should still be borne in mind as an alternative with emergencies or when intravenous access is not attainable.

The selection and insertion of the most appropriate device for IV therapy are based on a number of key factors (Fig. 3.2):

3.2 Short Peripheral Intravenous Cannula (PIVC)

A short peripheral intravenous cannula (PIVC) is a catheter less than 7.5 cm in length, most commonly inserted in the veins of the hand, forearm or region of the antecubital fossa. PIVCs are used for the infusion of non-irritating, non-vesicant treatments and are a consideration for placement when qualifying treatments are expected to last for less than 5 days. Solutions with high osmolarity are considered irritants or vesicants based on the response of the tissue to the solution. Irritating or vesicant medications and those with an osmolarity greater than 900 mOsm require larger veins for maximum haemodilution to avoid complications and should not be routinely given through a PIVC (Gorski et al. 2016). Irritating medications administered through a PIV should be avoided except in urgent situations, and the device should be replaced as soon as warranted due to patient condition. Complications associated with the use of irritating medications or solutions through catheters with peripheral terminal tip placement include phlebitis, thrombosis, occlusion and other complications arising from damage or inflammation of the vein wall. Dwell time is based on clinically indicated removal (Gorski et al. 2016; Rickard et al. 2012a). Peripheral cannulae are removed when a complication occurs or when therapy is completed.

3.3 Extended Dwell Peripheral (EDP) Cannula

An extended dwell cannula is a peripheral cannula measuring less than 8 cm but designed with a longer cannula (3–7.5 cm) to facilitate ultrasound-guided placement, deeper vein access and longer dwell (Castro and Allison 2012; Gorski et al. 2016). Placement varies but is preferred in the veins of the forearm or upper arm with a catheter long enough to ensure at least two-thirds of the catheter length will reside in the vein after insertion. Infusate considerations and dwell time are the same as with peripheral cannula (INS 2016). EDP may, at times, be considered a midline catheter depending on length and placement location.

3.4 Midline Catheter

A midline catheter is a longer peripheral cannula most commonly inserted into the upper arm via the basilic, cephalic or brachial veins, with the internal terminal tip located below the level of the axilla, distal to the shoulder (Gorski et al. 2016; Adams et al. 2016; Moureau and Chopra 2016). Midline catheter length ranges from 8 cm up to 20 cm. Midline should not extend to the axillary vein or enter the chest. As with short peripheral IV catheters, midline catheters are not used if the osmolarity of prescribed solution is greater than 900 mOsm or the solution is considered irritating or vesicant. Haemodilution, which aids in protecting the vein from damage caused by irritating solutions, occurs at a lower rate in the smaller peripheral veins; therefore, irritating medications are not recommended for non-central placement. Characteristics of certain medications and their level of irritation can be mitigated with dilution resulting in lower concentrations of the irritant. Insertion of a midline catheter is performed in a sterile manner. Midline catheters are available in different lengths, materials (i.e. silicone or polyurethane) and differing insertion methods (i.e. over the needle peel-away, accelerated Seldinger, Seldinger). A midline catheter is considered appropriate when therapy extends beyond 2 days up to approximately 14 days; however, dwell time of a midline catheter does not often exceed 4 weeks and follows clinically indicated removal (Chopra et al. 2015). Optimal dwell time for a midline catheter is unknown and based on complications or clinical need for removal with completion of treatment (O'Grady et al. 2011a, b).

3.5 Central Venous Access Device

A central venous access device (CVAD) is a catheter or implanted port where the tip terminates in the vena cava either superior or inferior depending on upper or lower extremity placement.

The types of CVADs are:

- Peripherally inserted central catheters (PICCs)
- Non-tunnelled devices
- Tunnelled devices
- Implantable ports

CVADs facilitate the delivery of medications and solutions into larger central vessels providing greater haemodilution, reducing the risk of chemical phlebitis and ensuring rapid distribution and clinical effect. The advantages of CVAD are that they can be used to infuse any medication. The disadvantages are the potentially life-threatening insertion-related complications (RCN 2005; Scales 2008) of air embolism, haemorrhage, pneumothorax and post-insertion thrombosis or infection.

3.5.1 Peripherally Inserted Central Catheter (PICC)

A PICC is a central venous cannula inserted through peripheral veins of the extremities or neck with the tip residing in the distal portion of the superior vena cava (SVC) or inferior vena cava (IVC) (Gorski et al. 2016). Any PICC positioned with the terminal tip outside the SVC/IVC is considered malpositioned and is not considered a PICC as the termination is no longer central. PICCs are indicated for patients receiving IV therapy for periods greater than 5 days or when irritating medications or solutions are required (Chopra et al. 2015). As a centrally positioned catheter, PICCs can be used to administer any type of fluid or medication. Terminal catheter tip is confirmed via electrocardiogram (ECG) positioning method, x-ray or fluoroscopic guidance verifying SVC IVC placement prior to use. Complications associated with PICCs include most commonly infection, thrombosis and occlusion. Dwell time is based on clinically indicated removal when a central line is no longer necessary or when a complication develops; optimal dwell time is unknown (O'Grady et al. 2011a, b).

3.5.2 Non-tunnelled Acute Care Catheter

Non-tunnelled acute care catheters are inserted via percutaneous access into the internal jugular, subclavian, axillary or femoral veins and are typically used for patients in acute care requiring critical access. As with all central catheters, the terminal tip is positioned in the SVC/IVC. Available in standard polyurethane, silicone and antimicrobial materials, and configured as single, dual, triple and quad lumens, these catheters are commonly used in critical care areas. Dwell time is often limited to 7–14 days since this is one of the highest-risk catheters and risk of infection increases with the number of days the catheter is in situ (Maki et al. 2006). Dialysis catheters are intentionally excluded from this discussion.

3.5.3 Tunnelled Long-Term Catheter

A tunnelled long-term catheter (neck, chest or groin) is a device that exits the vein in one location and is tunnelled under the skin to a separate exit site, where it emerges from underneath the skin. These catheters are held in place by a Dacron cuff adherent to the catheter, just underneath the skin at the exit site. The exit sites of tunnelled CVADs are most commonly located on the chest to facilitate catheter care. Passing the catheter under the skin in a tunnel may minimize bacterial movement along the insertion tract of the catheter into the vein. The tunnel also provides stability by anchoring the catheter with a Dacron cuff around the catheter positioned just under the skin in the tunnel and adherent within fibrous and subcutaneous tissue. Owing to their more invasive and permanent nature, tunnelled catheters are generally used for patients who require nutritional support or long-term venous access. Removal of tunnelled catheter requires dissection of the adherent cuff within the tunnel.

3.5.4 Subcutaneous Implanted Intravenous Port

Implanted ports considered a long-term CVAD are placed by surgical technique; they are positioned by creating a pocket in the subcutaneous tissue of the chest, arm, abdomen or leg, sliding the port into the pocket and connecting a centrally placed catheter to the port. The catheter, previously advanced into the SVC/IVC, is attached to the port by way of a clip or metal cuff that holds the catheter on the port entrance. Ports have a minimal maintenance when not in use; monthly flushing is all that is recommended to maintain patency (Camp-Sorrell 2011). Implanted ports have a lower risk of infection compared to other external tunnelled and non-tunnelled central lines (Maki et al. 2006). The insertion of a port allows a patient to have minimal body image change owing to the implanted nature of the device with minimal visibly. Physical activity is not impaired with ports; swimming is allowed when the port is not accessed. The disadvantages of ports include some anxiety and discomfort associated when port is accessed with a Huber needle. Training is recommended for the nurse unfamiliar with the steps of port access. The first access should be supervised by another professional familiar with the procedure, along with a review of the hospital policy and instructions for use of the device.

3.6 Other VAD Selection Factors

3.6.1 Quality of Infusate

The characteristics of the infusate can dictate device selection. Solution or medication concentration, level of irritation, vasoactivity and chemical makeup will determine whether the medication is compatible with peripheral devices or requires a CVAD (Alexander and Hankins 2009; Gorski et al. 2016; Stranz 2002).

3.6.2 Length of Therapy

The duration of intravenous therapy impacts appropriate device selection (Chopra et al. 2015). The use of a peripheral intravenous catheter (PIVCs) for peripherally compatible medications in the short term is appropriate; however extended duration of therapy with PIVCs would not be suitable even if the medication is peripherally compatible. PIVC usage would come under scrutiny if the duration of use is intended to exceed 14 days due to the ongoing need for device replacement related to device failure (Wallis et al. 2014).

Those factors determining the length of time a patient will remain in an acute care bed include speed of diagnosis, initiation of treatment, consistent administration of treatment and response to treatment plan. Whilst evaluation of the diagnosis and treatment plan is ongoing, factors such as failed vascular access and delays in administration of medications are variables that impact the evaluation of adequate patient response to the treatment.

Kokotis, in her publication of 2005, described the impact of reduced length of stay as an area of cost reduction dependent on reliable drug infusion via a reliable vascular access device from the onset of therapy resulting in outcome improvement and the potential reduction on length of stay for the facility (Kokotis 2005). In a study conducted at Brigham and Women's Hospital/ Harvard Medical School in Boston, Robinson et al. found the institution of a peripherally inserted central catheter (PICC) team using bedside ultrasound for placement reduced their cost of placement and reduced delays in patient discharge resulting in a savings to the hospital estimated at $950,000 (Robinson et al. 2005). In another study conducted by the University of Michigan, savings with length of stay reductions were minimal, at 3% or less, since the highest cost is at the beginning of the stay (40%) and average cost per day at the end of hospitalization was $304 (Taheri et al. 2000).

Based on the savings with Robinson's group, the reductions from early placement of bedside PICCs by a specialized team resulted in earlier discharges, adding up to significant savings to the facility. Initiation of a process to select those patients most at risk as length of stay outliers, those spending more than 6 days in acute care, has the greatest potential of improving the outcomes for the patient and resulting in decreased length of stay.

Vessel Health and Preservation utilizes evidence to support the best choice of VAD based on expected duration of treatment and infusate characteristics of peripheral compatibility or irritating nature of medication (Babu et al. 2016; Chopra et al. 2015). The knowledge of device selection algorithms can help prevent common problems with peripheral devices such as phlebitis and infiltration but also more serious complications that include bloodstream infection and thrombosis (Moureau and Chopra 2016).

3.6.3 Patient Assessment for Device Selection

Reducing risk and unnecessary harm in the hospital environment begins with assessment of the patient's condition, history, risk assessment and relative vessel health (Figs. 3.3 and 3.4). Matching the patient's current state of health with the need for intravenous access prevents unnecessary IV restarts, reduces medication delays, is economically efficient and provides for optimal outcomes.

There are specific patient conditions that may increase the risk of complications or require special treatment or knowledge when placing vascular access devices. Knowing these risk triggers in advance and planning for specialized treatment for placement of devices when these risks are present provide for safer vascular access and better outcomes for the patient. The recommendations presented here are consistent with published guidance from organizations such as the Joint Commission, the National Patient Safety Goals (NPSG), the Centers for Disease Control and Prevention, the Institute for Healthcare Improvement, the Infusion Nurses Society, the American Society of Diagnostic and Interventional Nephrology, the Oncology Nursing Society and the Society for Healthcare Epidemiology of America (SHEA) strategies (Camp-Sorrell and Matey 2017; Gorski et al. 2016; Hoggard et al. 2008; IHI 2012; Joint Commission 2017; O'Grady et al. 2011a, b).

When selecting a vascular access device, it is important to:

- Minimize the size of the catheter and select the smallest and shortest catheter possible to achieve infusion requirements without complications
- Select the fewest number of lumens; fewer lumens equal less risk for infection

Patient MRN: Age: _____ Admission Date: __________ Discharge Date: _______

LOS:______ Diagnosis List: 1.________________ 2.______________ 3.__________________

Infusions: 1.______________ 2.___________ 3.___________ 4._____________ 5.____________

- Daily assessment of device need documented for each day? **Yes / No**
- Documentation of device choice based on assessment of patient need and risk factors? **Yes / No**
- Documentation of vein health prior to device insertion? **Yes / No**
- Catheter / Vein Ratio Documentation? **Yes / No**
- Assessment for Right Device with in 24 hours? **Yes / No**

Vascular Access Risk Factor Selection: Check all that apply

☐ **Limited Arm Use: CVA, Mastectomy, Trauma**	☐ **Age > or = 65 years**
☐ **Renal Failure**	☐ **History of multiple IV attempts for one successful IV**
☐ **Steroid Use**	☐ **Metastatic Disease**
☐ **Diabetes**	☐ **Antibiotic Infusion**
☐ **HTN**	☐ **Chemotherapy Infusion**
☐ **IV Drug Use**	☐ **Continuous IV Drip**
☐ **Failed IV Access in < 24 hours**	☐ **Parenteral Nutrition**
☐ **Previous Central Line Use**	☐ **Blood Product Transfusion**

Device Data:

Device	Attempts	Date of Insertion	Date of Removal	Dwell Time	Complication Type	Reason for Removal

Fig. 3.3 Patient assessment and VHP audit data collection tool (used with permission N. Moureau, PICC Excellence)

- Select the largest vessel possible to maximize dilution of medications with a terminal tip location appropriate to that medication and risk
- Consider the risk associated with insertion of a particular device and patient condition given the patient's vascular access needs to determine risk/benefit ratio
- Select location and/or extremity with healthiest veins
- Select the device that is least invasive but most appropriate for treatment and duration
- Evaluate for renal dysfunction (creatinine greater than 2.0 or GFR <59 mL/min/1.73 m^2) and avoid the use of the cephalic veins (preserve for future fistula formation)
- Seek to accomplish required device placement within 24–48 h of admission
- Use multidisciplinary approach when performing patient evaluation

3.6.4 Evaluation of Patient Risk Factors

Once the best vascular access device has been indicated based on the diagnosis, required therapies and duration of therapy, the patient is assessed to determine if there are any additional risk factors that contraindicate that device or require special placement considerations for the person/department placing the device (Figs. 3.5 and 3.6).

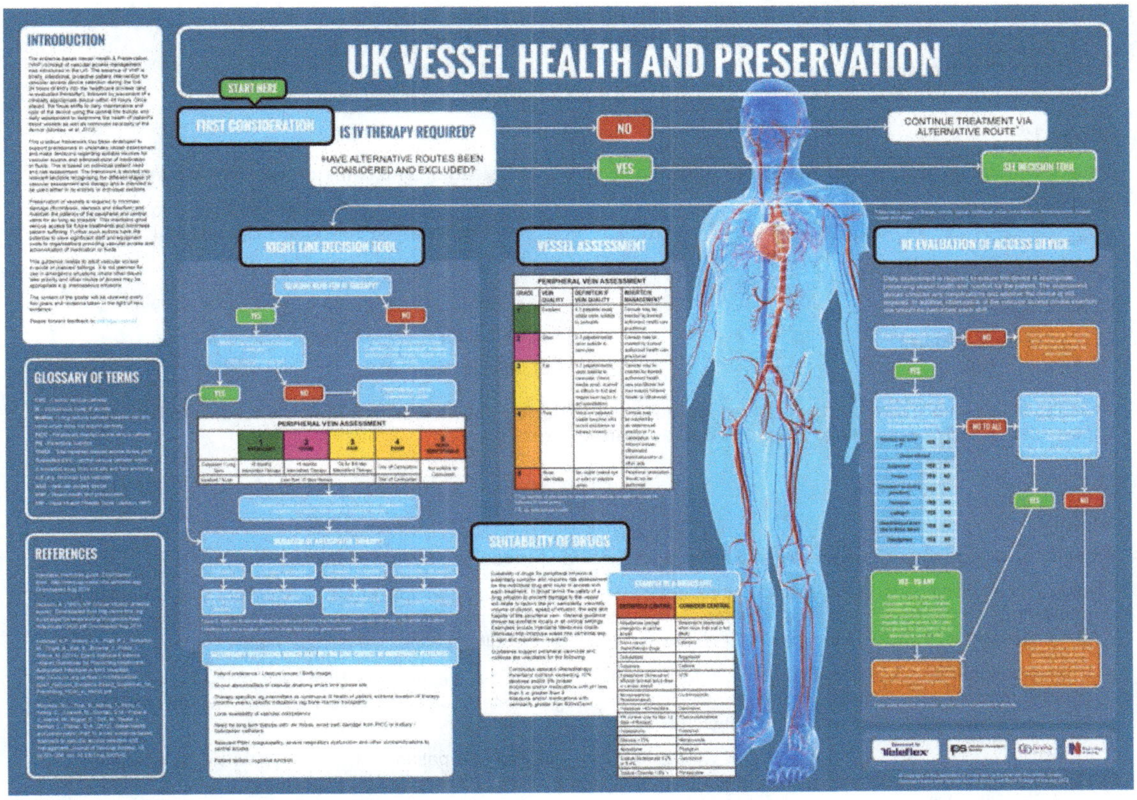

Fig. 3.4 UK vessel health and preservation (used with permission of Carole Hallam and the Infection Prevention Society)

3.6.5 Stage 1 Assessment: Skin Condition (Fig. 3.5)

The most substantial barrier to infection available to any patient is his own skin. When the skin is healthy and intact and free of disease, breaks or other trauma, it provides an occlusive covering preventing bacteria from entering the body. Any break in the skin anywhere on the body provides a portal of entry for bacteria on the skin to enter the body and begin to colonize with the potential to cause infection.

When venous access is required, a puncture is made through the skin and then into the vein. The puncture site now provides a portal of entry for bacteria to enter the body and move directly into the bloodstream along the path of the catheter or directly from within the catheter. To limit the number of bacteria entering the bloodstream, antiseptics are used on the skin to reduce and kill the bacteria around the intended site prior to the venipuncture. Additionally, an occlusive dressing is used to act as a temporary protective skin layer in conjunction with an extra chlorhexidine-impregnated sponge if desired. For these procedures to provide effective protection, they must be performed correctly. The antiseptics must be allowed to dry, and the skin integrity must be intact. In other words, the skin must be healthy enough to withstand the frictional scrub of an antiseptic, and it must be strong enough to allow a dressing to adhere to it in an occlusive manner.

When assessing a patient for risk factors prior to placement of a venous access device, the following factors should be considered:

- Are there skin conditions such as lacerations, abrasions, rashes or psoriasis that prevent an intended site from being accessed?
- Is the skin around the intended insertion site in a condition to safely manage punctures, abrasive cleaning and an occlusive dressing (free from haematomas, skin tears, burns or other forms of skin breakdown)?

Vessel Health and Preservation Protocol
Right Patient Tool – Risk Factors

Directions: Check all that apply.
These risk factors may require a referral or a consult for a vascular access specialist to place indicated device.

Stage 1:

Patient conditions require clinician to use with skin access, vein selection, and catheter size determination.

❑ Elderly skin/loss of elasticity
❑ Abrasions
❑ Psoriasis, skin breakdown
❑ Rash or allergies
❑ Long-term steroid use
❑ Small peripheral veins accommodating 22g or smaller while still allowing 50% space around catheter
❑ Diabetes
❑ History of cancer treatment to peripheral veins
❑ Dehydration or fluid restrictions
❑ Malnutrition

These conditions are known to commonly require multiple restarts. Any patient requiring 2 or more restarts within 24 hours should automatically be referred to Stage 2 and a vascular access consultation.

Stage 2:

Patient conditions require extra care and referral to Vascular Access Specialist for consultation.

❑ High volume fluid needs: blood or blood by-products, intravenous medications, antibiotics, pain meds, TPN/PPN, chemotherapy, inotropes, other types (list not inclusive)
❑ Limited peripheral access due to single side mastectomy, chest or neck surgery, amputation of arms, infection, cellulitis, fistula, trauma or Injury, bums, hematomas, obesity >250lbs
❑ Circulatory status: Stroke, hemiparesis, thrombosis to upper extremity, sign of illegal drug use, elevated INR, fistulas or shunts, severe dehydration or edema/fluid overload, DVT
❑ Previous complications: presence of CVC, frequent IV restarts, history of poor access, hourly blood & draws, required central line access in past
❑ Critical factors: Acuity, life sustaining infusions, inotropes, unstable cardiac status, confirmed MI, arrhythmia, respiratory compromise
❑ Pediatric patient: less than 8 years old, child with high activity level (Pediatric specialist)
❑ Creatinine levels >2.0. Requiring nephrologist OK prior to PICC line placement.

Do not attempt to place device yourself. Refer to Vascular Access Specialist for consultation and placement.

Stage 3:

Patient conditions require clinician to refer patient to Interventional Radiology or Surgeon for placement of any vascular access device.

❑ History of radiology access placement
❑ Renal failure requiring Dialysis catheter
❑ Upper extremity DVT

Do not attempt to place device yourself. Refer to Interventional Radiology or Surgeon for placement.

Fig. 3.5 Right patient tool—risk factors (used with permission of Teleflex)

Some conditions may contraindicate the use of certain venous access devices. The following conditions which affect skin integrity should cause the clinician to pause, consider complications that may be triggered by the condition and determine if another device or site should be chosen based on the patient's individual skin presentation:

- Elderly skin/loss of elasticity
- Geriatric patients
- Lacerations
- Abrasions
- Haematomas
- Psoriasis
- Rash or allergies
- Long-term steroid use (causes thinning of the skin)
- Diabetes
- History of cancer treatment to peripheral veins
- Dehydration or fluid restrictions
- Malnutrition

Remember, the skin is the patient's most substantial barrier to protection from infection. Inserting a vascular access device breaks that

Vessel Health and Preservation Protocol Right Line Contraindication Tool

Place patient label here

Use this tool to determine any risk factors or contraindications that may prevent use of the "right line" as determined by PAGE 1 of the Right Line Tool.

PIV INDICATED UNLESS:	Choose this device instead
❑ Infection, injury or surgery that interferes with access	Internal Jugular or CVC
❑ Meds/fluids that are known irritants	PICC
❑ Continuous infusion of vesicant meds	PICC
❑ Meds as chemotherapeutic agents	PICC
❑ Thrombosis/Clots	CVC
❑ Mastectomy (same side)	CVC
❑ Peripheral neuropathy	Internal Jugular

PIV INDICATED UNLESS:	Choose this device instead
❑ Therapy required for > 4 weeks	PICC
❑ Irritating or vesicant medications	PICC
❑ Fluids that exceed 900mOsm	PICC
❑ Vancomycin is considered an irritant	PICC
❑ Thrombosis/Clots	CVC

PIV INDICATED UNLESS:	Choose this device instead
❑ Thrombosis, peripheral neuropathy, circulatory impairment	CVC
❑ Cellulitis, injury to one or both arms	CVC
❑ History of CVA, mastectomy, upper extremity fistulas	CVC
❑ Fistula; Renal Failtue or Creatinine >2.0	Internal Jugular

PIV INDICATED UNLESS:	Choose this device instead
❑ Elevated INR	Reconsider PICC or PIV
❑ Central or deep vein thrombosis (DVT)	Reconsider PICC or PIV
❑ Low platelet level (50,000)	Reconsider PICC or PIV
❑ Critical status of patient exceeds risk	Reconsider PICC or PIV
❑ Ventilator	Reconsider PICC or PIV
❑ Tracheotomy	Reconsider PICC or PIV
❑ Existing Dialysis Catheter	PIV hand vein or Internal Jugular
❑ Elevated Creatinine >2.0	Internal Jugular

TIPS

- **Always use the smallest device that will administer treatment.**
- **Use the least number of lumens, single when possible.**
- **Consider vein size and catheter size to fit without tourniquet.**
- **Total size of the catheter lumen should not exceed 50% of the vein size.**
- **Each morning complete Daily Assessment for VHP to determine IV device necessity.**
- **Remove IV devices as soon as possible (ASAP).**
- **During ANTT cleanse hubs with frictional scrub before each access to prevent contamination.**
- **When any cap is removed from a catheter or intravenous tubing always apply a sterile cap, never reuse same cap.**
- **Flush all intravenous devices well (10-20ml) after any blood draws.**

❑ No Contraindications present ❑ Device Contraindicated ❑ Device Contraindicated ____________________

Person determining contraindication of device: ____________________

Fig. 3.6 Right line contraindication tool (used with permission of Teleflex)

barrier. Prior to puncturing the skin, pause and consider if this is the best place on the patient's body to break that barrier, and if so, determine how to adequately provide protection to limit the number of bacteria entering the body at that site.

In addition to evaluating skin integrity, consider risks associated with bacterial concentration on various parts of the body. Bacteria are present in differing colony counts throughout the body based on temperature, hair follicles and sebaceous glands. Lower counts of bacteria are present on cooler structures such as the arms and legs. As you move from the extremities toward the main trunk of the body, temperatures increase along with bacterial counts. Because the main body is warmer and usually covered by clothing, bacterial counts are approximately twice that of the extremities. Places such as the groin, the axilla and even the neck have high bacterial counts. When selecting the best insertion site with the lowest risk based on bacterial counts, start from the extremities, and move inward. The groin carries the highest count of bacteria followed by the neck, then the chest and, last, the extremities, with the lowest count.

As with all evaluations of risk, there are many factors to consider when selecting the best site for vascular access selection; integrity of the skin, bacterial counts, risk with insertion and underlying structures all play a part in determining a safe access site for the patient.

3.6.6 Stage 2 Assessment: Vein Conditions and Special Requirements

Once the integrity of the skin has been evaluated, the patient's health history and vasculature must be assessed. Although the skin may appear to be relatively healthy and able to withstand abrasive cleaning and the application of an occlusive dressing, the underlying anatomy may tell a different story.

Certain patient conditions may contraindicate the use of an otherwise indicated device or may require special placement of the device by a vascular access specialist (Fig. 3.5). Any time a patient has a limited extremity, has small peripheral veins or veins that the clinician cannot visualize, expects to receive treatment for more than 5 days or has any other limiting factors, the patient should be referred to a vascular access specialist. The specialist can assess the veins using ultrasound to determine the optimal access site and device for that individual patient. Some additional factors requiring special attention include:

3.6.7 Limited Peripheral Access

A patient with limited peripheral access due to chronic treatments, a mastectomy, breast cancer, chest or neck surgery, amputation of the arms, infection or cellulitis anywhere along the arms, a fistula, trauma or injury needs special assessment for a device that will last the full length of therapy. Patients with multiple IV attempts, high INRs, low platelets or haematomas may require assessment and placement of device by a specialist. Obese patients are particularly challenging and require a specific plan for maintaining access.

3.6.8 High-Volume Fluid Needs

Those patients with high-volume fluid needs require a larger catheter to support the volume of the fluid. Placement of a larger catheter requires an ultrasound assessment of the patient's venous anatomy to determine the optimal access site based on the size of the veins. When administering blood/blood by-products and certain medications (antibiotics, pain meds, TPN/PP, chemotherapy, inotropes), the risk to the patient is higher if the device malfunctions thus necessitating larger vein access.

3.6.9 Circulatory Status

Patients with signs of poor circulation, peripheral neuropathy, a history of stroke, hemiparesis, fistulas or shunts that restrict flow, recurrent thrombosis or other conditions that impact circulation require vascular access performed in such a way as to avoid the affected area(s). These patients may require ultrasound assessment to determine the safest location and vascular access device.

3.6.10 Previous Complications

Those patients who have previously experienced complications with vascular access devices are more likely to have additional complications. Simply the presence of a CVC increases the risk of complications. Patients who require frequent IV restarts, have poor access and need hourly blood draws or other multiple line accesses may require assessment by a specialist for the best device.

3.6.11 Critical Factors

Intensive care patients require many forms of access to accommodate a variety of high-risk medications and solutions. Any patient needing more than two access points for intravenous medications should have a plan for the best access device rather than relying on the access device of the moment. Many types of life-sustaining infusions or inotropes for patients with unstable cardiac status, confirmed MI, arrhythmias or respiratory compromise frequently need a device for longer than 5 days and thus meet the recommendation for consideration of a central venous catheter. Evaluation of a patient's condition and critical status lends itself to early planning to select the right line for the patient to allow treatment access over the full length of therapy.

3.6.12 Other Conditions

Certain conditions place a patient at greater risk for complications with access devices. Patients with chronic conditions such as haematologic and oncologic disease where risk of coagulopathy is great, history of illegal drug use or multiple devices can all lead to challenges with vascular access choices. PICCs may or may not be appropriate for those patients with peripheral injury or overuse. Careful consideration for the right line, in conjunction with the therapy and length of treatment, is paramount with this patient population.

3.6.13 Paediatric Patients

Patients under the age of 8 are particularly challenging for vascular access. Avoiding the trauma of multiple attempts and developing a clear plan for the best device for the patient are most important for paediatric patients. Clinicians with paediatric experience may perform access easily but may or may not be trained with central venous catheter access. Vascular access specialists can perform assessments and aid in the selection of the right line for the patient's treatment.

3.6.14 Stage 3 Assessment: Interventional Radiology Placements

Some patients have predisposing conditions that do not allow for peripheral placement of a device or have a history of difficulty with peripheral or central placement. These patients are candidates for referral to interventional radiology or to a surgeon for placement of a dialysis catheter, tunnelled device or implanted port. The focus for renal patients is on internal jugular placement with avoidance of the subclavian or use of arm veins that may inhibit later fistula placement as with PICCs (Hoggard et al. 2008). Some specific conditions include:

- Renal failure patient requiring dialysis catheter (creatinine >2.0 or GFR <60 mL/min/1.73 m^2)
- Patient with upper extremity deep vein thrombosis
- Patients with a history of radiology access placement
- Contraindication of both extremities
- Bilateral mastectomy/lymph node dissection
- Patient with multiple IV drugs/lumen access
- Unsuccessful PICC access attempt(s)

Because these patients may have limitations and do not have veins or extremities available or their extremities do not provide a safe and healthy option for access, the patients require a centrally inserted vascular access device which must be placed by a surgeon or by interventional radiology.

The focus of the Vessel Health and Preservation Protocol is to provide timely, intentional, proactive patient intervention for vascular access device selection during the first hours of entry into an acute care facility with device placement of the most appropriate catheter within the first days of treatment. Performing risk assessment prior to placement of an indicated device allows the clinician to check for risk factors, critical conditions, acuity, contraindications and infusion needs confirming this patient is indeed the right patient

Table 3.1 Vein identification scale for inserter selection (modified) (used with permission of the Infection Prevention Society (Hallam et al. 2016))

Grade	Vein quality	Definition of vein quality	Type of inserter needed
1	Excellent	4–5 palpable/easily visible veins suitable to cannulate	Clinician trained and competent to insert PIVCs
2	Good	2–3 palpable/visible veins suitable to cannulate	Clinician trained and competent to insert PIVCs
3	Fair	1–2 palpable/visible veins suitable to cannulate (veins may be small, scarred or difficult to find and may require heat to aid vasodilation)	Advanced/specialized training
4	Poor	Veins *not* palpable/visible (requires visualization technology, ultrasound/infrared)	Advanced/specialized training in visualization technology
5	Not identifiable	No visible veins (unable to palpate or identify veins suitable for cannulation)	Advanced/specialized training in visualization technology

for the specified access device. Performing a risk assessment also determines whether the clinician can initiate the vascular access device or if the patient should be referred to a vascular access specialist to perform the procedure (Table 3.1).

3.6.15 Peripheral Versus Central Venous Access Devices (CVAD vs PIVC)

Determination of patient need for peripheral or central cannulation is focused primarily on the characteristics of the treatment medications and secondarily on the duration of treatment as was previously discussed and represented in Figs. 3.7 and 3.8. Other factors may also be considered for selection such as outpatient treatment requiring reliable access, patient-specific contraindications as in renal failure, history of complications and those factors previously discussed.

The use of peripherally inserted central catheters (PICCs) has grown substantially in recent years. Increasing use has led to the realization that PICCs are associated with important complications, including thrombosis and infection. Moreover, some PICCs may not be placed for clinically valid reasons. Defining appropriate indications for insertion, maintenance and care of PICCs is thus important for patient safety. An international panel was convened that applied the RAND/UCLA Appropriateness Method to develop criteria for the use of PICCs (Chopra et al. 2015). After systematic review of the literature, scenarios related to PICC use, care and maintenance were developed according to patient population (e.g. general hospitalized, critically ill, cancer, kidney disease), indication for insertion (infusion of peripherally compatible infusates vs vesicants) and duration of use (≤5 days, 6–14 days, 15–30 days or ≥31 days). Within each scenario, appropriateness of PICC use was compared with that of other venous access devices. After a review of 665 scenarios, 253 (38%) were rated as appropriate, 124 (19%) as neutral/uncertain and 288 (43%) as inappropriate. For peripherally compatible infusions, PICC use was rated as inappropriate when the proposed duration of use was 5 or fewer days. Midline catheters and ultrasonography-guided peripheral intravenous catheters were preferred to PICCs for use between 6 and 14 days. In critically ill patients, non-tunnelled central venous catheters were preferred over PICCs when 14 or fewer days of use were likely. In patients with cancer, PICCs were rated as appropriate for irritant or vesicant infusion, regardless of duration. The panel of experts used a validated method to develop appropriate indications for PICC use across patient populations. These criteria can be used to improve care, inform quality improvement efforts and advance the safety of medical patients.

Prior to the selection and insertion of a vascular access device, an understanding of the indications for that device should be clear. Simple indications would include the need to administer IV fluids, whereas more specific need for parenteral nutrition would indicate a CVAD. CVADs are indicated when peripheral infusion is contraindicated due to treatment with irritating solutions and risk of phlebitis, longer dwell time is expected, frequent blood draws or there is a critical need for vasopressors, anticoagulants, insulin infusions or other dedicated infusions.

3.6.16 Home vs Inpatient Treatment

Patients requiring continuation of treatment from inpatient facility to home or outpatient care have considerations for the type of device inserted. The needs of the home care patient take into account reliability of the catheter, availability of trained clinicians to provide care, minimal number of lumens and consideration for the cost of maintenance. Patient preference is a necessary consideration for the type of VAD since patients may be responsible for some or all therapy administration. The patient receives informed consent and information on device options and types, risk with positive and negative components of each and specific indications for certain devices based on the need and therapy.

3.7 Device-Specific Features

Peripheral and central cannula and ports have specific features and indications that may make one more suitable than another when patient factors are taken into consideration (Figs. 3.6, 3.7, and 3.8). Catheter materials vary with polyurethane and silicone being predominant. Improvements in polyurethane and similar components have added increased flexibility, variations in lumen size, valved and non-valved catheters and impregnation of antibiotic or anti-

Device Type	Proposed Duration of Infusion			
	≤5 d	6–14 d	15–30 d	≥31 d
Peripheral IV catheter	No preference between peripheral IV and US-guided peripheral IV catheters for use ≤5 d			
US-guided peripheral IV catheter	US-guided peripheral IV catheter preferred to peripheral IV catheter if proposed duration is 6–14 d			
Nontunneled/acute central venous catheter	Central venous catheter preferred in critically ill patients or if hemodynamic monitoring is needed for 6–14 d			
Midline catheter	Midline catheter preferred to PICC if proposed duration is ≤14 d			
PICC		PICC preferred to midline catheter if proposed duration of infusion is ≥15 d		
Tunneled catheter				PICC preferred to tunneled catheter and ports for infusion 15–30 d
Port				

Appropriate | Neutral | Inappropriate | Disagreement

Fig. 3.7 Device recommendations for peripherally compatible infusions (The Michigan Appropriateness Guide for Intravenous Catheters (MAGIC) Recommendations) (Chopra et al. 2015)

Device Type	Proposed Duration of Infusion			
	≤5 d	6–14 d	15–30 d	≥31 d
Peripheral IV catheter				
US-guided peripheral IV catheter				
Nontunneled/acute central venous catheter	Central venous catheter preferred in critically ill patients or if hemodynamic monitoring is needed for 6–14 d			
Midline catheter				
PICC		PICC rated as appropriate at all proposed durations of infusion		
Tunneled catheter		Tunneled catheter neutral for use ≥15 d	No preference between tunneled catheter and PICC for proposed durations ≥15 d	
Port				No preference among port, tunneled catheter, or PICC for ≥31 d

Appropriate | Neutral | Inappropriate | Disagreement

IV – intravenous: PICC – peripherally inserted central catheter; US – ultrasonography.

Fig. 3.8 Venous access device MAGIC recommendations for infusion of non-peripherally compatible infusates (Chopra et al. 2015)

septic components (Pittiruti et al. 2014). CVADs with antimicrobial properties may be the best choice for patients with compromised immunity or a propensity for infection (Kramer et al. 2017). Antithrombotic catheters may reduce risk of deep vein thrombosis (DVT) or other types of occlusions (Kleidon et al. 2018). As with any material and foreign matter placed into the body, patient sensitivities to the material may cause reactions (i.e. latex or chlorhexidine allergy). Review of evidence is necessary to measure the value of features and price of products for patient use.

Higher risk is associated with multi-lumen cannula (Chopra et al. 2014; Dobbins et al. 2003; O'brien et al. 2013; Trerotola et al. 2010). Single lumen catheters should be the default for all patients unless indications for added lumen are specified (Byrne and Penwarden 2018). Using single lumen vs multi-lumen catheters has saved millions of dollars and reduced infection and thrombosis rates (O'brien et al. 2013). When multi-lumen catheters are necessary in the case of critically ill patients, consideration should be given to use of antimicrobial catheters. In critically ill patients, it is often difficult to predict evolving need for number of lumens; therefore in acute stage of critical illness, practice is often to accept higher number of lumens and consider de-escalating as the patient stabilizes. The addition of a lumen solely for blood sampling is considered inappropriate (Chopra et al. 2015). There is an overriding principle that unused lumens pose unacceptable risks of infection and should be avoided. Therefore, adopt a practice of 'least number of lumens possible'.

3.7.1 Indications for Multi-lumen Catheters

- Dedicated lumen for parenteral nutrition or vasopressors
- Drug compatibilities/incompatibilities—particularly an issue in critical care patients who

are often receiving multiple infusions of vasoactive agents

- Need for specific lumens for specific functions (i.e. haemodynamic monitoring)
- Medications with irritating characteristics, high osmolarity, vesicants and other solutions that require central administration

3.7.2 Catheter Size

Principles of catheter length and gauge/calibre influence flow (Nifong and Mcdevitt 2011). Poiseuille's equation and application to VAD selection are pertinent to the type of therapy needed (i.e. larger calibre/shorter length equates to increased flow rate). In critically ill patients, the need for fluid resuscitation and emergency care warrants larger calibre cannula to facilitate treatment. Effectively there needs to be a balance between the optimum flow dynamics for the catheter to fulfil its intended role, and the effect of its presence causes as a foreign body within the vessel (Piper et al. 2018).

The best solution for the 'right device' is often a multidisciplinary decision involving the vascular access specialist (VAS), the bedside nurse responsible for administering the therapy and when appropriate the patient. Rather than looking at only a single admission, the patient and VAS may identify an ongoing need for more permanent access moving to a tunnelled catheter of subcutaneously implanted port.

3.7.3 Dialysis, Apheresis and Other Pulmonary Arterial Catheters

Other types of catheters may be used for specific disease states or condition. Patients with chronic renal failure may require dialysis with a large bore catheter inserted through the internal jugular vein allowing high flow rates that facilitate exchange of blood. In a similar process, apheresis catheter are large bore, often tunnelled under the skin to promote stability and long-term use, promoting the process of whole blood removal for therapeutic or donor purposes. Samples of apheresis blood are processed into components such as platelets, plasma, white blood cells, red blood cells or stem cells. Another type of catheter used for pressure readings in the heart is pulmonary artery catheter. This type of catheter is positioned in the pulmonary artery (i.e. Swan-Ganz or right heart catheter) and used in the management of acute myocardial infarction and other critical conditions providing cardiac hemodynamic monitoring.

3.8 Conclusion

The most convenient intravenous device is not always the most efficient in facilitating the completion of the treatment plan. Intentional assessment and selection of VADs based on the patient, treatment, device and clinician provider factors combine to indicate a reliable VAD resulting in the best outcomes for the patient. The types of devices and indications for use are summarized in the Vascular Access Dashboard as shown in Fig. 3.9.

Our goal is to make the vascular access device decision-making process easier and more standardized thereby reducing variations in care, avoiding delays in treatment and increasing patient satisfaction. Developing an organized approach to vascular access device selection provides the educational, regulatory and clinical outcomes necessary for establishing and maintaining reliable access for the delivery of the treatment plan. Patient safety and preservation of vessel health is our goal. The use of the Vessel Health and Preservation program allows for the reduction of variations in care and increases positive patient outcomes.

Vascular Access Dashboard

Device	PIV	USGPIV	MIDLINE	PICC	CVC non-tunnelled	Antimicrobial CVC	Tunnelled CVC	PORT
Indications	Immediate Intravenous access, general Infusions. Treatment with peripher-ally compatible infusion. Forearm placement more reliable	Difficult access patient (DIVA) with 1 or more attempts Treatment 5 days or less than 14 days (transition to midline). Requires longer peripheral catheter	Difficult access patient (DIVA) less than 14 days. More reliable than USGPIV and may be more appropriate in ICU setting	Central Catheter indications for peripher-ally incompat-ible Infusions/ irritants, vesicants, vasoactive medications. Measure vein size to approximate catheter to vein ratio of less than 45%	Central catheter indications. Critically ill patients requiring vasopressors, haemodynamic monitoring. Subclavian preferred for lower infection risk.	Antimicrobial catheters reduce incidence of infections and may be most appropriate for ICU patients. Central catheter indications. For high risk patients or those with history of infections.	Central catheter indications. Longer term treatment for Parenteral nutrition, cancer, other	Central catheter indications. Longer term treatment for Parenteral nutrition, cancer, other
Treatment	Peripherally compatible infusions	Peripherally compatible infusions	Peripherally compatible infusions	Peripherally incompatible infusions or based on duration	Peripherally incompatible infusions or based on duration	Peripherally Incompatible Infusions with history of infection	Peripherally incompatible infusions and based on duration	Peripherally Incompatible infusions and based on duration
Duration	Treatment 5 days or less. Clinically indicated removal policy may extend time if required and without complications for less than 6 days	Treatment less than 6 days or up to 14 days. Clinically indicated removal policy may extend time if required and without complications	Treatment exceeding 6 days and less than 14 days. Clinically indicated removal policy may extend time if required and without complications	Treatment with any infusion greater or equal to 15 days up to 30 days. Difficult access patient greater than 6 days Preference for midline with less than 15 days. Any duration for peripherally incompatible Infusions.	Treatment 6-14 days. Any duration for peripher-ally incompat-ible infusions. Preferred device for critically ill/unstable patients or if haemodynamic monitoring is needed.	Treatment up to 30 days. May be appropriate for catheter exchanges. Applies to PICC and chest Inserted CVC (CICC)	Treatment 15-30 days or longer	Treatment 15-30 days or longer
Contra-indications	Circulatory impairment, or hemiparesis. For chronic renal failure (CKD) patients insertion focused on dorsum of the hand.	Circulatory impairment, or hemiparesis. For chronic renal failure (CKD) patients insertion focused on dorsum of the hand.	Circulatory impairment, or hemiparesis, history of upper extremity deep vein thrombosis. Not appropriate for CKD patients	Greater risk of thrombosis with unstable, hypercoagu-lable or patients with history of thrombosis.	Coagulopathies and other patient specific contrain-dications.	Sensitivity to chlorhexidine or other impregna-tions.	Without availability of trained inserter	Morbid obesity, coagulopathies
RISK LEVEL	0.2-0.5/1000 catheter days	0.2-0.5/1000 catheter days	0.2-0.8/1000 catheter days	2.1/1000 cath-eter days Higher risk in Intensive Care areas	2-5/1000 catheter days	1.2-1.6/1000 catheter days	1.6/1000 cath-eter days	0-0.4/1000 catheter days

References

1. Ajenjo MC, Morley JC, Russo AJ, McMullen KM, Robinson C, Williams RC, Warren DK (2011) Peripherally inserted central venous catheter-associated bloodstream infections in hospital-ized adult patients. Infect Control Hosp Epidemiol. 32(21): 125-30.
2. Chopra V. Anand S. KreinSL et al., (2012) Bloodstream infec-ton, venous thrombosis, and peripherally inserted central catheters: reappraising the evidence. Am J Med. 125(8): 733-41.
3. Maki DG. Kluger DM. Crnich CJ (2006) The risk of blood-stream infection in adult with different intravascular devices: a systematic review of 200 published prospective studies. Mayo Clin Proc, 81(9): 1159-71.
4. Pikwer A, Åkeson J. Lindgren S (2012) Complications asso-ciated with peripheral or central routes for central venous cannulation. Anaesthesia, 67(1): 65-71.
5. Deutsch GB. Sathyanarayana SA, Singh N et al. (2014) Ultra-sound-guided placement of midline catheters in the surgical intensive care unit: a cost-effective proposal for timely central line removal. J Surg Res, 191(1): 1-5.
6. Wilson TJ, Stetler WR, Fletcher JJ (2013) Comparison of cath-eter-related large vein thrombosis in centrally inserted versus peripherally inserted central venous lines in the neurological intensive care unit. Clin Neurol Neurosurg. 115(7): 879-82.
7. Anderson NR (2004) Midline catheters: the middle ground of intravenous therapy administration. J Infus Nurs, 27(5): 313-21.
8. Simonov M, Pittirutl M, Rickard CM, Chopra V (2015) Navigating venous access: a guide for hospitalists.J Hosp Med, 10(71) 471-8.

Fig. 3.9 Vascular access dashboard (used with permission N. Moureau, PICC Excellence)

Case Study

Mrs. Smith is a 76-year-old with complicated pneumonia. Her treatment process includes administration of irritating intravenous medications for at least 7 days. A short peripheral catheter was initially inserted and has infiltrated within just a few hours of insertion. Mrs. Smith has few visible veins, is a small woman and is receiving non-irritating medications.

What is the best device to consider that would facilitate completion of the treatment plan?

Following vein assessment, it was apparent that veins of the lower arm/forearm were not suitable for intravenous access. A midline catheter was selected as the best device and placed with ultrasound guidance into the basilic vein. The patient received medication infusions without interruption for 7 days completing the course of treatment. The midline catheter was removed, and the patient discharged to home.

Summary of Key Points

1. VAD selection is optimal when individualized for the patient based on treatment plan, medication types, duration and patient-specific factors.
2. Understanding the types and available options of VAD is key to selection for each patient.
3. Collaborative practice with device selection including the patient results in long-term solutions that work for all.
4. Vessel Health and Preservation process is designed to guide the clinician to select the lowest-risk device option for the patient by applying research and guidelines such as MAGIC for device appropriateness.
5. Multi-lumen devices are associated with increased complications and should only be inserted when absolutely necessary.

References

Alexander M, Hankins J. Infusion nursing: an evidence-based approach: Elsevier Health Sciences; 2009.

Babu S, Bennett J, Binks R, Fee P, Fox B, Johnston A, Klein A, Langton J, Mclure H, Tighe S. Association of Anaesthetists of Great Britain and Ireland: safe vascular access 2016. Anaesthesia. 2016;71:573–85.

Byrne D, Penwarden L. Selection of single-versus double-lumen peripherally inserted central catheters and the influence on alteplase use. J Infus Nurs. 2018;41:118–21.

Camp-Sorrell D. Access device guidelines: recommendations for nursing practice and education. 2nd ed. Oncology Nursing Society; 2011. p. 170.

Camp-Sorrell D, Matey L. Access device standards of practice for oncology nursing. Pittsburg: Oncology Nursing Society; 2017.

Castro S, Allison R. Use of midline (extended dwell peripheral IV) device improves patient safety and saves costs compared to PICCs. Poster presented at Association for Vascular Access Annual Scientific Meeting, San Antonio, TX, October 2012.

Chopra V, Ratz D, Kuhn L, Lopus T, Lee A, Krein S. Peripherally inserted central catheter-related deep vein thrombosis: contemporary patterns and predictors. J Thromb Haemost. 2014;12:847–54.

Chopra V, Flanders SA, Saint S, Woller SC, O'Grady NP, Safdar N, Trerotola SO, Saran R, Moureau N, Wiseman S, Pittiruti M, Akl EA, Lee AY, Courey A, Swaminathan L, Ledonne J, Becker C, Krein SL, Bernstein SJ, Michigan Appropriateness Guide for Intravenous Catheters Panel. The Michigan appropriateness guide for intravenous catheters (MAGIC): results from a multispecialty panel using the RAND/UCLA appropriateness method. Ann Intern Med. 2015;163:S1–40.

Dobbins BM, Catton JA, Kite P, Mcmahon MJ, Wilcox MH. Each lumen is a potential source of central venous catheter-related bloodstream infection. Crit Care Med. 2003;31:1688–90.

Gorski L, Hadaway L, Hagle M, Mcgoldrick M, Orr M, Doellman D. Infusion therapy: standards of practice. J Infus Nurs. 2016;39(Suppl 1):S1–S159.

Gorski, et al. 2016 (for the INS reference).

Hallam C, Weston V, Denton A, Hill S, Bodenham A, Dunn H, Jackson T. Development of the UK Vessel Health and Preservation (VHP) framework: a multi-organisational collaborative. J Infect Prev. 2016;17:65–72.

Hoggard J, Saad T, Schon D, Vesely T, Royer T. Guideline for venous access in patients with chronic kidney disease: a Position Statement from the American Society of Diagnostic and Interventional Nephrology Clinical Practice Committee and the Association for Vascular Access. Semin Dial. 2008;21:186–91.

IHI. How-to-guide: prevent central line-associated bloodstream infections. 2012.

Joint Commission. National patient safety goals: the Joint Commission Accreditation Program: Hospital. 2017.

Kleidon T, Ullman AJ, Zhang L, Mihala G, Chaseling B, Schoutrop J, Rickard CM. How does your PICCOMPARE? A pilot randomized controlled trial comparing various PICC materials in pediatrics. J Hosp Med. 2018;13(8):517–25.

Kokotis K. Cost containment and infusion services. J Infus Nurs. 2005;28:S22–32.

Kramer RD, Rogers MA, Conte M, Mann J, Saint S, Chopra V. Are antimicrobial peripherally inserted central catheters associated with reduction in central line–associated bloodstream infection? A systematic review and meta-analysis. Am J Infect Control. 2017;45:108–14.

Maki DG, Kluger DM, Crnich CJ. The risk of bloodstream infection in adults with different intravascular devices: a systematic review of 200 published prospective studies. Mayo Clin Proc. 2006;81:1159–71.

Moureau N, Chopra V. Indications for peripheral, midline, and central catheters: summary of the Michigan appropriateness guide for intravenous catheters recommendations. J Assoc Vasc Access. 2016;21:140–8.

Nifong T, Mcdevitt T. The effect of catheter to vein ratio on blood flow rates in a simulated model of peripherally inserted central venous catheters. Chest. 2011;140:140–53.

O'brien J, Paquet F, Lindsay R, Valenti D. Insertion of PICCs with minimum number of lumens reduces complications and costs. J Am Coll Radiol. 2013;10:864–8.

O'Grady N, Alexander M, Burns L, Dellinger E, Garland J, Heard S, Lipsett P, Masur H, Mermel L, Pearson M, Raad I, Randolph A, Rupp M, Saint S. Guidelines for the prevention of intravascular catheter-related infections, 2011. Centers for Disease Control; 2011a. p. 1–83.

O'Grady N, Alexander M, Burns L, Dellinger E, Garland J, Heard S, Lipsett P, Masur H, Mermel L, Pearson M, Raad I, Randolph A, Rupp M, Saint S, Healthcare Infection Control Practices Advisory Committee (HICPAC). Centers for Disease Control Guidelines for the prevention of intravascular catheter-related infections. Clin Infect Dis. 2011b;52:e162–93.

Piper R, Carr PJ, Kelsey LJ, Bulmer AC, Keogh S, Doyle BJ. The mechanistic causes of peripheral intravenous catheter failure based on a parametric computational study. Sci Rep. 2018;8:3441.

Pittiruti M, Emoli A, Porta P, Marche B, Deangelis R, Scoppettuolo G. A prospective, randomized comparison of three different types of valved and non-valved peripherally inserted central catheters. J Vasc Access. 2014;15:519–23.

RCN. Standards for infusion therapy. 4th ed. London: Royal College of Nursing; 2005. p. 1–94.

Rickard CM, Webster J, Wallis MC, Marsh N, McGrail MR, French V, Foster L, Gallagher P, Gowardman JR, Zhang L, McClymont A. Routine versus clinically indicated replacement of peripheral intravenous catheters: a randomised controlled equivalence trial. Lancet. 2012;380(9847):1066–74.

Robinson M, Mogensen K, Grudinskas G, Kohler S, Jacobs D. Improved care and reduced costs for patients requiring peripherally inserted central catheters: the role of bedside ultrasound and a dedicated team. J Parenter Enter Nutr. 2005;29:374–9.

Scales K. Intravenous therapy: a guide to good practice. Br J Nurs. 2008;17(Suppl 8):S4–12.

Stranz M. Adjusting PH and osmolarity of infusion solutions: what is reasonable? NAVAN Annual Conference, January, 1–5. 2002.

Taheri P, Butz D, Greenfield L. Length of stay has minimal impact on the cost of hospital admission. J Am Coll Surg. 2000;191:123–30.

Trerotola S, Stavropoulos S, Mondschein J, Patel A, Fishman N, Fuchs B, Kolansky D, Kasner S, Pryor J, Chittams J. Triple-lumen peripherally inserted central catheter in patients in critical care unit: prospective evaluation. Radiology. 2010;256:312.

Wallis MC, Mcgrail MR, Webster J, Gowardman JR, Playford G, Rickard CM. Risk factors for PIV catheter failure: a multivariate analysis from a randomized control trial. Infect Control Hosp Epidemiol. 2014;35:63–8.

Part II

The Importance of Right Education

4

VAD Inserter: Training and Education

Evan Alexandrou, Nicholas Mifflin, and Peter J. Carr

Abstract

Optimal vascular access insertion and management requires clinicians to have appropriate education and skill on the best procedural techniques or be supervised during the process of acquiring the necessary education. The second quadrant of the Vessel Health and Preservation (VHP) model requires a qualified inserter, a clinician who has undertaken a comprehensive clinical and vascular assessment and is applying the latest evidence and guidelines to select the most appropriate device for patient treatment, leading to the successful insertion of a peripheral or central VAD. Appropriate device selection and number of necessary lumens are a determination made according to lowest risk for patient insertion and potential for infection, in conjunction with the needs of the therapy. Selection of the best vascular access for the patient also requires an understanding of the most appropriate intravascular device to be used, influenced by infusate characteristics to be administered and the length of anticipated dwell, which in turn, influences the most appropriate vessel and anatomical position for device placement.

Keywords

VAD training · VAD education · Training requirements · Core competencies for validation · Training recommendations Simulation training · Checklists · Rating scales

E. Alexandrou (✉)
School of Nursing and Midwifery, Western Sydney University, Penrith, NSW, Australia

Central Venous Access and Parenteral Nutrition Service—Liverpool Hospital, Liverpool, NSW, Australia

Menzies Health Research Institute—Alliance for Vascular Access Teaching and Research (AVATAR) Group, Griffith University, Brisbane, QLD, Australia

Faculty of Medicine, South West Sydney Clinical School, University of New South Wales Australia, Sydney, NSW, Australia
e-mail: e.alexandrou@westernsydney.edu.au

N. Mifflin
School of Nursing and Midwifery, Western Sydney University, Penrith, NSW, Australia

Central Venous Access and Parenteral Nutrition Service—Liverpool Hospital, Liverpool, NSW, Australia
e-mail: Nicholas.Mifflin@health.nsw.gov.au

P. J. Carr
HRB Clinical Research Facility Galway, National University of Ireland Galway, University Hospital Galway, Galway, Ireland

4.1 Introduction

Insertion of the right device and the right inserter encompass the second stage of the VHP process. Selection of the inserter and application of infection prevention principles are contributing factors for patient safety. Vascular access specialists and teams' function to aid in selection and insertion of the most appropriate device. Ensuring the insertion is performed by a trained and qualified clinician with ultrasound skills reduces insertion and post insertional complications. The training, education and competency necessary to become a qualified VAD inserter are discussed throughout the rest of this chapter.

4.2 The Need for Adequate Education

Insertion of IV devices is a highly technical, high-risk procedure with greater risk to patients when CVADs are inserted and used (Chopra et al. 2015). The successful insertion of vascular devices relies on clinician expertise which is determined by training, credentialing and procedural volume. Historically, clinical expertise was seen as synonymous with the medical profession. Technically advanced vascular access such as central venous catheter (CVC) placement was the domain of the medical practitioner. However, clinical practice is continuously evolving; patient complexity, technology and hospital workload demands have spurred new clinical subspecialties that are changing the boundaries of traditional clinical work, where the medical practitioner is not necessarily at the centre of all clinical procedures (Dowling et al. 1995; Williams et al. 1997; Alexandrou et al. 2010).

According to the US Food and Drug Administration (FDA) in a survey of 1988 and subsequent investigations by a Central Venous Catheter Working group, over 55% of all vascular access-related complications were attributable to healthcare workers (Scott 1988). Whilst these data are dated, this investigation indicated lack of training and validation of competency as a direct cause of complications. In current literature, this concept of training and validation is illustrated in both newer ultrasound practices and with infection reduction methods (Primdahl et al. 2016; Rusche et al. 2001). Insufficient understanding of evidence-based assessment, selection, insertion and management of peripheral and central venous access devices leaves the patient at risk for more serious complications and the added trauma associated with frequent replacement of catheters (Rickard et al. 2013).

Comprehensive education on VAD insertion including competency assessment has shown to reduce procedural complications in comparison to minimal or no education (Alsaad et al. 2017; Evans et al. 2010; Sherertz et al. 2000). Procedural load plays a significant role in successful vascular device insertion, and the number of devices placed is a known modifiable risk factor (Alexandrou et al. 2014; Eisen et al. 2006; Sherertz et al. 2000). The number of devices placed can increase clinician experience and confidence. Studies have reported that experienced CVAD inserters who have inserted more than 50 catheters have half the complication rate of CVAD inserters who have inserted less than 50 catheters (McGee and Gould 2003).

Inadequate training and education on vascular access theory and techniques can expose patients to unnecessary iatrogenic complications (Alexandrou et al. 2010; Castro-Sánchez et al. 2014; Scott 1988). The insertion of central venous access devices (CVADs) by operators with minimal experience or supervision can pose significant risk to patient safety (Alexandrou et al. 2010, 2014; Hamilton 2005). Serious adverse outcomes have been reported from procedural complications related to CVAD insertion that have contributed to patient morbidity and mortality (Carr et al. 2018). These complications can include mechanical and infectious complications as well as thrombotic complications (McGee and Gould 2003). The most critical insertion-related complications include pneumothorax, nerve damage and major artery puncture and may occur in up to one in six catheter insertions (Eisen et al. 2006; Taylor and Palagiri 2007). Patients with previous cannulation attempts, history of surgery at the site of proposed cannulation, obesity and a lack of operator expertise have all been documented as influencing factors for CVAD insertion complication risk (Nayeemuddin et al. 2013).

The right education and training in VAD insertion have a positive impact on reducing central line-associated bloodstream infectious complications (Coopersmith et al. 2002; Sherertz et al. 2000). The primary goal of VHP is to reduce risk associated with the insertion and management of VADs; this can be achieved through infection prevention education. The Centers for Disease Control (CDC) endorse education as a necessary component of infection prevention (O'Grady et al. 2011). Additionally, the CDC recommends that education by specialist teams results in the best outcomes for CVAD insertion and management. An increased risk of device infection is associated with unskilled, inexperienced or unqualified inserters. Successful insertion of VADs relies on operator knowledge, expertise and application of evidence-based guidelines shown to reduce complications (Babu et al. 2016; Mourad et al. 2010).

There has been significant improvement in the health outcomes of patients in recent decades, most notably through the advancements in technology and evidenced-based treatment (Loveday et al. 2014; Teramoto et al. 2017). In contrast, the increasing complexity of patient comorbidity and specialised procedural skills required to treat such patients has also attributed to adverse procedural outcomes and a need for more training (Barach and Johnson 2006; Pronovost et al. 2002). Vascular access device (VAD) placement is one such procedural skill that has become an essential component to many therapies yet carries risks which can lead to serious adverse patient outcomes contributing to morbidity and mortality (Eisen et al. 2006; McGee and Gould 2003; Miliani et al. 2017).

4.3 The Right Education: Insertion Training

It is worth recognising that people learn in different ways, and having some understanding of these concepts will allow the educator to plan the most effective way to assist learning (Taylor and Hamdy 2013). Significance of patient safety and fairness to novice clinicians has seen the paradigm of "see one, do one, teach one" evolve significantly into models of required educational components for CVAD placement (Davidson et al. 2012; Lenchus 2010; Moureau et al. 2013; Rodriguez-Paz et al. 2009). It is clear that standardized, structured approaches incorporating education, supervision and simulation to teach procedures improve knowledge and skill acquisition, increase learner confidence and reduce complications in clinical practice (Herrmann-Werner et al. 2013).

Comprehensive vascular access training should consist of didactic lectures, skills acquisition in a simulated environment and supervised application with patient insertions (Marschall et al. 2014; Troianos et al. 2011). Competency assessment in VAD insertion in a simulated environment before patient insertion should be a basic patient safety goal in every healthcare facility (Davidson et al. 2012). It is still not uncommon, however, for trainees to undertake invasive procedures with minimum or no supervision as is the case with many ultrasound-guided peripheral catheter insertions. It is also not uncommon for supervisors to be junior and inexperienced with risk mitigating strategies (Lenhard et al. 2008). All of these factors contribute to or reduce the level of risk for the patient requiring vascular access insertion and management.

4.4 Right Education for PIVC Success

Successfully inserting a PIVC on the first attempt preserves veins and enhances the concept of vessel health and preservation. This immediate success with insertion can impact patient wellbeing and experience, in addition to the probability of concluding treatment without complication. Insertion success and lack of complications are influenced by a variety of clinical variables and include clinician, patient-specific, products and technology as well as ergonomic and environmental factors (Carr et al. 2016a; Chopra et al. 2012).

Many international clinical guidelines include recommendations for various aspects of PIVC insertion and care (Gorski et al. 2016; Loveday et al. 2014; O'Grady et al. 2011). Despite such guidance, PIVC insertion can be difficult (Riker et al. 2011; van Loon et al. 2016; Yen et al. 2008), time consuming, anxiety producing (Dougherty and Lamb 2014) and painful for the patient (Fields et al. 2014). Clinicians are required to be competent (and in some cases, certified) to perform a range of functions regarding the insertion of a PIVC that include assessment of the potential insertion site, proficiency with the insertion procedure and ability to maintain the device post insertion and perform surveillance to detect complications or loss of function (Moureau et al. 2013; Moureau 2017).

Studies report wide-ranging variability of first-time insertion success: between 2 and 81%. Patients may be subjected to two or more attempts when a traditional landmark/palpation-guided insertion approach is used (Aulagnier et al. 2014; Carr et al. 2010; Witting 2012). The use of ultrasound to guide insertion may improve these rates, but as yet, ultrasound is inconsistently used for PIVC insertions. Given the variability in first-time insertion success, there is an opportunity to address this clinical phenomenon and improve outcomes for patients.

The literature suggests some patient factors that increase the risk of insertion failure (Carr et al. 2016b; Fields et al. 2014; Maki and Ringer 1991; Sebbane et al. 2013). Failure within this literature base is attributed to the skill of the inserter; experience and knowledge of ultrasound; catheter length and amount within the vein, depth and size of the vein; ability to guide needle and catheter deeply into the vein; and various patient factors. However, there has been little research on how these risk factors can then potentially be used to assess the degree of insertion difficulty, i.e. the likelihood of PIVC insertion success prior to insertion. Such guidance would be useful in identifying high-risk patients to target with interventions that may prevent insertion failure. The VHP framework incorporates the peripheral vein visual inspection process, identifying anticipated levels of difficulty by the condition of veins (Hallam et al. 2016).

Avoiding scheduled PIVC insertions and opting for clinically indicated removal have been predicted to save tens of millions of dollars for facilities each year (Tuffaha et al. 2014). Furthermore, considering the patient experience and satisfaction with care, improving the patient journey with better vascular access protocols should be a priority for hospital administrators (Moureau et al. 2012). Achieving greater first-time insertion success in addition to increasing the functional dwell time of inserted PIVCs through a standardised vascular access bundle could potentially support such an endeavour, saving money and impacting positively on the patient experience (Cooke et al. 2018; Larsen et al. 2017). In addition, capturing relevant insertion and post insertion data points prospectively in a digital first strategy through a clinical database could conceivably answer a variety of clinical questions and inform local hospitals of their baseline and continuous data points (Davis 2011).

Given that documentation of PIVCs is often not percieved as a clinical concern (Castro-Sánchez et al. 2014), when outcomes are poorly recorded in the medical chart or computer record, greater emphasis is required to stress the usefulness of vascular access data recording. Such a concept, when underpinned by VHP, could revolutionise the decision-making for vascular access science in addition to contributing to a continuous data cycle to inform hospitals of actual and potential outcomes.

4.5 Approaches to Training

Depending on available resources, an online web-based approach to training may serve to replace or support traditional face-to-face educational lectures and has been proven as an acceptable alternative (Chenkin et al. 2008; Moureau et al. 2013). Online training is potentially advantageous in that it can be standardised and accessible almost anywhere, at any time. Incorporating video as a tool to demonstrate procedures and techniques has been a common inclusion within successful programmes (Evans et al. 2010; Nguyen et al. 2014).

Simulation-based training for teaching procedures is shown to improve skill acquisition, increase learner confidence and reduce complications in clinical practice (Hirvela et al. 2000). Simulators used in vascular access training range from highly technical interactive mannequins, to partial task trainers replicating anatomical structures and to simulators incorporating virtual reality. Whilst equipment like this can be expensive, effective high-fidelity phantoms may be produced with readily accessible items such as poultry breasts fitted with drains for comparatively little cost (Loukas et al. 2011; Moureau et al. 2013; Rippey et al. 2015).

Approaches to training should be based on a curriculum that clearly defines the cognitive knowledge and technical skill required to undertake ultrasound-guided vascular access (Schmidt and Kory 2014; Troianos et al. 2011). An international evidence-based consensus task force established through the World Congress of Vascular Access recommends 6–8 h of didactic education, 4 h hands-on training on inanimate models and 6 h hands-on training on normal human volunteers for appreciation of normal ultrasound anatomy (Moureau et al. 2013). Training is then followed by supervised insertions, guided by experienced clinicians giving feedback for improvement. The number of procedures required to achieve competence in real-time ultrasound-guided vascular access is unspecified due to the variables in knowledge and skill acquisition between individuals (Moureau et al. 2013; Troianos et al. 2011).

Technical performance in vascular access is typically assessed using checklists or global rating scales. Procedures in vascular access are generally comprised of a number of sequential steps, thus making assessment possible using a checklist (Moureau et al. 2013). Although global rating scales can be contentious, they can be a better indicator of procedural competency compared to checklist assessment (Ma et al. 2012; Moureau et al. 2013). Clinicians performing high-risk procedures such as vascular access insertions require periodic competency assessment, determined by each facility, but recommended as part of annual or biennial credentialing.

The following sections reflect core competencies necessary for undertaking catheter insertion safely based on the VHP philosophy and minimal training requirements (Moureau et al. 2013):

1. Anatomy and physiology of relevant body systems
2. Ultrasound for insertion and assessment
3. Central venous device tip location
4. Infection control and ANTT
5. Device selection and indications
6. Insertion procedures, complication prevention, evaluation and management
7. Care and maintenance practices along with needle-free connectors and securement devices
8. Qualification and competency
9. Simulation training
10. Anatomical models
11. Objective grading and proficiency
12. Examination and competency
13. Supervised instruction
14. Didactic or web-based training
15. Developing clinical competence
16. Education for children and neonates

4.5.1 Anatomy and Physiology

A working knowledge of anatomy and physiology is essential for those undertaking vascular access procedures to minimise complications (Bannon et al. 2011; Moureau et al. 2013). Traditionally, it was the presumed location of a blood vessel, the correlation between surface anatomical landmarks and deep anatomical structures that would guide percutaneously inserted VAD (Bannon et al. 2011). Ultrasound guidance is advantageous in that it provides an "inside view" of deep anatomical structures but requires anatomical knowledge to manipulate both transducer and insertion needle avoiding complications from cannulation of incorrect vessels (Bannon et al. 2011; Troianos et al. 2011). Understanding both normal and variant anatomies enables clinicians to safely complete procedures and identify complications such as misplaced catheters should they occur (Bannon et al. 2011; Moureau et al. 2013).

4.5.2 Use of Ultrasound

Ultrasound for vascular access is not a new concept and has been used in clinical practice for decades. Over time ultrasound has become widely accepted as a means to improve procedural success rates and reduce associated complications and is now included in many practice guidelines (Moore 2014; Moureau et al. 2013; Troianos et al. 2011). Notwithstanding a multitude of evidence showing the benefit of using ultrasound guidance for vascular access, success is not guaranteed through mere placement of a transducer on the patient (Lamperti et al. 2012; Moore 2014). The clinician must have an understanding of ultrasound physics, mechanisms of image acquisition and optimization and artefacts and ultimately be able to interpret 2D images representing 3D anatomical structures. When novice clinicians first begin to practise using ultrasound and align the ultrasound probe and the needle over the vein of the phantom, it is common to see the probe moving to the side, in the direction that the clinician's head turns. When using ultrasound, the ultrasound screen should be placed directly in front of the clinician so that only a glance ahead to look at the screen is needed; this placement reduces sideways movement of the probe. Additionally, there are required practical aspects that include hand-eye coordination and manual dexterity to allow manipulation of the transducer and needle according to what is being viewed on the image display (Moureau et al. 2013; Troianos et al. 2011).

To derive the maximum advantage using ultrasound, real-time guidance for vessel access must be preceded by vascular assessment with ultrasound. Ultrasound assessment of vessels allows one to establish the best site for insertion, ensuring the right vessel is chosen, accounting for size, patency and risk minimisation as was discussed in previous chapters. These factors taken together emphasise the need to understand the theory of Virchow's triad and the effects of catheter to vessel ratio. Ultrasound enables placement and management of VADs for difficult access patients, those morbidly obese, intravenous drug users and other chronically ill patients with limited access. Being a user-dependent technology, specific education and training are required for successful implementation into practice (Lamperti et al. 2012; Moureau et al. 2013; Troianos et al. 2011).

Ultrasound, as an aid to vascular assessment and needle guidance, results in greater success and fewer complications than blind or landmark insertions for both peripheral cannula and central venous catheter insertions (Chinnock et al. 2007; Mahler et al. 2010). Patients with poor vasculature, difficult-to-access peripheral veins and comorbidities that inhibit cannula insertion require technology to reduce the number of attempts required to gain access (Sou et al. 2017). For central venous catheters, GAVeCeLT (Italian Group for Venous Access Devices) recommended the use of US during CVC insertions for six different purposes: (1) US evaluation of all veins available, (2) choice of the vein on the basis of rational US-based criteria, (3) real-time US-guided venipuncture, (4) US-based control of guidewire/catheter orientation during the procedure, (5) US-based control of pleura-pulmonary integrity after axillary or subclavian vein puncture and (6) transthoracic echocardiography for verification of the position of the tip of the catheter at the end of the procedure. Ultrasound, when training and competency is provided, has demonstrated reduced time required to obtain access, greater first-attempt success and increased patient satisfaction (Bauman et al. 2009; Costantino et al. 2005; Mills et al. 2007; Stein et al. 2009; White et al. 2010; Woo et al. 2009).

Doctors and nurses alike have begun to use ultrasound for peripheral and central access of veins. With training specific to ultrasound-guided peripheral cannulae (USGPIV) access, publications support education of 0–3 h and supervised insertions of 0–25 insertions (Blaivas and Lyon 2006; Rose and Norbutas 2008; Schoenfeld et al. 2011; Stein et al. 2009; White et al. 2010; Witting et al. 2010). The literature reflects an increased number of insertion attempts associated with USGPIV when minimal training is received: 6–10 attempts in 3 publications with varying success levels from 0 to 100% (Miles et al. 2012; Stein et al. 2009; Sou et al. 2017). Following USGPIV insertion, failure rates vary within 1 and

24 h and often reflect shorter dwell time than traditionally placed peripheral cannula (Dargin et al. 2010; Keyes et al. 1999; Miles et al. 2015). Education and supervision provided prior to novice attempts coupled with longer catheters and Seldinger-wired insertions report higher success and longer cannula dwell with fewer complications that result in cannula failure (Elia et al. 2012; Harvey and Cave 2011; Mahler et al. 2010). Validation of competency by a supervisor for 5–15 attempts following training resulted in fewer attempts and reduced complications (Adhikari et al. 2010; Moore 2013; Schoenfeld et al. 2011; White et al. 2010).

4.5.3 Catheter Tip Position

Insertion site selection and final catheter tip position are both influential factors in the incidence of catheter-related complications (Gorski et al. 2016; Loveday et al. 2014). A well-placed centrally inserted device should have its tip reside deep in the SVC, ideally at the cavo-atrial junction (CAJ). Such placement permits parallel positioning of the device to the vessel wall in an area of high blood flow (Babu et al. 2016; Moureau et al. 2013). Catheter tips located in more cephalad regions of the SVC are associated with an increased risk of thrombotic complications (Luciani et al. 2001; Moureau 2013a). Clinicians should be mindful that catheters are subject to movement associated with patient position and respiration and consider this at the time of insertion to ensure optimal tip placement (Babu et al. 2016; Forauer and Alonzo 2000).

4.5.4 Infection Prevention

A working knowledge of infection prevention practices for device insertion is a critical training requirement. Breaching a patient's skin to obtain vascular access carries inherent risks including the possibility of infection. Catheter-related bloodstream infection (CRBSI) is a serious, potentially life-threatening complication associated with central venous access device insertion and management. CRBSI can stem from extraluminal contamination, where organisms migrate from the point of insertion to the catheter, to intraluminal contamination involving direct transfer of organisms to the catheter hub, and contamination may also occur via haematogenous seeding of organisms from other infected sites (Loveday et al. 2014; Moureau 2014; O'Grady et al. 2011). CRBSI contributes to morbidity and mortality as well as burdening healthcare institutions with significant financial costs and increased length of stay as noted in the guidelines. Additional information on infection prevention is provided in subsequent chapters.

4.5.5 Insertion Technique

Education on insertion of intravenous devices covers direct puncture, Seldinger and modified Seldinger techniques, with incorporation of ultrasound to provide a greater degree of safety, and application of sterile practices with maximal barrier precautions specific to CVAD insertions. Knowledge of procedures specific to each product is part of the educational process in keeping with manufacturer instructions for use. In the chapters that follow, additional details of device insertion, post insertion management and device maintenance are provided for both adults and children.

4.6 Insertion and Post Insertion Bundles

Once the vascular access device is inserted, the challenge is to maintain it, avoiding failure and complication. Ensuring the VAD does not succumb to failure is a clinical concern as this can lead to a disruption in treatment. Various assessment tools exist to assess VAD failure but are heavily focused on infection or phlebitis as the precursor to infection (Carr et al. 2017). One of the largest clinical observational studies on PIVC has pragmatically classified PIVC failure into three types: (1) infective/phlebitis, (2) occlusion/infiltration and (3) accidental dislodgement (Marsh et al.

2018). In the adult population, it is recognised that at least 25–69% of PIVCs fail before the end of treatment from complications such as occlusion, phlebitis, dislodgement, infection and infiltration (Marsh et al. 2018; Wallis et al. 2014). Device failure can lead to a reduced therapeutic effect of prescribed medicines and an increased length of hospital stay, thus interrupting the patient care processes and clinical pathways (Barton et al. 1998). Complications can be painful and even lead to nerve injury and disability (Stevens et al. 2012). Whilst research has focused on post insertion interventions to avoid failure, there has been little evidence on the link between insertion procedural aspects and future device failure.

Evidence-based recommendations for vascular access procedures and ongoing care and maintenance of devices are abundant in the literature (Chan et al. 2015; Entesari-Tatafi et al. 2015). The use of checklists or "bundles" that record compliance with Surgical-ANTT and infection prevention practices can reduce catheter-associated bloodstream infection (CABSI) (Collaborative 2011; Pronovost et al. 2006). Bundles focus on grouping key principles of practice designed to limit procedural risk and mitigate complications and therefore improve patient care (Collaborative 2011; Moureau 2013b; Pronovost et al. 2006). A collaborative quality improvement project in intensive care units (ICUs) to promote aseptic insertion of central venous lines (CVADs) was performed to identify specific educational needs. A checklist was used to record compliance with all aspects of aseptic CVAD insertion, with maximal sterile barrier precautions for clinicians ("clinician bundle") and patients ("patient bundle"). Central line-associated bloodstream infections (CLABSI) were identified and reported using a standard surveillance definition. Many ICUs were found lacking in the organisation and staff to support quality improvement and audit. Results demonstrated that compliance with all aspects of aseptic CVAD insertion significantly reduces the risk of CRBSI.

Developing any PIVC insertion bundle requires a stepped process: firstly, to identify the appropriate variables and, secondly, to identify the risk factors for insertion failure. From these, arguments can be made for appropriate device placement. If we assume the data collection strategy includes specific clinician data points, then assumptions on the right clinician can occur. Once evaluated for validity, reliability, clinical utility, clinical acceptability and usability, widespread formal implementation can occur.

Despite the evolution of insertion bundles, better methodological standardised definitions of what constitutes the right device, what ensures insertion success and what reduces post insertion complications will improve the current paucity of high-level evidence for this area of vascular access science. Application of insertion bundles may be enhanced when specialty teams are involved with insertion and care of VADs.

Previous examples of framework or clinical decision strategies, such as bundles and specialised teams for vascular access, have evidenced improved patient experiences with appropriate device placement resulting in longer device function to the end of treatment and reduced length of hospital stay (Barton et al. 1998). However, this approach lacks robust analysis and validation, and evidence is almost 20 years old where replication studies to support these data have not been found. Ideally, prospective and clinically relevant data from a patient group make it generalizable to that population (Hendriksen et al. 2013).

The widely recognised study conducted out of Michigan, known as the Keystone ICU project, tested the impact on CRBSI, the bundle approach for insertion of CVADs with five key interventions in intensive care units: hand hygiene, selection of the lowest risk device for the treatment, skin disinfection with alcoholic chlorhexidine, maximum sterile barriers and procedure for CVAD insertion and evaluation for device necessity daily (Pronovost et al. 2006). Each of the interventions was an evidence-based recommendation of the Center for Disease Control (CDC). The study demonstrated significant reduction of CRBSI across all participating ICUs based on the group of interventions (O'Grady et al. 2011; Pronovost et al. 2006).

Post insertion, devices are accessed frequently for the purposes of administering and monitoring treatment, and each access presents an opportunity

Table 4.1 Example of a bundle used to reduce the risk of CRBSI during the insertion process

Aseptic central venous access devices	
Patient bundle	Clinician bundle
• Select lowest risk device for patient and treatment	• Scrub hands for at least 2 min prior to insertion of CVAD
• Prepare procedure site with 2% alcoholic chlorhexidine	• Wear hat, mask, and eyewear
• Maximum sterile barrier with full sterile sheet draping for patient	• Don't sterile gloves and gown
• Verify position of CVAD through imaging, ECG or transducer	• Maintain Surgical-ANTT throughout with observer

for microorganisms to be introduced into the bloodstream (The Joint Commission 2013). It must be acknowledged that poor application of post insertion care often results in complications including device failure and infection (Davis 2011; O'Grady et al. 2011; Wallis et al. 2014). The bundled approach (Table 4.1) has been proven to reduce the rate of CRBSI primarily by the maintenance of sterility during the insertion phase (Burrell et al. 2011; Moureau 2013a).

Bundles are used in a variety of acute specialties and can assist the clinician in improving the safety and quality of healthcare delivery and thus improve clinical and patient outcomes. Defined by the Institute of Healthcare Improvement as "a group of interventions related to a disease process that, when executed together, results in better outcomes than when implemented individually" and a "structured way of improving care processes and patient outcomes, a small, straightforward set of evidence-based practices—generally **three to five**—that, when performed collectively and reliably, have been proven to improve patient outcomes".

Examples of bundles of care include the Institute for Healthcare Improvement's 5 Million Lives Campaign (McCannon et al. 2007) for central venous catheter and ventilator bundles and severe sepsis bundle (Levy et al. 2010). In the absence of an appropriate service delivery for vascular access (i.e. vascular access specialist team), bundles of care for vascular access aim to improve outcomes by promoting best evidence-based interventions. Ideally the components are based on Level 1 evidence, and each component must be performed at point of care.

Is the PIVC clinically indicated? The vascular access literature reveals evidence of inappropriate device selection and one bundle component that, in the pre-insertion phase may be suggested, is a component which asks, is this device clinically indicated or not? (Chopra et al. 2015; Ricard et al. 2013). Examples for PICCs include the MAGIC calculator and app for appropriate PICC use (Michigan MAGIC, www.improvepicc.com). Recently, a systematic scoping review on tools, rules and algorithms for approaches to PIVC insertion identified that few well-validated, reliable tools exist for PIVC insertion, but this is perhaps owing to the variety of clinical disciplines which perform PIVCs (Carr et al. 2017).

Admittedly, VHP could be accused of not being evidence based; however, it is a conceptual framework that underpins a series of relationships with vascular access, similar to the bundle approach, and, as a result, is available for adoption and validation. Equally, there are gaps, or rather opportunities, to develop bundles of care for vascular access that will enhance the concepts of the VHP framework. Ideally, any bundle should represent insertion and post insertional phases of the vascular access device and alert healthcare professionals when clinical concerns occur. This means pre-insertion, insertion and post insertion bundles must be aware of the clinical symptoms that may occur which demand further critique and common sense considerations.

Case Study

A 178 kg female was admitted to acute care with gastritis, nausea and vomiting. Unable to initiate PIVC, a specialist was contacted. An ultrasound-guided PIVC was placed for medication administration. Following the insertion, the laboratory verified an appendicitis and the need for more reliable access for surgery. The vascular access specialist, also trained for midline placement, inserted a midline in the cephalic vein of the right arm.

Summary of Key Points

1. Patients have the right to the most qualified inserter for every insertion.
2. Inserters with training, experience and verified competency have the lowest rate of complications.
3. Minimal education and training requirements are necessary for clinicians who insert central venous access devices (Moureau et al. 2013).
4. Competency assessment is a measure of performance necessary to ensure safe practice and should be performed initially and at scheduled intervals.

References

Adhikari S, Blaivas M, Morrison D, Lander L. Comparison of infection rates among ultrasound-guided versus traditionally placed peripheral intravenous lines. J Ultrasound Med. 2010;29(5):741–7.

Alexandrou E, Spencer TR, Frost SA, Parr MJ, Davidson PM, Hillman KM. A review of the nursing role in central venous cannulation: implications for practice policy and research. J Clin Nurs. 2010;19(11–12):1485–94.

Alexandrou E, Spencer T, Frost S, Mifflin N, Davidson P, Hillman K. Central venous catheter placement by advanced practice nurses demonstrates low procedural complication and infection rates—a report from 13 years service. Crit Care Med. 2014;42(3):536–43. https://doi.org/10.1097/CCM.0b013e3182a667f0.

Alsaad AA, Bhide VY, Moss JL Jr, Silvers SM, Johnson MM, Maniaci MJ. Central line proficiency test outcomes after simulation training versus traditional training to competence. Ann Am Thorac Soc. 2017;14(4):550–4.

Aulagnier J, Hoc C, Mathieu E, Dreyfus JF, Fischler M, Guen M. Efficacy of AccuVein to facilitate peripheral intravenous placement in adults presenting to an emergency department: a randomized clinical trial. Acad Emerg Med. 2014;21(8):858–63.

Babu S, Bennett J, Binks R, Fee P, Fox B, Johnston A, et al. Association of Anaesthetists of Great Britain and Ireland: safe vascular access 2016. Anaesthesia. 2016;71(5):573–85.

Bannon MP, Heller SF, Rivera M. Anatomic considerations for central venous cannulation. Risk Manag Healthc Policy. 2011;4:27.

Barach P, Johnson J. Understanding the complexity of redesigning care around the clinical microsystem. Qual Saf Health Care. 2006;15(Suppl 1):i10–6.

Barton A, Danek G, Johns P, Coons M. Improving patient outcomes through CQI: vascular access planning (the clinical impact of cost reduction). J Nurs Care Qual. 1998;13(2):77–85.

Bauman M, Braude D, Crandall C. Ultrasound-guidance vs. standard technique in difficult vascular access patients by ED technicians. Am J Emerg Med. 2009;27(2):135–40. https://doi.org/10.1016/j.ajem.2008.02.005.

Blaivas M, Lyon M. The effect of ultrasound guidance on the perceived difficulty of emergency nurse-obtained peripheral IV access. J Emerg Med. 2006;31(4):407–10. https://doi.org/10.1016/j.jemermed.2006.04.014.

Burrell A, McLaws M, Murgo M, Calabria E, Pantle A, Herkes R. Aseptic insertion of central venous lines to reduce bacteraemia. Med J Aust. 2011;194(11):583–7.

Carr PJ, Glynn RW, Dineen B, Kropmans TJ. A pilot intravenous cannulation team: an Irish perspective. Br J Nurs. 2010;19(Suppl 10):S19–27.

Carr PJ, Higgins NS, Cooke ML, Mihala G, Rickard CM. Vascular access specialist teams for device insertion and prevention of failure. Cochrane Database Syst Rev. 2018;(3).

Carr PJ, Rippey JC, Budgeon CA, Cooke ML, Higgins N, Rickard CM. Insertion of peripheral intravenous cannulae in the emergency department: factors associated with first-time insertion success. J Vasc Access. 2016a;17(2):182–90.

Carr PJ, Rippey JC, Cooke ML, Bharat C, Murray K, Higgins NS, et al. Development of a clinical prediction rule to improve peripheral intravenous cannulae first attempt success in the emergency department and reduce post insertion failure rates: the Vascular Access Decisions in the Emergency Room (VADER) study protocol. BMJ Open. 2016b;6(2):e009196.

Carr PJ, Higgins NS, Rippey J, Cooke ML, Rickard CM. Tools, clinical prediction rules, and algorithms for the insertion of peripheral intravenous catheters in adult hospitalized patients: a systematic scoping review of literature. J Hosp Med. 2017;12(10):851–8.

Castro-Sánchez E, Charani E, Drumright LN, Sevdalis N, Shah N, Holmes AH. Fragmentation of care threatens patient safety in peripheral vascular catheter management in acute care—a qualitative study. PLoS One. 2014;9(1):e86167. https://doi.org/10.1371/journal.pone.0086167.

Chan M-C, Chang C-M, Chiu Y-H, Huang T-F, Wang C-C. Effectiveness analysis of cross-functional team to implement central venous catheter care bundle. J Microbiol Immunol Infect. 2015;48(2):S90.

Chenkin J, Lee S, Huynh T, Bandiera G. Procedures can be learned on the web: a randomized study of ultrasound-guided vascular access training. Acad Emerg Med. 2008;15(10):949–54.

Chinnock B, Thornton S, Hendey GW. Predictors of success in nurse-performed ultrasound-guided cannulation. J Emerg Med. 2007;33(4):401–5. https://doi.org/10.1016/j.jemermed.2007.02.027.

Chopra V, Anand S, Krein S, Chenoweth C, Saint S. Bloodstream infection, venous thrombosis, and peripherally inserted central catheters: reappraising the evidence. Am J Med. 2012;125(8):733–41. https://doi.org/10.1016/j.amjmed.2012.04.010.

Chopra V, Flanders S, Saint S, Woller S, O'Grady N, Safdar N, et al. The Michigan Appropriateness Guide for Intravenous Catheters (MAGIC): results from a multispecialty panel using the RAND/UCLA appropriateness method. Ann Intern Med. 2015;163(6 Suppl):S1–40. https://doi.org/10.7326/M15-0744.

Collaborative N. Aseptic insertion of central venous lines to reduce bacteraemia. Med J Aust. 2011;194(11):583–7.

Cooke M, Ullman AJ, Ray-Barruel G, Wallis M, Corley A, Rickard CM. Not "just" an intravenous line: consumer perspectives on peripheral intravenous cannulation (PIVC). An international cross-sectional survey of 25 countries. PLoS One. 2018;13(2):e0193436.

Coopersmith CM, Rebmann TL, Zack JE, Ward MR, Corcoran RM, Schallom ME, et al. Effect of an education program on decreasing catheter-related bloodstream infections in the surgical intensive care unit. Crit Care Med. 2002;30(1):59–64.

Costantino TG, Parikh AK, Satz WA, Fojtik JP. Ultrasonography-guided peripheral intravenous access versus traditional approaches in patients with difficult intravenous access. Ann Emerg Med. 2005;46(5):456–61. https://doi.org/10.1016/j.annemergmed.2004.12.026.

Dargin JM, Rebholz CM, Lowenstein RA, Mitchell PM, Feldman JA. Ultrasonography-guided peripheral intravenous catheter survival in ED patients with difficult access. Am J Emerg Med. 2010;28(1):1–7. https://doi.org/10.1016/j.ajem.2008.09.001.

Davidson I, Lok C, Dolmatch B, Gallieni M, Nolen B, Pittiruti M, et al. Virtual reality: emerging role of simulation training in vascular access. Paper presented at the Seminars in Nephrology. 2012.

Davis J. Central line associated bloodstream infection: comprehensive, data-driven prevention. Pennsylvania Patient Safety Authority. Pa Patient Saf Advis. 2011;8(3):100–4.

Dougherty L, Lamb J, editors. Principles of intravenous therapy. Oxford: Wiley; 2014.

Dowling S, Barrett S, West R. With nurse practitioners, who needs house officers? Br Med J. 1995;311(7000):309–13.

Eisen LA, Narasimhan M, Berger JS, Mayo PH, Rosen MJ, Schneider RF. Mechanical complications of central venous catheters. J Intensive Care Med. 2006;21(1):40–6.

Elia F, Ferrari G, Molino P, Converso M, De Filippi G, Milan A, Apra F. Standard-length catheters vs long catheters in ultrasound-guided peripheral vein cannulation. Am J Emerg Med. 2012;30(5):712–6. https://doi.org/10.1016/j.ajem.2011.04.019.

Entesari-Tatafi D, Orford N, Bailey MJ, Chonghaile MNI, Lamb-Jenkins J, Athan E. Effectiveness of a care bundle to reduce central line-associated bloodstream infections. Med J Aust. 2015;202(5):247–9.

Evans LV, Dodge KL, Shah TD, Kaplan LJ, Siegel MD, Moore CL, et al. Simulation training in central venous catheter insertion: improved performance in clinical practice. Acad Med. 2010;85(9):1462–9.

Fields JM, Piela NE, Au AK, Ku BS. Risk factors associated with difficult venous access in adult ED patients. Am J Emerg Med. 2014;32(10):1179–82.

Forauer AR, Alonzo M. Change in peripherally inserted central catheter tip position with abduction and adduction of the upper extremity. J Vasc Interv Radiol. 2000;11(10):1315–8.

Gorski L, Hadaway L, Hagle M, McGoldrick M, Orr M, Doellman D. Infusion therapy: standards of practice. J Infus Nurs. 2016;39(Suppl 1):S1–S159.

Hallam C, Weston V, Denton A, Hill S, Bodenham A, Dunn H, Jackson T. Development of the UK Vessel Health and Preservation (VHP) framework: a multi-organisational collaborative. J Infect Prev. 2016;17(2):65–72. https://doi.org/10.1177/1757177415624752.

Hamilton H. A nurse-led central venous vascular access service in the United Kingdom. J Assoc Vasc Access. 2005;10(2):77–80.

Harvey M, Cave G. Ultrasound-guided peripheral venous cannulation using the Seldinger technique. Emerg Med J. 2011;28(4):338. https://doi.org/10.1136/emj.2010.100602.

Hendriksen J, Geersing G, Moons K, De Groot J. Diagnostic and prognostic prediction models. J Thromb Haemost. 2013;11:129–41.

Herrmann-Werner A, Nikendei C, Keifenheim K, Bosse HM, Lund F, Wagner R, et al. "Best practice" skills lab training vs. a "see one, do one" approach in undergraduate medical education: an RCT on students' long-term ability to perform procedural clinical skills. PLoS One. 2013;8(9):e76354.

Hirvela E, Parsa C, Aalmi O, Kelly E, Goldstein L. Skills and risk assessment of central line placement using bedside simulation with 3-dimensional ultrasound guidance system. Crit Care. 2000;28:A78.

Keyes LE, Frazee BW, Snoey ER, Simon BC, Christy D. Ultrasound-guided brachial and basilic vein cannulation in emergency department patients with difficult intravenous access. Ann Emerg Med. 1999;34(6):711–4.

Lamperti M, Bodenham AR, Pittiruti M, Blaivas M, Augoustides JG, Elbarbary M, et al. International evidence-based recommendations on ultrasound-guided vascular access. Intensive Care Med. 2012;38(7):1105–17.

Larsen E, Keogh S, Marsh N, Rickard C. Experiences of peripheral IV insertion in hospital: a qualitative study. Br J Nurs. 2017;26(19):S18–25.

Lenchus JD. End of the "see one, do one, teach one" era: the next generation of invasive bedside procedural instruction. J Am Osteopath Assoc. 2010;110(6):340–6.

Lenhard A, Moallem M, Marrie RA, Becker J, Garland A. An intervention to improve procedure education for internal medicine residents. J Gen Intern Med. 2008;23(3):288–93.

Levy MM, Dellinger RP, Townsend SR, Linde-Zwirble WT, Marshall JC, Bion J, et al. The Surviving Sepsis Campaign: results of an international guideline-based performance improvement program targeting severe sepsis. Intensive Care Med. 2010;36(2):222–31.

Loukas C, Nikiteas N, Kanakis M, Georgiou E. Evaluating the effectiveness of virtual reality simulation training in intravenous cannulation. Simul Healthc. 2011;6(4):213–7.

Loveday H, Wilson J, Pratt R, Golsorkhi M, Tingle A, Bak A, et al. EPIC3: national evidence-based guidelines for preventing healthcare-associated infections in NHS Hospitals in England. J Hosp Infect. 2014;86(Suppl 1):S1–70. https://doi.org/10.1016/s0195-6701(13)60012-2.

Luciani A, Clement O, Halimi P, Goudot D, Portier F, Bassot V, et al. Catheter-related upper extremity deep venous thrombosis in cancer patients: a prospective study based on Doppler US. Radiology. 2001;220(3):655–60.

Ma IW, Zalunardo N, Pachev G, Beran T, Brown M, Hatala R, McLaughlin K. Comparing the use of global rating scale with checklists for the assessment of central venous catheterization skills using simulation. Adv Health Sci Educ. 2012;17(4):457–70.

Mahler SA, Wang H, Lester C, Conrad SA. Ultrasound-guided peripheral intravenous access in the emergency department using a modified Seldinger technique. J Emerg Med. 2010;39(3):325–9. https://doi.org/10.1016/j.jemermed.2009.02.013.

Maki D, Ringer M. Risk factors for infusion-related phlebitis with small peripheral venous catheters: a randomized controlled trial. Ann Intern Med. 1991;114(10):845–54.

Marschall J, Mermel L, Fakih M, Hadaway L, Kallen A, O'Grady N. Strategies to prevent central line–associated bloodstream infections in acute care hospitals: 2014 update. Infect Control Hosp Epidemiol. 2014;35(Suppl 2):S89–107.

Marsh N, Webster J, Larson E, Cooke M, Mihala G, Rickard C. Observational study of peripheral intravenous catheter outcomes in adult hospitalized patients: a multivariable analysis of peripheral intravenous catheter failure. J Hosp Med. 2018;13(2):83–9.

McCannon CJ, Hackbarth AD, Griffin FA. Miles to go: an introduction to the 5 Million Lives Campaign. Jt Comm J Qual Patient Saf. 2007;33(8):477–84.

McGee D, Gould M. Preventing complications of central venous catheterization. N Engl J Med. 2003;348(12):1123–33.

Miles G, Salcedo A, Spear D. Implementation of a successful registered nurse peripheral ultrasound-guided intravenous catheter program in an emergency department. J Emerg Nurs. 2012;38(4):353–6. https://doi.org/10.1016/j.jen.2011.02.011.

Miles G, Newcomb P, Spear D. Comparison of dwell-times of two commonly placed peripheral intravenous catheters: traditional vs. ultrasound-guided. Open J Nurs. 2015;5(12):1082.

Miliani K, Taravella R, Thillard D, Chauvin V, Martin E, Edouard S, et al. Peripheral venous catheter-related adverse events: evaluation from a multicentre epidemiological study in France (the CATHEVAL Project). PLoS One. 2017;12(1):e0168637.

Mills CN, Liebmann O, Stone MB, Frazee BW. Ultrasonographically guided insertion of a 15-cm catheter into the deep brachial or basilic vein in patients with difficult intravenous access. Ann Emerg Med. 2007;50(1):68–72. https://doi.org/10.1016/j.annemergmed.2007.02.003.

Moore C. An emergency department nurse-driven ultrasound-guided peripheral intravenous line program. J Assoc Vasc Access. 2013;18(1):45–51.

Moore CL. Ultrasound first, second, and last for vascular access. J Ultrasound Med. 2014;33(7):1135–42.

Mourad M, Kohlwes J, Maselli J, Auerbach AD, MERN Group. Supervising the supervisors—procedural training and supervision in internal medicine residency. J Gen Intern Med. 2010;25(4):351–6.

Moureau N. Catheter-related infection and thrombosis: a proven relationship. A review of innovative PICC technology to reduce catheter-related infection and thrombosis. 2013a. http://www.chlorhexidinefacts.com/docs/Relationship_of_Catheter_Related_Infection_Thrombosis_WP_2012-1261.pdf.

Moureau N. Safe patient care when using vascular access devices. Br J Nurs. 2013b;22(2):S14, S16, S18 passim. https://doi.org/10.12968/bjon.2013.22.Sup1.S14.

Moureau N. Catheter-associated bloodstream infection prevention: what is missing? Br J Healthc Manag. 2014;20(11):502–10.

Moureau NL. Vessel health and preservation: vascular access assessment, selection, insertion, management, evaluation and clinical education. Doctor of Philosophy by Publication (PhD) Thesis and Exegesis (PhD Doctorate), Griffith University. 2017. https://www120.secure.griffith.edu.au/rch/items/e6aea329-fae8-4c41-aa3f-6b4f80298977/1/(gu1507011216006).

Moureau N, Trick N, Nifong T, Perry C, Kelley C, Carrico R, et al. Vessel health and preservation (Part 1): a new evidence-based approach to vascular access selection and management. J Vasc Access. 2012;13(3):351–6. https://doi.org/10.5301/jva.5000042.

Moureau N, Lamperti M, Kelly L, Dawson R, Elbarbary M, van Boxtel J, Pittiruti M. Evidence-based consensus on the insertion of central venous access devices: definition of minimal requirements for training. Br J Anaesth. 2013;110(3):333–46.

Nayeemuddin M, Pherwani A, Asquith J. Imaging and management of complications of central venous catheters. Clin Radiol. 2013;68(5):529–44.

Nguyen B-V, Prat G, Vincent J-L, Nowak E, Bizien N, Tonnelier J-M, et al. Determination of the learning curve for ultrasound-guided jugular central venous catheter placement. Intensive Care Med. 2014;40(1):66–73.

O'Grady N, Alexander M, Burns L, Dellinger E, Garland J, Heard S, et al. Centers for Disease Control Guidelines for the prevention of intravascular catheter-related infections. Clin Infect Dis. 2011;52(9):e162–93.

Primdahl S, Todsen T, Clemmesen L, Knudsen L, Weile J. Rating scale for the assessment of competence in ultrasound-guided peripheral vascular access—a Delphi Consensus Study. J Vasc Access. 2016;17(5):440–5.

Pronovost P, Wu AW, Dorman T, Morlock L. Building safety into ICU care. J Crit Care. 2002;17(2):78–85.

Pronovost P, Needham D, Berenholtz S, Sinopoli D, Chu H, Cosgrove S, et al. An intervention to decrease catheter-related bloodstream infections in the ICU: keystone project. N Engl J Med. 2006;355(26):2725–32.

Ricard J-D, Salomon L, Boyer A, Thiery G, Meybeck A, Roy C, et al. Central or peripheral catheters for initial venous access of ICU patients: a randomized controlled trial. Crit Care Med. 2013;41(9):2108–15.

Rickard CM, Webster J, Playford EG. Prevention of peripheral intravenous catheter-related bloodstream infections: the need for routine replacement. Med J Aust. 2013;199(11):751–2.

Riker MW, Kennedy C, Winfrey BS, Yen K, Dowd MD. Validation and refinement of the difficult intravenous access score: a clinical prediction rule for identifying children with difficult intravenous access. Acad Emerg Med. 2011;18(11):1129–34.

Rippey JC, Blanco P, Carr PJ. An affordable and easily constructed model for training in ultrasound-guided vascular access. J Vasc Access. 2015;16(5):422–7.

Rodriguez-Paz J, Kennedy M, Salas E, Wu A, Sexton J, Hunt E, Pronovost P. Beyond "see one, do one, teach one": toward a different training paradigm. Qual Saf Health Care. 2009;18(1):63–8.

Rose JS, Norbutas CM. A randomized controlled trial comparing one-operator versus two-operator technique in ultrasound-guided basilic vein cannulation. J Emerg Med. 2008;35(4):431–5. https://doi.org/10.1016/j.jemermed.2007.11.009.

Rusche J, Besuner P, Partusch S, Berning P. CE test: competency program development across a merged healthcare network. J Nurs Staff Dev. 2001;17(5):241–2.

Schmidt GA, Kory P. Ultrasound-guided central venous catheter insertion: teaching and learning. Intensive Care Med. 2014;40(1):111–3.

Schoenfeld E, Boniface K, Shokoohi H. ED technicians can successfully place ultrasound-guided intravenous catheters in patients with poor vascular access. Am J Emerg Med. 2011;29(5):496–501. https://doi.org/10.1016/j.ajem.2009.11.021.

Scott WL. Complications associated with central venous catheters: a survey. Chest. 1988;94(6):1221–4.

Sebbane M, Claret P-G, Lefebvre S, Mercier G, Rubenovitch J, Jreige R, et al. Predicting peripheral venous access difficulty in the emergency department using body mass index and a clinical evaluation of venous accessibility. J Emerg Med. 2013;44(2):299–305.

Sherertz RJ, Ely EW, Westbrook DM, Gledhill KS, Streed SA, Kiger B, et al. Education of physicians-in-training can decrease the risk for vascular catheter infection. Ann Intern Med. 2000;132(8):641–8.

Sou V, Mcmanus C, Mifflin N, Frost SA, Ale J, Alexandrou E. A clinical pathway for the management of difficult venous access. BMC Nurs. 2017;16:64.

Stein J, George B, River G, Hebig A, McDermott D. Ultrasonographically guided peripheral intravenous cannulation in emergency department patients with difficult intravenous access: a randomized trial. Ann Emerg Med. 2009;54(1):33–40. https://doi.org/10.1016/j.annemergmed.2008.07.048.

Stevens R, Mahadevan V, Moss A. Injury to the lateral cutaneous nerve of forearm after venous cannulation: a case report and literature review. Clin Anat. 2012;25(5):659–62.

Taylor DC, Hamdy H. Adult learning theories: implications for learning and teaching in medical education: AMEE Guide No. 83. Med Teach. 2013;35(11):e1561–72.

Taylor RW, Palagiri AV. Central venous catheterization. Crit Care Med. 2007;35(5):1390.

Teramoto T, Tsuchikane E, Yamamoto M, Matsuo H, Kawase Y, Suzuki Y, et al. Successful revascularization improves long-term clinical outcome in patients with chronic coronary total occlusion. IJC Heart Vasc. 2017;14:28–32.

The Joint Commission. Preventing central line–associated bloodstream infections: useful tools, an international perspective. 2013.

Troianos CA, Hartman GS, Glas KE, Skubas NJ, Eberhardt RT, Walker JD, Reeves ST. Guidelines for performing ultrasound guided vascular cannulation: recommendations of the American Society of Echocardiography and the Society of Cardiovascular Anesthesiologists. J Am Soc Echocardiogr. 2011;24(12):1291–318.

Tuffaha HW, Rickard CM, Webster J, Marsh N, Gordon L, Wallis M, Scuffham PA. Cost-effectiveness analysis of clinically indicated versus routine replacement of peripheral intravenous catheters. Appl Health Econ Health Policy. 2014;12(1):51–8. https://doi.org/10.1007/s40258-013-0077-2.

van Loon FH, Puijn LA, Houterman S, Bouwman AR. Development of the A-DIVA scale: a clinical predictive scale to identify difficult intravenous access in adult patients based on clinical observations. Medicine. 2016;95(16):e3428.

Wallis M, McGrail M, Webster J, Marsh N, Gowardman J, Playford E, Rickard C. Risk factors for peripheral intravenous catheter failure: a multivariate analysis of data from a randomized controlled trial. Infect Control Hosp Epidemiol. 2014;35(1):63–8. https://doi.org/10.1086/674398.

White A, Lopez F, Stone P. Developing and sustaining an ultrasound-guided peripheral intravenous access program for emergency nurses. Adv Emerg Nurs J. 2010;32(2):173–88.

Williams S, Dale J, Glucksman E, Wellesley A. Senior house officers' work related stressors, psychological distress, and confidence in performing clinical tasks in accident and emergency: a questionnaire study. BMJ. 1997;314(7082):713.

Witting MD. IV access difficulty: incidence and delays in an urban emergency department. J Emerg Med. 2012;42(4):483–7.

Witting MD, Schenkel SM, Lawner BJ, Euerle BD. Effects of vein width and depth on ultrasound-guided peripheral intravenous success rates. J Emerg Med. 2010;39(1):70–5. https://doi.org/10.1016/j.jemermed.2009.01.003.

Woo M, Frank J, Lee A, Thompson C, Cardinal P, Yeung M, Beecker J. Effectiveness of a novel training program for emergency residents in ultrasound-guided insertion of central venous catheters. Can J Emerg Med (CJEM/JCMU). 2009;11(4):343–8.

Yen K, Riegert A, Gorelick MH. Derivation of the DIVA score: a clinical prediction rule for the identification of children with difficult intravenous access. Pediatr Emerg Care. 2008;24(3):143–7.

5

VAST: Definitions and Usage

Peter J. Carr and Nancy L. Moureau

Abstract

Patients admitted to hospital are exposed to invasive procedures and will receive various interventions from different professional roles all with different levels of experience: some with limited experience and some with extensive experience. In simple terms, an orthopaedic surgeon fixes your broken bones, a cardiologist attends to your heart, a geriatrician focuses on elderly patient care, and a vascular surgeon focuses on vascular surgery. Yet, which vascular access device is inserted influences the clinical outcomes within each of these select specialties. Insertion procedures and care and maintenance are shared by a variety of healthcare professional disciplines, all with a variety of experience, guided by local policy frameworks. Because of this interdisciplinary sharing, responsibility becomes fragmented, and ownership of outcomes is lacking leading to increased patient safety risks. This chapter will firstly identify the various definitions that make up a vascular access specialist team (VAST) and secondly the variety of evidence supporting the concept and what empirical guidelines say about it. Finally, it explores the use of a vascular access specialist teams to promote unity in patient care and assurance that only well-trained clinicians who are qualified to select, insert and care for VADs can do so, promoting greater patient safety and positive patient outcomes.

Keywords

Vascular access specialists · Vascular access teams · Benefits of VAST

5.1 Introduction

The scale of healthcare is arguably as big as any major industry with up to 85% of individuals worldwide seeking healthcare services once a year and a quarter of those exceeding four visits yearly (Rosen et al. 2018). Vascular access and intravenous therapy devices are a massive contributor to the invasive device market with annual worldwide use of VADs in the billions (Alexandrou et al. 2018). Yet the request, assessment and insertion of a VAD, the care and maintenance and, indeed, the removal of VADs are shared by a variety of healthcare professional disciplines.

When a patient is admitted to hospital, they are invariably exposed to a variety of invasive VAD procedures. Many will receive clinical interventions from

P. J. Carr (✉)
HRB Clinical Research Facility Galway, National University of Ireland Galway,
University Hospital Galway, Galway, Ireland
e-mail: peter.carr@nuigalway.ie

N. L. Moureau
Menzies Health Institute, Alliance for Vascular Access Teaching and Research (AVATAR) Group, Griffith University, Brisbane, QLD, Australia
e-mail: nancy@piccexcellence.com

different professional roles, all with different levels of experience following specific professional guidelines. Such a strategy is best represented as an interdisciplinary sharing method: one entity for insertion and another for care and maintenance. This process has resulted in responsibility for VADs being fragmented and this process identified as an increased patient safety risk (Castro-Sanchez et al. 2014). Specialist medical care is not so fragmented, for example, in specific healthcare domains of cardiology, orthopaedics, paediatrics and others all providing a higher level of quality care within their area of specialization. Therefore, it is important that highly skilled clinicians or specialists are available to improve VAD outcomes, ideally adopting a vessel health preservation (VHP) approach (Moureau and Carr 2018).

VAD practice is not yet globally accepted to be one that demands a specialist healthcare profession to ensure maximum patient safety with their use. It is often described as a generic skill or a clinical procedure absorbed into other competing clinical responsibilities and professional domains. Despite the pervasive use of VADs and associated technologies, the ownership of its term as a specialty or specialist team is in its infancy (Davis et al. 2016). This means high-level evidence for the specialty and teams is also lacking (Carr et al. 2018). Notwithstanding this reality, it is worth exploring the contribution of a vascular access specialist and team approach has made to patient's health and on the patient experience. Moreover, how a team approach can be adopted into a future where a safety science culture is likely to become commonly accepted in healthcare (Marshall et al. 2013) and where it can demonstrate sustained value as an authority on vascular access quality and safety (Dixon-Woods et al. 2013). The adoption and use of VHP and VAST will add important and timely insights into a concept eager for clinical validation.

5.2 Vascular Access Teams Defined

A vascular access team is the grouping of healthcare professionals whose primary role is to assess, insert, manage, perform surveillance, analyse their service data and solve clinical concerns and where possible remove VADs. The antecedents to a vascular access team were generalist nurses and medical doctors performing the insertion of VADs, be it peripheral or central catheters, with the latter overwhelmingly performed by medical doctors. However, the emergence of the peripherally inserted central catheter (PICC) has seen the adoption of PICC services, with the majority of PICC insertions led by the nursing workforce (Chopra et al. 2017a, b). Insertion of peripheral intravenous catheters (PIVC) has long been in the scope of nursing throughout most of the world, and this was recently validated (Alexandrou et al. 2018), and while physicians such as anaesthetists commonly place central venous catheters (CVC), nurses have increasingly assumed the role for PICCs and Midline insertions.

VADs are inserted under a plethora of health service models, medical only for central devices and nursing for other peripherally inserted devices; the adoption of a vascular access team could promote collegiate responsibility and lead to proactive decision-making, as opposed to developing a solution arising from an avoidable clinical problem. One recent example in the literature with regard to a difficult intravenous access patient cohort, identifies how a team approach can improve insertion outcomes in this specific patient population (Sou et al. 2017). An additional accepted term within a team approach includes the title vascular access specialist; referring to an individual clinician, (Marsh et al. 2018) with much variation in their description, professional role and clinical privileges. What is likely an encouraging phenomenon is that vascular access teams and specialists working within them appear to be initiated from a service context less clinical trial evidence. There is an opportunity for fuller scientific evaluation; both quality improvement and clinical research methods to evaluate the impact of the vascular access team concept. As a result a stronger empirically valid definitions of the team concept is likely to evolve. In future, the merging of healthcare and clinical disciplines such as surveillance scientists (Devries, 2016) within a team will signal a new era for vascular access science. Moreover, a patient included model of care that accepts the most appropriate device inserted and managed by a group of clinical experts analysing standardised data is likely to inform and provide the highest quality of care.

5.3 Vascular Access Specialist Defined

Consensus regarding the term vascular access as a specialty is beginning to assume prominence in the literature (Davis et al. 2016), but it is fair to say it is a term that is not regularly used in hospitals worldwide. However, *vascular access specialist* is emerging as an accepted term in the literature (Chopra et al. 2017a, b). Adoption of this term and approach will likely occur, and one hopes it is introduced with appropriate evidence using appropriate methodologies. If we acknowledge and accept the necessity of VADs in current medical treatment, then by reason the use of vascular access specialists within a team will likely evolve into an established entity within the future of healthcare.

5.4 Evidence Supporting Vascular Access Specialist Team

In the 1980 the first controlled clinical trials investigating the impact of intravenous teams was reported with a primary outcome identifying the team approach reduced phlebitis (Tomford et al. 1984). Over a decade later, another clinical study asked the same question with similar results (Soifer et al. 1998). Both studies favoured the adoption and implementation of intravenous (IV) teams into clinical practice as a strategy to negative outcomes of IVs for reduced infection and phlebitis. In 2008 results from a dedicated IV team revealed a high percentage of sustained first-time insertion success (Carr et al. 2010).

Conceptually a vascular access specialist team (VAST) should be underpinned with the highest level of evidence (Carr et al. 2018). However, VAST can be accused of compromising VHP principles of right device selection in vascular access decision-making as some VASTs perform only PIVC insertion, some only PICCs and/or CVADs. Moreover, if a VAST approach focuses on an insertion-only model, it may limit the available time to follow up and troubleshoot VAD issues. Despite prospective studies revealing better insertion outcomes and reduced complications, many services require greater evidence to expand into a team approach and justify the economic benefit (Bolton 2009; Hadaway et al. 2013). Furthermore, economically, the team approach appears to be more cost-effective (Robinson et al. 2005), as it is associated with greater first-time insertion success as well as reducing length of hospital stay, improving efficiency with supplies and reducing device complications. In addition, Cochrane reviews on the subject matter identify few controlled clinical trials on vascular access teams and specialists. Only one current trial on the World Health Organization's clinical trials registry was identified with one registered clinical trial awaiting publication (Carr et al. 2018).

As a result, uncertainties exist, and the efficacy or credibility of VASTs is limited to pre- and post-descriptive, observational and prospective studies on this subject. Moreover, when viewed individually, it is unclear from the limited, dated, underpowered randomized controlled trials (RCTs) available to date which vascular access insertion model is most effective. Specifically, in relation to RCTs, it is unclear if the specialist/team is superior or equivalent to one with multiple clinicians inserting VADs. Table 5.1 displays a selection of benefits for healthcare facilities in adopting a VAST approach.

Table 5.1 Why healthcare facilities should adopt a VAST

Centralizes an approach to the co-ordination of VAD care
Create and sustain a consistent approach to VAD underpinned by safety science
Lead the implementation of multimodal initiatives to improve VAD outcomes
Interpret VAD data to monitor clinician performance and policy compliance
Establish VAST as the clinical lead and hospital authority on VAD standards
VAST will improved the patient experience
VAST will use fewer VADs based on fewer attempts
VAST will evaluate products and technology prior to clinical adoption
VAST would lead clinical simulation, education and training of VAD
VAST will promote patient education and ensure a patient safety culture is maintained
VAST is more likely to integrate visualization technologies that promote greater insertion success and reduce complications
VAST can assist with implementation and translation of new evidence

5.5 What the Guidelines Recommend

Scientific reports substantiate clinical guidelines and the variety published promote the concept of specialty training for healthcare professionals; the team approach and an improvement in the process of vascular access (Bodenham et al. 2016; Gorski et al. 2016; O'Grady et al. 2011; Royal College of Nursing 2016; Pittiruti and Scoppettuolo 2017). Regardless of the lack of high-quality interventional data to support strong recommendations for a VAST and the different terminology used to describe a team or group of specialist inserters, major clinical guidelines endorse their adoption where possible. Infusion Nursing Standards (INS) define an infusion team as one with a scope for clinical care that *consists of a variety of activities related to the safe insertion, delivery and maintenance of all infusion and vascular access therapies including fluids and medications, blood and blood components and parenteral nutrition* and acknowledge that dedicated infusion teams report better insertion success and reduce device complication (Gorski et al. 2016). INS adds that the VAST also provides a role for product evaluation and education resource, as well as a source to collect meaningful data (Gorski et al. 2016). Specifically, with regard to insertion, a European clinical manual for the insertion of PICCs and Midlines suggests that dedicated venous access teams lead to significant advantages, namely, safety, cost-effectiveness and efficiency (Pittiruti and Scoppettuolo 2017). This group also suggested VAST collaboration with hospital pharmacy was important, thus highlighting another discipline involved in VHP. The Centers for Disease Control 2011 guidelines reference "IV Teams" and suggest the team approach leaves no doubt as to their effectiveness in reducing the incidence of CRBSI (O'Grady et al. 2011). However, there is also contradictory evidence in the CDC guideline that supports ward-based nurse to performing dressing changes, as opposed to a dedicated infusion team demonstrating a cost saving of $90,000 per year (Abi-Said et al. 1999). A more recent guideline from the Association of Anaesthetists of Great Britain and Ireland, titled *Safe Vascular Access*, recommend hospitals to develop a process to ensure patients receive effective, timely and safe vascular access (Bodenham et al. 2016). Conceivably, this could mean the development of specialist vascular access training and or a VAST approach adopting the principles of VHP (Hallam et al. 2016). Adopting such a strategy it appears would be necessary as the current systems for vascular access are variable. As a result, a lack of clinical consistency for patient outcomes occurs (Bodenham et al. 2016).

5.6 Benefits of Vascular Access Specialist Team

Identifying who is best qualified to insert and manage vascular devices could likely lead to adaption of better outcomes for patients, see Table 5.2. For example, difficult IV access and central venous catheter insertion are generally associated with surgeons, anaesthetics and intensivist, yet this group does not routinely perform CVC dressing changes. In following up the impact of initial insertion decisions on post-insertion complications, a better approach could reduce complications (Carr et al. 2017). Modification of insertion practice to promote dressing integrity could lead to a reduction of catheter-related infection as evidenced in a large intensive care study (Timsit et al. 2012).

Table 5.2 Patients benefit from a VAST

Patients will have their VAD assessment and insertion performed or proctored by a VAST experienced clinician
Patients will be able to enter a shared decision-making concept understanding alternative devices can be used ensuring the right device is used
The likelihood a VAD will be inserted on the first attempt is very high
Post-insertion complications will be reduced leading to uninterrupted therapy
Improved patient experience
Dedicated point of care resource to troubleshoot VAD issues or patient queries
Could be exposed to having better products and technology used to improve clinical outcomes

Important publications, including one RCT, describe the effectiveness of nurses inserting acute CVCs and tunnelled devices; despite evidence of equivalent or better outcomes, they are also economically more efficient with high patient satisfaction scores (Boland et al. 2003; Hamilton 2005; Yacopetti et al. 2010).

Given the variety of disciplines and practices involved in the process required for VAD insertion and care, it's illogical for hospital not to incorporate a version of VAST. Expecting the current process of new clinicians to perform invasive procedures and without appropriate, consistent and recurrent training (Carr et al. 2011) or to accomplish a specific training scheme serves the clinician and educators not the patient (Moureau et al. 2013). In essence, patients want fewer attempts (Cooke et al. 2018). The best evidence to date is that insertion attempts are reduced with team or with specialist qualifications. Ensuring VASTs are better resourced and evolve to invite a wide variety of clinical disciplines and professional roles into it will surely strengthen its cause and will hopefully translate into stronger clinical outcomes and evidence.

5.7 Summary

VHP is a pathway that begins with assessment of patient veins and selection of the lowest-risk device to deliver the treatment plan. Integration of research and guidelines into VHP is designed to result in the best outcomes for patients, allowing completion of treatment with fewer VADs, less cost, fewer supplies and less time while limiting complications. With a thorough knowledge base of types of VADs available, criteria for use and training for insertion, clinicians are better able to meet the needs of patients in a safe and efficient manner. Specially trained clinicians with protected time and defined clinical roles working in a VAST are better equipped to provide consultation for appropriate device, maintain first-time success with device insertion and report the lowest risk of complications with invasive VAD procedures.

Case Study

A hospital in the inner city noted a steady increase in CLABSI. All CVADs were placed by doctors either surgeons or in radiology department. In addition, multiple PIVC-related infections were noted over the past 12 months. A committee was established to study the problem as well as complaints of excessive PIVC attempts, complications associated with PIVCs and long wait time for CVADs. The committee noted a high total purchase rate for PIVCs equating five catheters per patient admission for the year (catheters purchased/patients admitted = catheters per patient admission). Supplies and cost per placement were evaluated to be approximately $24.65 per PIVC attempt. PIVC failure rate was approximately 55% within the first 48 h. Observations identified fragmentation, inconsistency and frequent breaks in aseptic technique during PIVC and CVAD insertions. A determination was made to develop training and education for insertion, vein selection, appropriate use of supplies, Aseptic Non Touch Technique (ANTT) and care and maintenance with all VADs. Evaluation of published research pointed to added benefits of establishing specialists for insertion. A pilot study was created within a unit of the hospital with the highest complications. The unit was staffed with a trained vascular access specialist. After 3 months improvement was noted in patient satisfaction, reduced use of supplies and complication reduction by more than 65% in CVADs and 82% in PIVCs. Catheter usage for the study unit was reduced to less than two catheters per patient admission. PIVC failure rate was reduced to less than 20% in 72 h. The data from the pilot study demonstrated significant cost saving calculated and presented to the Chief Financial Officer. Plans for expansion of the specialist model for other units were proposed and accepted by administration.

Summary of Key Points

1. Patients have the right to the most qualified inserter for every insertion; hospitals should therefore consider vascular access teams.
2. In future, vascular access teams will likely evolve to include an assessment; insertion and post insertion clinical resource.
3. Respected clinical guidelines recommend the vascular access team/specialist approach despite limited empirical evidence.
4. There is an opportunity for the vascular access team to disrupt and become a new innovation in healthcare.
5. Vascular access teams are possibly the best advocate to translate and implement the VHP concept.

References

Abi-Said D, Raad I, Umphrey J, Gonzalez V, Richardson D, Marts K, Hohn D. Infusion therapy team and dressing changes of central venous catheters. Infect Control Hosp Epidemiol. 1999;20:101–5.

Alexandrou E, Ray-Barruel G, Carr PJ, Frost S, Inwood S, Higgins N, Lin F, Alberto L, Mermel L, Rickard CM. Use of short peripheral intravenous catheters: characteristics, management, and outcomes worldwide. J Hosp Med. 2018;13.

Bodenham A, Babu S, Bennett J, Binks R, Fee P, Fox B, Johnston A, Klein A, Langton J, Mclure H. Association of Anaesthetists of Great Britain and Ireland. Safe vascular access 2016. Anaesthesia. 2016;71:573–85.

Boland A, Haycox A, Bagust A, Fitzsimmons L. A randomised controlled trial to evaluate the clinical and cost-effectiveness of Hickman line insertions in adult cancer patients by nurses. Health Technol Assess. 2003;7(36):iii, ix–x, 1–99. NCCHTA.

Bolton D. Writing a business case for the expansion of service: expanding the IV therapy team, from start to finish. J Infect Prev. 2009;10:S27–32.

Carr PJ, Glynn RW, Dineen B, Kropmans TJ. A pilot intravenous cannulation team: an Irish perspective. Br J Nurs. 2010;19:S19–27.

Carr PJ, Glynn RW, Dineen B, Devitt D, Flaherty G, Kropmans TJ, Kerin M. Interns' attitudes to IV cannulation: a KAP study. Br J Nurs. 2011;20:S15–20.

Carr P, Higgins N, Cooke M, Mihala G, Rickard C. Vascular access specialist teams for device insertion and prevention of failure. Cochrane Database Syst Rev. 2014;2014.

Carr PJ, She GN, Pickersgill H, Bessley T, Murray K, Jackson G, Ho K, Litton E. The state of the art of central venous catheter care in the intensive care unit of a tertiary hospital; A quality initiative and call to action. Aust Crit Care. 2017;30:112.

Carr PJ, Higgins NS, Cooke ML, Mihala G, Rickard CM. Vascular access specialist teams for device insertion and prevention of failure. The Cochrane Library. 2018.

Castro-Sanchez E, Charani E, Drumright L, Sevdalis N, Shah N, Holmes A. Fragmentation of care threatens patient safety in peripheral vascular catheter management in acute care—a qualitative study. PLoS One. 2014;9:e86167.

Chopra V, Kuhn L, Ratz D, Shader S, Vaughn VM, Saint S, Krein SL. Vascular access specialist training, experience, and practice in the United States. J Infus Nurs. 2017a;40:15–25.

Chopra V, Kuhn L, Ratz D, Winter S, Carr PJ, Paje D, Krein SL. Variation in use of technology among vascular access specialists: an analysis of the PICC1 survey. J Vasc Access. 2017b;18:243–9.

Cooke M, Ullman AJ, Ray-Barruel G, Wallis M, Corley A, Rickard CM. Not "just" an intravenous line: consumer perspectives on peripheral intravenous cannulation (PIVC). An international cross-sectional survey of 25 countries. PLoS One. 2018;13:e0193436.

Davis L, Owens A, Thompson J. Defining the specialty of vascular access through consensus: shaping the future of vascular access. J Assoc Vasc Access. 2016;21:125–30.

DeVries M, Valentine M, Mancos P. Protected clinical indication of peripheral intravenous lines: successful implementation. J Assoc Vasc Access. 2016;21(2):89–92

Dixon-Woods M, Leslie M, Tarrant C, Bion J. Explaining Matching Michigan: an ethnographic study of a patient safety program. Implement Sci. 2013;8:70.

Gorski L, Hadaway L, Hagle M, Mcgoldrick M, Orr M, Doellman D. Infusion therapy: standards of practice. J Infus Nurs. 2016;39(Suppl 1):S1–S159.

Hadaway L, Dalton L, Mercanti-Erieg L. Infusion teams in acute care hospitals: call for a business approach: an infusion nurses society white paper. J Infus Nurs. 2013;36:356–60.

Hallam C, Weston V, Denton A, Hill S, Bodenham A, Dunn H, Jackson T. Development of the UK Vessel Health and Preservation (VHP) framework: a multi-organisational collaborative. J Infect Prev. 2016;17:65–72.

Hamilton H. A nurse-led central venous vascular access service in the United Kingdom. J Assoc Vasc Access. 2005;10:77–80.

Marsh N, Webster J, Larsen E, Genzel J, Cooke M, Mihala G, Cadigan S, Rickard CM. Expert versus generalist inserters for peripheral intravenous catheter insertion: a pilot randomised controlled trial. Trials. 2018;19(1).

Marshall M, Pronovost P, Dixon-Woods M. Promotion of improvement as a science. Lancet. 2013;381:419–21.

Moureau NL, Carr PJ. Vessel Health and Preservation: a model and clinical pathway for using vascular access devices. Br J Nurs. 2018;27:S28–35.

Moureau N, Lamperti M, Kelly L, Dawson R, Elbarbary M, Van Boxtel J, Pittiruti M. Evidence-based consensus on the insertion of central venous access devices: definition of minimal requirements for training. Br J Anaesth. 2013;110:333–46.

O'Grady N, Alexander M, Burns L, Dellinger E, Garland J, Heard S, Lipsett P, Masur H, Mermel L, Pearson M, Raad I, Randolph A, Rupp M, Saint S, Healthcare Infection Control Practices Advisory Committee (HICPAC). Centers for Disease Control Guidelines for the prevention of intravascular catheter-related infections. Clin Infect Dis. 2011;52:e162–93.

Pittiruti M, Scoppettuolo G. Gavecelt manual of PICC and midline: indications, insertion, management, Italy. Edna S.p.A.; 2017.

Robinson M, Mogensen K, Grudinskas G, Kohler S, Jacobs D. Improved care and reduced costs for patients requiring peripherally inserted central catheters: the role of bedside ultrasound and a dedicated team. J Parenter Enter Nutr. 2005;29:374–9.

Rosen MA, Diazgranados D, Dietz AS, Benishek LE, Thompson D, Pronovost PJ, Weaver SJ. Teamwork in healthcare: key discoveries enabling safer, high-quality care. Am Psychol. 2018;73:433.

Royal College of Nursing. Standards for infusion therapy. In: Denton A, editor. . London: Royal College of Nursing; 2016.

Soifer N, Borzak S, Edlin B, Weinstein R. Prevention of peripheral venous catheter complications with an intravenous therapy team: a randomized controlled trial. Arch Intern Med. 1998;158:473–7.

Sou V, Mcmanus C, Mifflin N, Frost SA, Ale J, Alexandrou E. A clinical pathway for the management of difficult venous access. BMC Nurs. 2017;16:64.

Timsit J, Bouadma L, Ruckly S, Schwebel C, Garrouste-Orgeas M, Bronchard R, Calvino-Gunther S, Laupland K, Adrie C, Thuong M. Dressing disruption is a major factor for catheter-related infections. Crit Care Med. 2012;40:1707–14.

Tomford JW, Hershey CO, Mclaren CE, Porter DK, Cohen DI. Intravenous therapy team and peripheral venous catheter—associated complications: a prospective controlled study. Arch Intern Med. 1984;144:1191–4.

Yacopetti N, Alexandrou E, Spencer T, Frost S, Davidson P, O'sullivan G, Hillman K. Central venous catheter insertion by a clinical nurse consultant or anaesthetic medical staff: a single-centre observational study. Crit Care Resusc. 2010;12:90–5.

Part III

Cardiovascular Insertion

6

Insertion and Device Selection

Steve Hill

Abstract

The way in which clinicians practice the art and science of vascular access insertion and management is subject to change as more information and research are made available regarding the implications of practices. The goal is ever to minimize complications while administering the necessary treatment for the patient. In this chapter, we explore standards of practice, uncovering the causes of complications to reinforce best practice. The underlying principle of vessel health and preservation, the act of placing the Right device at the Right time for the Right patient™ (Teleflex, Raleigh, North Carolina, USA), is the aim. However, without the right insertion practice, the "Rights" included in the VHP model become unattainable.

Keywords

Peripheral intravenous cannula · Central venous catheter · Seldinger technique Guidewire · Number of attempts · Local anesthetic · Jugular · Axillary · Femoral veins Insertion · Complications · Malposition Securement

S. Hill (✉)
The Christie NHS Foundation Trust, Manchester, UK

Precision Vascular and Surgical Services Ltd, Manchester, UK
e-mail: info@precisionvascular.co.uk; steve.hill@christie.nhs.uk

6.1 Introduction to Insertion

Selection of the right device, right inserter, and insertion technique encompasses the second stage in quadrant 2 of the VHP process. Appropriate device selection and number of necessary lumens are determinations made according to lowest risk for patient insertion and potential for infection in conjunction with the needs of the therapy. Selection of the inserter and application of infection prevention principles are contributing factors for patient safety. The technique chosen for insertion is dependent on the device selected, whether peripheral or central, and the indications dictated by patient and treatment factors. The use of technology for visualization during insertion and tip positioning of central catheters aids in reducing insertional and post-insertional complications.

6.2 Appropriateness in Device Selection

According to the Society for Healthcare Epidemiology of America (SHEA), intravenous devices, specifically CVADs, should be inserted only when clinically indicated (Marschall et al. 2014). Evidence for indications specific to VADs was not available until 2016. The Michigan Appropriateness Guide for Intravenous Catheters (MAGIC) was developed by an international panel of experts to establish indications and contraindications for VAD usage (Chopra et al. 2015). MAGIC guidelines suggest that shorter PIVC, 1–6 cm, be inserted for treatment up to 5 days, with longer length catheters (4–6 cm) used with ultrasound guidance and treatment from 6 to 14 days. Local policy should advocate removal when clinically indicated; routine scheduled replacement of a peripheral catheter is no longer needed (Rickard et al. 2012).

The designation of patients with difficult venous access (DIVA), as a patient who has experienced one or more failed attempts or has unidentifiable veins, necessitates higher-level insertion and the use of ultrasound or other visualization technology as a recommended next step to gaining successful access (Gorski et al. 2016). Some patients receive the designation DIVA through chronic illness resulting in recurrent admissions and repeated VAD. It is important that healthcare organizations have strategies in place to initiate optimal practice when a patient is readmitted with DIVA to avoid subjecting the patient to multiple insertion attempts. Highlighting the patient as DIVA means the patient ideally is escalated to a VAD specialists, anesthetics, or other higher skill level clinician to receive the optimal VAD selection, visualization technologies, and insertion consistent with their current presentation and treatment.

6.3 Optimal Peripheral Cannula Insertion

PIVCs are the most commonly placed vascular access device, with over a billion sold worldwide each year, but their failure rate lies between 35 and 50% (Bertoglio et al. 2017). PIVCs are still the default vascular access device in many institutions, even when other alternatives may be more suitable for the indicated therapy. This may be because of limited resources in terms of the availability of skilled staff to perform a more advance insertion, staff availability to provide ultrasound-guided cannula insertion, or the lack of availability of ultrasound or vein viewing technology.

In the absence of skilled vascular access teams/specialists, an environment may be created where a PIVC seems the easy, fast, and predominant solution, regardless of other options. Nursing staff and junior doctors are often the frontline providers and clinicians initiating IV treatment and inserting PIVC. Failed attempts at this stage may result in escalation to a more experienced colleague and then, perhaps another before eventually, an expert such as an anesthetist provides the final successful access after many attempts. Such journeys for patients are sadly not uncommon, reflected in the VADER study by Carr et al. (2016) who identified the overwhelming device of choice of emergency department colleagues was for a PIVC and identified documentary evidence that many devices were failing to the last 3 days (Carr et al. 2015). Identified in that study, PIVC first-time success ranged from 18 to 86% among clinical staff in pediatric and adult populations, but specialist vascular access insertion teams can achieve 98–99% first-time insertion success.

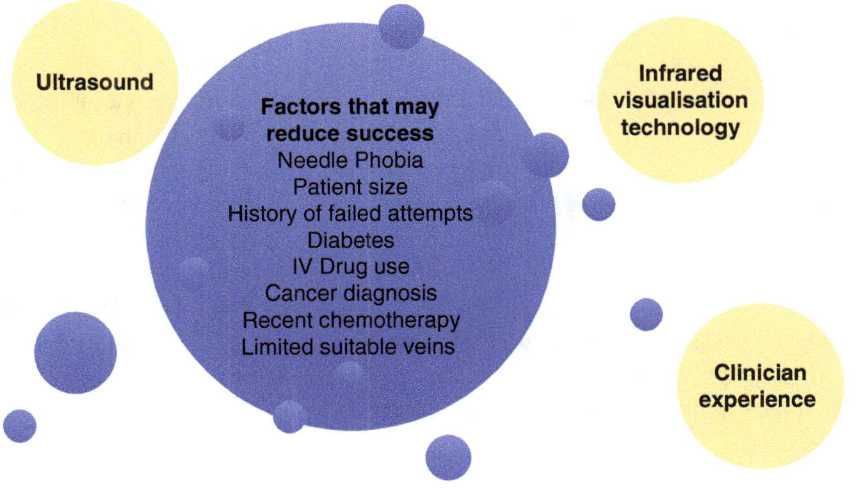

Fig. 6.1 Factors enhancing first time access success rates. Using factors identified in the VADER study; Carr et al. (2015). Factors listed in black text reduce chances of first-time access success; factors listed in red text enhance the chances of first-time access success (Carr et al. 2016)

As shown in Fig. 6.1, inhibitors to first-time success include age, needle phobia, patient size, previous history of failed attempts, recent hospital admission, diabetes, intravenous drug use, cancer diagnosis, and recent chemotherapy. Factors that may enhance first-time access success include ultrasound and other vessel locating devices and the clinician's experience (number of PIVC procedures the clinician has previously performed).

6.4 Selection of an Insertion Site for PIVC Cannulation

6.4.1 Vein Characteristics

When performing an ultrasound assessment of veins for cannulation, look for veins that are palpable and bouncy and refill quickly following compression (Weinstein 2007). The vein selected should be straight, long enough to house the catheter, and more than double the diameter of the catheter (Dougherty and Lister 2011). Avoid veins with bifurcations, tortuosity, and thrombosis. The lower arm area of the forearm is associated with decreased pain, greater stability to reduce accidental removal, and increased dwell time (Gorski INS 2016). The veins can be selected by visualization/palpation or ultrasound assessment (Larue 2000; Mcdiarmid et al. 2017). Some of the steps detailed in the Marsden Manual (Dougherty and Lister 2015) include placing the tourniquet 6–8 in. above the site, tapping on the vein lightly to release histamines which cause dilatation, positioning the limb below the heart, and consideration for using a warm compress if necessary. PIVC can also be placed in the external jugular vein or veins in the foot for emergent use or when used for less than 4 days.

6.4.2 Skin Considerations

The skin and tissue integrity changes from patient to patient and can be a factor affecting VAD insertion success. These differences in skin integrity are perceptible to the clinician through tactile feedback and subtle pressure variations as the needle passes through the skin, tissues, and venous wall. The amount of pressure required to pass through the skin and tissues and enter the vein is influenced by the patient's skin integrity and the quality and sharpness of the access needle. Many factors determine skin and tissue integrity, but age is a universal common denominator. As we age, the structural stability of the skin and tissues inevitably deteriorates. The amount and speed of deterioration vary and are subject to intrinsic and extrinsic factors such as a buildup of damaging waste products, cellular metabolism, and extrinsic environmental factors (Farage et al. 2013).

6.5 Safe Practices for Insertion

Attention to good practices with peripheral insertion focuses on vein selection, catheter choice, skin disinfection, and ANTT with insertion, stabilization of the catheter, and consideration for add-on extension tubing and flushing to confirm patency. Vein and catheter selections are discussed in previous sections. Skin disinfection is best performed with a 70% alcohol and greater than 0.5% chlorhexidine solution (O'Grady et al. 2011). Disinfection of the access point is also necessary with each flush and infusion. ANTT applies to all aspects of insertion, access for infusions, and care of the cannula and surrounding areas.

Hand hygiene is performed immediately prior to any patient contact and just before an insertion procedure. Following handwashing apply clean or sterile gloves for insertion of any intravenous device, sterile gloves for arterial and central access. Consider the use of strategies for improving visualization of veins (e.g., warm towels, warm blankets, palpation, augmentation, transillumination, ultrasound, infrared). Specific recommendations that follow for peripheral cannula insertion can be applied that lead to improved outcomes for the patient (Bertoglio et al. 2017).

6.6 Recommendations for PIVC Insertion

- A PIVC is clinically indicated for administration of medical intravenous treatment.

- Use a PIVC of appropriate size/gauge and length for the patient, the vein size, and treatment indications.
- Select a vein in the forearm as the preferred location; avoid areas of insertion near joints (i.e., wrist, fingers, antecubital fossa); insert two or more centimeters away from a joint or mobile area.
  - Clean skin with alcoholic chlorhexidine or other approved disinfecting agents.
  - Consider extended dwell cannula, catheter length of 2–6 cm as the preferred length for ultrasound-guided insertion when duration of treatment exceeds 3 days.
  - Consider the use of PIVC with added extension or integrated extension.
  - Stabilize the cannula with securement device prior to transparent dressing application.

6.7 Patient Assessment and Insertion

- Hand hygiene performed immediately prior to PIVC insertion.
- Clean or sterile glove use during insertion procedure for operator and patient protection.
- Apply strategies for improving venous access vein visualization (e.g., warm towels/blankets, palpation, augmentation).
- Single use of single patient tourniquet applied to the upper arm to dilate veins.
- Most appropriate insertion site selected and marked (mid-forearm preferred, avoiding other contraindicated areas as with mastectomy or dialysis fistula sites).
- Insertion vein assessed by palpation and when necessary infrared visualization or ultrasound evaluation.
- Disinfect skin with 70% alcoholic chlorhexidine for 30 s and allow to dry completely.
- Perform cannula access/insertion using Surgical-ANTT or Standard-ANTT.
- No more than two attempts per clinician and new cannula with each attempt.
- Flush PIVC with sterile 0.9% sodium chloride to verify correct vein placement and patency. Consider the use of 0.9% sodium chloride prefilled syringes.
- Use positive pressure flushing technique of push pause, and follow correct clamping sequence for needle-free connectors.
- Use adequate strategies to guard against backflow or reflux. Consider neutral or anti-reflux displacement needle-free connector to reduce complications (Elli et al. 2016; Hull et al. 2018).

6.7.1 Needle Design and Quality

In addition to skin integrity, needle quality and design impact the clinical device insertion experience. Features and benefits of new equipment and catheters need to be evaluated objectively. To assess the needle for sharpness, consider how much external force is needed to advance the needle through the skin, tissues, and veins. Ultimately, the performance of the needle impacts ease of cannulating the vessel. Whether performing a peripheral or central insertion, the aim is to access the vein using a single wall puncture, minimizing damage to the vein. A needle that is not sufficiently sharp may cause undue tenting of the outer wall of the vessel as the clinician advances the needle for cannulation. Tenting reduces the diameter of the vessel at the point of cannulation through compression (see Figs. 6.2 and 6.3).

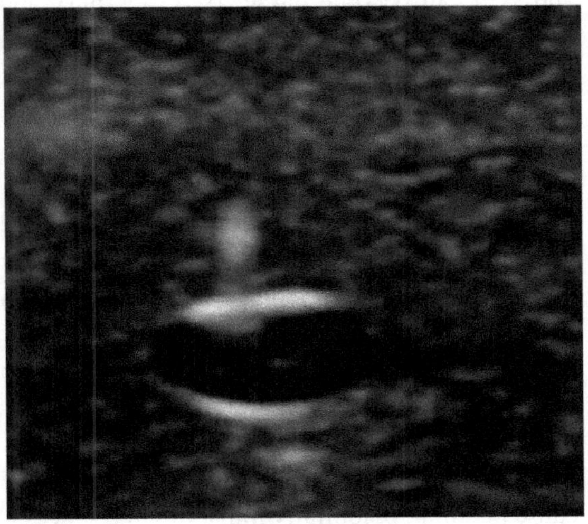

Fig. 6.2 Basilic vein needle tenting (used with permission S. Hill, Precision Vascular)

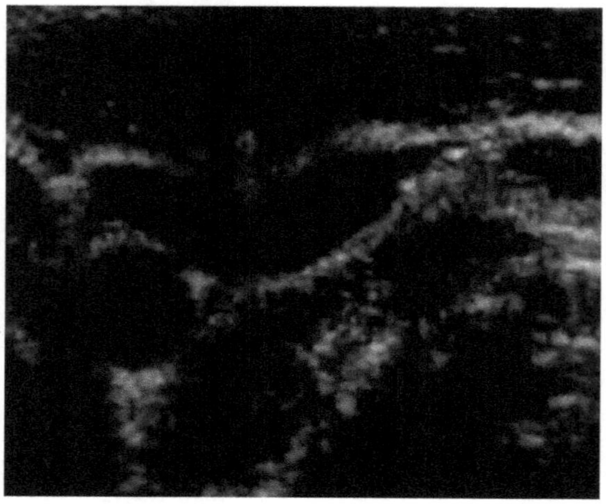

Fig. 6.3 Jugular vein needle tenting and compression (used with permission S. Hill, Precision Vascular)

The extra pressure that is then needed to puncture the vessel wall can lead to "overshooting" of the needle or passing the needle through the anterior and posterior wall in one movement, causing an unnecessary puncture in the back wall of the vein. This situation is avoidable and is not in keeping with the goals of vessel health and preservation. The clinician would then have to retract the needle until blood drips from the needle or until blood is aspirated into the syringe, establishing a good blood flow prior to guidewire advancement.

Patient factors may also influence needle selection (e.g., a patient with graft-versus-host disease). In some circumstances, the vessel walls and skin can become harder (scleroderma), and the quality and sharpness of the needle play an even more significant role in successful access. Similarly, the rigidity of the puncture needle is important when accessing deeper vessels. During insertion, micro movements are made as the needle tip passes from the surface of the skin toward the vein. As the clinician guides the needle in the direction of the vein, if slight changes in direction of the needle are needed, needle responsiveness becomes a factor. How responsive is the distal tip of the needle to clinician direction change/movement? Too much flexibility in the needle reduces the responsiveness at the needle tip and may cause bending, potentially impacting the successful puncture of the vessel. The quality and design of vascular access equipment can be determining factors in the success of the insertion procedure (Pearson and Rawlins 2005).

6.8 Additional Products

It is incumbent upon clinicians to be discerning in the selection of products. EPIC III guidelines (Loveday et al. 2014) recommend clinicians monitor product introduction and impact in clinical practice as follows:

> *The introduction of new intravascular devices or components should be monitored for an increase in the occurrence of device-associated infection. If an increase in infection rates is suspected, this should be reported to the Medicines and Healthcare Products Regulatory Agency in the UK.*

Following insertion of peripheral cannula, specific add-on devices may contribute to the reduction of catheter failure. Cannulas with adequate securement have fewer complications and longer dwell (Marsh et al. 2015). Manufactured securement devices including securement dressings have outperformed traditional tape and gauze and reduce the need to re-site the cannula. Another device included at the time of insertion is the short extension tubing that functions to reduce movement of the cannula at the insertion site and provide additional stress relief locations where the extension is taped to the arm (Bertoglio et al. 2017). Stabilizing the catheter and reducing movement in and around the insertion site promote longer dwell with reduced complications.

6.9 CVAD Insertion Preparation

Checklists, used help measure clinical performance and adherence to proper technique during a CVAD insertion, have been advocated for some time (Gorski et al. 2016; Pronovost et al. 2006). The Joint Commission (2009) sets out a template of critical steps to be included in the checklist including:

- Before the procedure: Perform a timeout to identify the patient and procedure establishing informed consent, check for allergy, have a pertinent history, and select the VAD with the lowest risk for the treatment ordered.

- During the procedure: Perform skin disinfection with alcoholic chlorhexidine or other approved agents, maintain Surgical-ANTT, confirm venous placement (ultrasound guidewire), aspirate each lumen and flush with physiologic solution (saline), and secure catheter.
- After the procedure: Verify terminal tip position, provide patient education, and ensure dressing is secure and date documented.

The National Safety Standards for Invasive Procedures (NatSSips) set out key steps necessary to underpin patient safety by standardizing processes that promote safety in patient care (England 2015). The concept of a never events was introduced in 2009, which includes core surgical never events such as retained foreign objects. Never events are considered wholly preventable, but by the provision of sequential procedural standards, and organizational standards, errors can be eliminated. The information that accompanies the scheduling of patients should include but not be limited to:

- Patient name
- Identification numbers, i.e., NHS number with or without hospital number
- Date of birth
- Gender
- Planned procedure
- Site and side of procedure if relevant
- Location of patient, e.g., ward or admissions lounge
- Further information that can be provided when relevant may include:
- NCEPOD classification of intervention
- Significant comorbidities
- Allergies, e.g., to latex or iodine
- Infection risk
- Any nonstandard equipment requirements or nonstock prostheses
- Body mass index
- Planned post-procedural admission to high dependency or intensive care facility

NatSSips follow the World Health Organization (WHO) safety checklist introduced in 2009 shown to improve patient safety and reduce complications and following the 2015 update now offer a more comprehensive safety approach (Pugel et al. 2015).

6.9.1 Insertion Environment

The environment and circumstances in which a vascular access device is placed can impact the outcomes of the procedure. For instance, devices placed in emergent settings are at higher risk for infections and complications than those placed electively (Tsotsolis et al. 2015). In the author's experience, the occasions in which complications have occurred have resulted from the clinician feeling pressured either by the procedure, circumstances of the day or both, and working in an unfamiliar environment. In the elective setting, there is a greater opportunity to create a more relaxed environment for the patient and for the clinician. Additionally, familiarity with equipment is essential. Using a compressive, inclusive procedure prep pack which may include the catheter allows the clinician to have a recognizable set up of equipment and creates an element of routine and adheres to normal practice, even in unfamiliar environments (Marschall et al. 2014; INS 2016).

It is important to ensure that the patient is placed in a position of comfort, and necessary analgesia is optimized if needed prior to the procedure. Clinician comfort is important, too, allowing for better focus and ability to maintain sterile procedure. Placing the ultrasound, ECG/navigation equipment in the line of site so the clinician can glance effortlessly from ultrasound to insertion site without twisting, turning, or having to alter the screen allows for optimal function and view.

6.9.2 Local Anesthetic

The effective use of anesthetic is a fundamental component of a successful procedure. It facilitates patient comfort at key stages, such as vein cannulation and passing the dilator into the skin. Firstly, the anesthetic should be infiltrated superficially under the surface of the skin with the bevel of the needle pointing upward. Blanching of the skin may be observed. Depending upon the depth of the vein, anesthetic may need to be infiltrated slightly deeper to ensure an adequately anesthetized pathway from the surface of the skin to the selected vein, making sure the dermatome nerve supply is adequately anesthetized while taking care to keep a safe distance from vascular and nerve branches.

Injecting the anesthetic may cause the tissues to swell, increasing the distance from the skin to vein. Applying mild pressure over the site allows the anesthetic to infiltrate the tissues close to the vein and help restore normal anatomy. Infiltration of the anesthetic should be cautiously administered using an advance, aspirate and inject method, ensuring that no blood is aspirated into the syringe. Higher gauge or smaller diameter needles increase the difficulty of aspirating blood, and deflection is also higher in smaller diameter needles (Reed et al. 2012). The infiltrated anesthetic works on nerve endings; the larger the nerve branch, the more difficult it is to anesthetize. Nerve structures within the arm should be identified prior to commencing the insertion and local anesthetic. Injecting anesthetic too close to the nerve bundle may cause paresthesia. Paresthesia caused by lidocaine should subside within 2 h of administration as the serum half-life of lidocaine is approximately 90 min (Becker and Reed 2006). The local anesthetic with the least toxic and/or the least risk for allergic reaction should be considered (RCN 2016). INS (2016) recommends removal of any peripheral catheter when there are reports of paresthesia-type pain, as the dwell of the catheter and fluid accumulation may lead to compression injuries (Gorski et al. 2016).

6.10 Seldinger Technique

We owe much of our vascular access practice to clinicians like Dr. Sven Ivar Seldinger, who originally described an over-wire technique of catheter insertion, using needle, a guidewire, and catheter. The technique includes access with a needle, advancement of a wire, needle removal, and catheter advancement over the wire. Initially, this technique was used in arterial cannulation; subsequent modifications saw it used in venous catheterization, and it is now seen in emergency medicine, CVC cannulation and percutaneous tracheal ventilation (Bishay et al. 2018). PICCs and Midlines are mainly inserted using a modified Seldinger technique, a standard 21-gauge needle and 0.018 guidewire followed by peel-away sheath and dilator. This approach allows the insertion of a catheter that is larger than the puncture site created by the access needle in the vessel. The initial puncture site is dilated and stretched as the peel-away introducer is inserted. This modification with the two-part dilator and peelable sheath is preferable to traditional approaches when PICCs were initially inserted by passing the PICC through a 14G cannula sheath, usually accessing antecubital veins and without ultrasound (Gabriel 2001). One of the advantages of the modification is avoidance of skin contact and reduction of catheter contamination during insertion. For patients with difficult venous access, ultrasound should be used to provide for better assessment, to enhance vein selection, to reduce access attempts, and to facilitate successful insertion (Gorski et al. 2016). Evidence underscores the increase in successful placement and improved outcome for those clinicians receiving education and precepted insertions when employing the use of ultrasound (Moore 2013).

Resistance during the guidewire advancement following cannulation may occur with Midline and PICC insertions. Guidewire resistance may be experienced at the needle bevel or further down the venous pathway and may be caused by several factors:

6.10.1 Guidewire Advancement Difficulties

- **Needle is not in the vein**—While a blood flashback was initially observed, it is possible that while the clinician is moving and reaching for the guidewire, the tip of the needle may move out of the vein. Secondly, it may be that the flash of blood was from the needle passing through the vein, but the needle was then inadvertently advanced through the back wall of the vessel (e.g., in a dehydrated patient), in which case a syringe (if not already being used) should be added to the needle and, while gently aspirating, slowly withdrawn until the needle tip enters the vein and blood is aspirated.

- **Bevel of the needle has not fully entered the vein**—This occurs when the needle tip has entered the vessel, allowing for a blood return, but the whole portion of the bevel has not entered the vein; therefore, a clear pathway for the guidewire has not been established. Slight advancement of the needle is needed.
- **Angle or position of the needle in the vein**—A steeper-angled needle approach is often needed in patients with increased body mass leading to a more difficult passage of the guidewire as it meets the posterior wall of the vessel and moves up the vein. Lowering the needle angle slightly may alleviate the resistance. Similarly, the proximity of the needle to the posterior vein wall may cause resistance as the wire attempts to negotiate passage through the acute angle and restricts space between needle tip and vein. Optimizing needle tip position within the vein will help to eliminate this problem.
- **Obstruction against a valve**—A valve can cause resistance of the guidewire advancement within the venous pathway. Other guidewire advancement difficulties are found with distorted vein system seen in patients with a history of IV drug abuse where veins can be tortuous, sclerosed, or thrombosed. Good ultrasound assessment is the key to ensure the optimal device and outcomes, along with acquiring patient history for which veins were not previously used during drug abuse.

6.10.2 Guidewire Check

The visualization of the guidewire once it has been inserted into the vein is an important safety check, but it is not infallible. The wire can be passed through the vein and then into the adjacent or underlying artery, and this is not always appreciated on ultrasound (Bowdle 2014). A singular static ultrasound view of the wire in the vein is insufficient; thorough visualization of the wire as it passes from the skin, through the tissues into the vein and then advances through the vein, is needed to exclude posterior wall puncture and to ensure arterial or extravenous placement has not occurred.

For all vascular access insertions, the ultimate aim is a single wall puncture on the first pass of the cannulating needle. However, this is not the reality in some situations and may be related to clinician skill, situational stress, working out of comfort zone, procedural fatigue, and anatomical presentation of the patient. If the view of the guidewire is unclear, movement of the outside portion of the wire may aid the view of the wire within the vein, but this should be reserved for when the wire cannot readily be seen, as the wire movement may increase friction on the intima. If there is doubt over the wire position, X-ray imaging should be obtained to ensure correct placement prior to advancing the dilator or advancing the catheter.

The National Safety Standards for Invasive Procedures view guidewire retention as a never event and set out requirements for organizations to establish policy, protocols, good education, and safe practices for practitioners (England 2015). Some manufacturers have placed a slight bend at the proximal end of the guidewire to help prevent guidewire advancement.

6.11 Number of Access Attempts

Eisen et al. (2006) analyzed 385 consecutive nontunneled CVC insertions undertaken on adult critically ill patients (Eisen et al. 2006). The authors identified that, with increasing attempts, the relative risk of complications increased accordingly and reported a rate of mechanical complications of 54% when two or more punctures were needed. Tsotsolis et al. (2015) identify the risk of one attempt at 4.3% and two or more attempts at 24% (Tsotsolis et al. 2015). The incidence of gaining first-time access to the vessel is considerably increased when using ultrasound. A randomized controlled trial (RCT) of 100 patients conducted by Karimi-Sari et al. (2014) compared landmark technique versus ultrasound-guided central venous catheter placements (Karimi-Sari et al. 2014). In this study, the mean access time, number of attempts, rate of first attempt success, and procedure success rates were all superior in the ultrasound group. Mehta et al. (2012) undertook a systematic review of US versus landmark approach of emergency physicians and identified IJ placements had a success rate of 93.9% versus 78.5% with landmark, and complications were 4.6% with US versus 16.9% with landmark technique (Mehta et al. 2013). Kornbau et al. (2015) confirmed that overall, the number of unsuccessful insertion attempts is the biggest predictor of complications and confirms that US has significantly reduced the incidence of immediate complications (Kornbau et al. 2015).

Tsotsolis et al. (2015) identified that inserter experience was of paramount importance. "A physician who has performed 50 or more catheterizations is half as likely to result in a mechanical complication as insertions by a physician who has performed fewer than 50 catheterisations" (Tsotsolis et al. 2015). A greater number of needle passes were also associated with increased risk. The authors quantified this as 1st pass risk at 4.3% and 2nd pass at 24% (see Fig. 6.4).

Tsotsolis explains that complications are largely related to three categories: patient factors, clinical factors, and catheter-related factors as illustrated in Fig. 6.5.

Our aim is to minimize trauma to the vessel, thereby reducing harmful effects and preserving the vessel for the future life of the patient. Thrombosis, infection, and mechanical-related complications can all be affected by the way we access veins. This is exemplified in the RCT performed by Li and colleagues (Li et al. 2014). The study involved 100 patients and included 50 blind insertions using a traditional 14G cannula passing the catheter through the cannula sheath and 50 insertions using MST with ultrasound guidance. The MST/ultrasound group showed higher migration rates but had lower unplanned removal, mechanical phlebitis, and incidence of thrombosis.

The rate of misplacement of catheters varies between VAD types and sites of insertion. Internal jugular, for instance, has lower instances of misplacement than axillary placements or PICCs. PICCs are reported to have three times greater risk of primary malposition than other CVADs (Gorski et al. 2016). PICCs must negotiate a longer distance from the insertion site to the

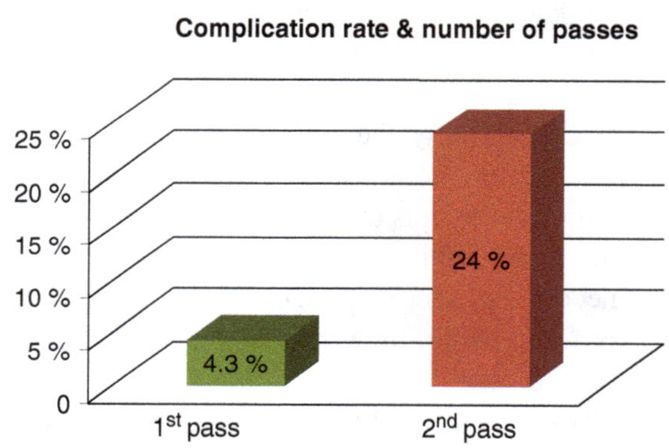

Fig. 6.4 A direct relationship between the number of access attempts and the risk of complication is identified (Tsotsolis et al. 2015)

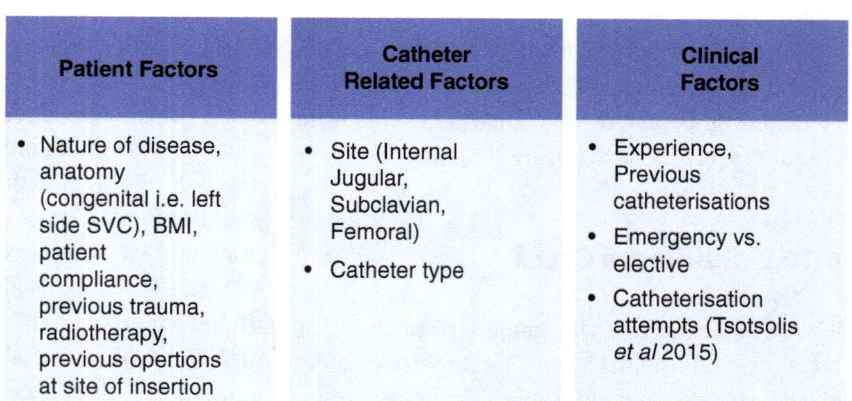

Fig. 6.5 Risk of complications is affected by patient factors, catheter-related factors, and clinical factors modified (Tsotsolis et al. 2015)

lower SVC and CAJ and may be inadvertently placed into a number of wrong veins on their journey. The most frequent malpositioning is the internal jugular vein. Inadvertent tip position into the jugular vein can be assessed using ultrasound during placement. Additionally, the catheter may be laid on the wall of the vein, which is not always readily visible with ultrasound. Close attention is needed to identify the hyperechogenic catheter. Using a sterile saline flush causes a saline swirl (microbubbles at catheter terminal end viewed with ultrasound). This "swirl" can be seen within the vein, also indicating that the tip has migrated into the internal jugular vein. Tip navigation and confirmation systems aid visualization of tip positioning into alternative veins so that corrective action can be undertaken immediately.

6.12 Conclusion

Insertion of a PIVC or CVAD is an invasive process that includes associated complications. Education and training on specific complications and methods to avoid those complications with insertion techniques will contribute to patient safety. VHP embraces consistent education for inserters in keeping with the Society for Healthcare Epidemiology of America recommendations (Marschall et al. 2014). Institutions are responsible to their patients to establish credentialing processes to ensure inserter safe practice. Initial training with supervision, precepting for ultrasound skill acquisition, insertion techniques for different devices, applications for each technique and device, competency assessment, and data collection on outcomes as measurement criteria are all necessary components of a high-quality program.

Case Study

Mrs. Jones, recently diagnosed with stage 4 lung cancer, required a CVAD for the administration of her vesicant chemotherapy treatment for 6 months. Following discussion with Mrs. Jones, a decision was made to insert a tunneled CVAD, and appointment was arranged with interventional radiology for placement. A specially trained nurse within the radiology department, with more than 10 years of experience and many hundreds of insertions, performed the insertion without complications. Mrs. Jones was satisfied with the procedure and thanked the inserter.

Summary of Key Points

1. The goal of vascular access is to minimize trauma to the vessel and preserve the vessel for the future life of the patient.
2. The number of unsuccessful insertion attempts is the biggest predictor of complications.
3. The number of insertions a clinician has performed directly affects the likelihood of first time access success. The more experience (e.g., >50), the more likely to gain access on first attempt.
4. Supervised or precepted insertions with ultrasound promote a higher percentage of success with subsequent insertions.

References

Becker DE, Reed KL. Essentials of local anesthetic pharmacology. Anesth Prog. 2006;53:98–109.

Bertoglio S, Van Boxtel T, Goossens GA, Dougherty L, Furtwangler R, Lennan E, Pittiruti M, Sjovall K, Stas M. Improving outcomes of short peripheral vascular access in oncology and chemotherapy administration. London: Sage Publications; 2017.

Bishay VL, Ingber RB, O'connor PJ, Fischman AM. Vascular access techniques and closure devices. In: IR playbook. Springer; 2018.

Bowdle A. Vascular complications of central venous catheter placement: evidence-based methods for prevention and treatment. J Cardiothorac Vasc Anesth. 2014;28:358–68.

Carr PJ, Rippey JC, Cooke ML, Bharat C, Murray K, Higgins NS, Foale A, Rickard CM. Development of a clinical prediction rule to improve peripheral intravenous cannulae first attempt success in the emergency department and reduce post insertion failure rates: the Vascular Access Decisions in the Emergency Room (VADER) study protocol. BMJ Open. 2016;6(2):e009196. https://doi.org/10.1136/bmjopen-2015-009196.

Carr PJ, Rippey JC, Cooke ML, Bharat C, Murray K, Higgins NS, Foale A, Rickard CM. Development of a clinical prediction rule to improve peripheral intravenous cannulae first attempt success in the emergency department and reduce post insertion failure rates: the Vascular Access Decisions in the Emergency Room (VADER) study protocol. BMJ Open. 2016;6:e009196.

Chopra V, Flanders S, Saint S, Woller S, O'grady N, Safdar N, Trerotola S, Saran R, Moureau N, Wiseman S, Pittiruti M, Akl E, Lee A, Courey A, Swaminathan L, Ledonne J, Becker C, Krein S, Bernstein S, Michigan Appropriateness Guide for Intravenous Catheters Panel. The Michigan Appropriateness Guide for Intravenous Catheters (MAGIC): results from a multispecialty panel using the RAND/UCLA appropriateness method. Ann Intern Med. 2015;163:S1–40.

Dougherty L, Lister S. The Royal Marsden Manual of clinical procedures. 7th ed. Oxford: Wiley-Blackwell; 2011.

Dougherty L, Lister S. The Royal Marsden manual of clinical nursing procedures. 9th ed. Wiley; 2015.

Eisen L, Narasimhan M, Berger J, Mayo P, Rosen M, Schneider R. Mechanical complications of central venous catheters. J Intensive Care Med. 2006;21:40–6.

Elli S, Abbruzzese C, Cannizzo L, Lucchini A. In vitro evaluation of fluid reflux after flushing different types of needleless connectors. J Vasc Access. 2016;17(5):429–34.

England N. National safety standards for invasie procedures (NatSSIPS). 2015;8:468–74. https://www.england.nhs.uk/wp-content/uploads/2015/09/natssips-safety-standards.pdf. Accessed 18 Aug 2018.

Farage MA, Miller KW, Elsner P, Maibach HI. Characteristics of the aging skin. Adv Wound Care. 2013;2:5–10.

Gabriel J. PICC securement: minimising potential complications. Nurs Stand. 2001;15:42–4.

Gorski LA, Hadaway L, Hagle M, McGoldrick M, Orr M, Doellman D. Infusion therapy standards of practice. J Infus Nurs. 2016;39(1 Suppl):S1–S159.

Hull G, Moureau N, Sengupta S. Quantitative assessment of reflux in commercially available needleless IV connectors. J Vasc Access. 2018;19(1):12–22.

Joint Commission. Improving America's Hospitals: the Joint Commission's Annual Report on Quality and Safety, Quality and Safety. NPSG. 2009;2–16.

Karimi-Sari H, Faraji M, Torabi SM, Asjodi G. Success rate and complications of internal jugular vein catheterization with and without ultrasonography guide. Nurs Midwifery Stud. 2014;3:e23204.

Kornbau C, Lee KC, Hughes GD, Firstenberg MS. Central line complications. Int J Crit Illn Inj Sci. 2015;5:170.

Larue GD. Efficacy of ultrasonography in peripheral venous cannulation. J Intraven Nurs. 2000;23:29–34.

Li J, Fan YY, Xin MZ, Yan J, Hu W, Huang WH, Lin XL, Qin HY. A randomised, controlled trial comparing the long-term effects of peripherally inserted central catheter placement in chemotherapy patients using B-mode ultrasound with modified Seldinger technique versus blind puncture. Eur J Oncol Nurs. 2014;18:94–103.

Loveday H, Wilson J, Pratt R, Golsorkhi M, Tingle A, Bak A, Browne J, Prieto J, Wilcox M. EPIC3: national evidence-based guidelines for preventing healthcare-associated infections in NHS hospitals in England. J Hosp Infect. 2014;86:S1–70.

Marschall J, Mermel L, Fakih M, Hadaway L, Kallen A, O'grady N, Pettis A, Rupp M, Sandora T, Maragakis L, Yokoe D. Strategies to prevent central line–associated bloodstream infections in acute care hospitals: 2014 update. Infect Control Hosp Epidemiol. 2014;35:753–71.

Marsh N, Webster J, Mihala G, Rickard C. Devices and dressings to secure peripheral venous catheters to prevent complications. Cochrane Database Syst Rev. 2015;12:CD011070.

Mcdiarmid S, Scrivens N, Carrier M, Sabri E, Toye B, Huebsch L, Fergusson D. Outcomes in a nurse-led peripherally inserted central catheter program: a retrospective cohort study. CMAJ Open. 2017;5:E535.

Mehta N, Valesky W, Guy A, Sinert R. Br Med J. 2012; 30(3). https://doi.org/10.1136/emermed-2012-201230

Mehta N, Valesky WW, Guy A, Sinert R. Systematic review: is real-time ultrasonic-guided central line placement by ED physicians more successful than the traditional landmark approach? Emerg Med J. 2013;30:355–9.

Moore C. An emergency department nurse-driven ultrasound-guided peripheral intravenous line program. J Assoc Vasc Access. 2013;18:45–51.

O'Grady N, Alexander M, Burns L, Dellinger E, Garland J, Heard S, Lipsett P, Masur H, Mermel L, Pearson M, Raad I, Randolph A, Rupp M, Saint S, Healthcare Infection Control Practices Advisory Committee (HICPAC). Centers for Disease Control Guidelines for the prevention of intravascular catheter-related infections. Clin Infect Dis. 2011;52:e162–93.

Pearson SD, Rawlins MD. Quality, innovation, and value for money: NICE and the British National Health Service. JAMA. 2005;294:2618–22.

Pronovost P, Needham D, Berenholtz S, Sinopoli D, Chu H, Cosgrove S, Sexton B, Hyzy R, Welsh R, Roth G. An intervention to decrease catheter-related bloodstream infections in the ICU. N Engl J Med. 2006;355:2725–32.

Pugel AE, Simianu VV, Flum DR, Dellinger EP. Use of the surgical safety checklist to improve communication and reduce complications. J Infect Public Health. 2015;8:219–25.

RCN. Standards for infusion therapy. 4th ed. Royal College of Nursing; 2016. p. 1–94.

Reed KL, Malamed SF, Fonner AM. Local anesthesia part 2: technical considerations. Anesth Prog. 2012;59:127–37.

Rickard C, Webster J, Wallis M, Marsh N, Mcgrail M, French V, Foster L, Gallagher P, Gowardman J, Zhang L, Mcclymont A, Whitby M. Routine versus clinically indicated replacement of peripheral intravenous catheters: a randomised controlled equivalence trial. Lancet. 2012;380:1066–74.

Tsotsolis N, Tsirgogianni K, Kioumis I, Pitsiou G, Baka S, Papaiwannou A, Karavergou A, Rapti A, Trakada G, Katsikogiannis N. Pneumothorax as a complication of central venous catheter insertion. Ann Transl Med. 2015;3:40.

Weinstein SM, editor. Plumers principles and practic of intravenous therapy. 8th ed. Philadelphia: JB Lippencott; 2007.

7

Catheter Tip Location

Steve Hill and Nancy L. Moureau

Abstract

This chapter provides insight into catheter tip location and review of vascular access devices from PIV to central venous non-tunnelled and tunnelled catheters, implanted ports and dialysis catheters. An overview of the guidelines related to tip location is discussed. The dynamic relationship between catheter tip location and how this influences complications during the procedure and post-insertion is examined. The various methods of confirming CVAD tip location are presented, including ECG (i.e. echocardiography) versus traditional means of X-ray, exploring patient implications of intraprocedural real-time tip location, reduced radiation dosage and incidence of manipulations. Case studies illustrating some of the challenges clinicians face when placing CVADs are incorporated into the discussion.

S. Hill
The Christie NHS Foundation Trust, Manchester, UK

Precision Vascular and Surgical Services Ltd, Manchester, UK
e-mail: info@precisionvascular.co.uk; steve.hill@christie.nhs.uk

N. L. Moureau (✉)
PICC Excellence, Inc., Hartwell, GA, USA

Menzies Health Institute, Alliance for Vascular Access Teaching and Research (AVATAR) Group, Griffith University, Brisbane, QLD, Australia
e-mail: nancy@piccexcellence.com

Keywords

Superior vena cava · Cavoatrial junction Tip location · Thrombosis · Arrhythmias Electrocardiogram · Terminal catheter tip Malposition · Complications · Central venous catheter

7.1 Introduction

A great deal of research, time and energy has gone into the subject of catheter tip position, yet it is still yielding debate and controversy. Many of the guidelines are united in placement of optimal tip position of a central venous access device. The associations are the Infusion Nursing Society (INS), Association of Anaesthetists of Great Britain and Ireland (AAGBI), European Society of Parenteral and Enteral Nutrition (ESPEN) and British Society for Haematology (BCSH) (Table 7.1).

The reason for the focus on tip position is that malposition of the catheter tip is associated with an increased risk of complications. These may occur at the time of insertion (atrial fibrillation, ventricular tachycardia or other arrhythmias, atrial wall damage, catheter malfunction) or post-insertion (catheter malfunction, vessel erosion, venous thrombosis). Misplacement of catheter does not only mean the incorrect vein but also includes catheters inserted in extra-venous positions such as in the arterial system, mediastinum,

Table 7.1 Guidelines for terminal tip placement (Gorski et al. 2016a; Pittiruti et al. 2009)

INS (2016)	Lower third of the superior vena cava or cavoatrial junction
AAGBI (2016)	Lower SVC upper right atrium
ESPEN (2006)	Lower third of the superior vena cava or at the atrio-caval junction
BCSH (2006)	Distal superior vena cava or upper right atrium

pleura, trachea, oesophagus, etc. (Gibson and Bodenham 2013). This chapter will focus on tip placement, controversies, guidelines and other considerations when selecting the tip position for centrally placed intravenous devices.

7.2 Vascular Access Device Terminal Tip Positioning

Correct terminal tip positioning of a vascular access device is determined by manufacturer specifications as well as regulatory and guideline evidence-based criteria. Indications for each VAD also contribute to the choice of device, function and tip position based on treatment plan.

- **Peripheral catheters** remain in the periphery with terminal tip below the level of the axillary vein for upper extremity placement. The terminal tip of a peripheral catheter does not enter the chest or torso and, therefore, does not require any verification following insertion (Gorski et al. 2016a).
- **Central venous access devices** (CVADs), as their name implies, are inserted with the terminal tip entering central circulation and advancing towards the heart. Except for haemodialysis catheters, terminal tip placement of all CVADs is in the vena cava. For upper extremity insertions, the terminal tip is advanced to the superior vena cava; for lower extremity insertions, the terminal tip is advanced to the inferior vena cava (Campisi et al. 2007; National Association of Vascular Access Networks 1998; Scott 1995; Vesely 2003).

7.3 Anatomy

A CVAD by definition has the distal tip of the catheter within the central veins. INS suggests that ideally a central venous catheter should have its tip situated in the lower third of the superior vena cava at or near the cavoatrial junction (Gorski et al. 2016a). Firstly, let's review venous anatomy relevant to tip placement; to consider tip position and recognise misplacement, we must be clear in our knowledge of the venous system. Venous structures, such as vein walls (tunica intima, tunica media and tunica adventitia), are thinner and more fragile than arteries, making them more prone to iatrogenic injury, and their longitudinal organisation of vein layers means that tears in the vein walls tend to extend longitudinally (Gibson and Bodenham 2013).

The larger venous vessels within the thorax relevant to vascular access include axillary, subclavian, brachiocephalic, internal jugular, superior vena cava, iliac, femoral and inferior vena cava (Fig. 7.1). In the adult, the superior vena cava's average length is 7 cm but varies from 5 to 11 cm (Verhey et al. 2008). The brachiocephalic veins, from the right side, is positioned at a steeper angle and is around 2.5 cm in length, and the left brachiocephalic around 6 cm in length joins the right brachiocephalic and the SVC at a less acute angle than the right brachiocephalic. CVAD insertions from the left brachiocephalic that are not long enough to drop down into the SVC can abut the wall of the SVC increasing the risk of thrombosis and erosion (Gibson and Bodenham 2013).

Other relevant vasculature also includes the azygos system which drains venous blood from the upper thorax and abdominal wall terminating in the SVC (Tortora and Derrickson 2006). The azygos vein drains some of the lumbar and posterior intercostal region and also connects to the posterior aspect of the IVC, level with the first or second lumbar vertebrae, to the IVC (Gibson and Bodenham 2013). Catheter tips placed in the azygos vein viewed on standard anterior-posterior X-ray can appear short at first glance, but with closer inspection and by performing a lat-

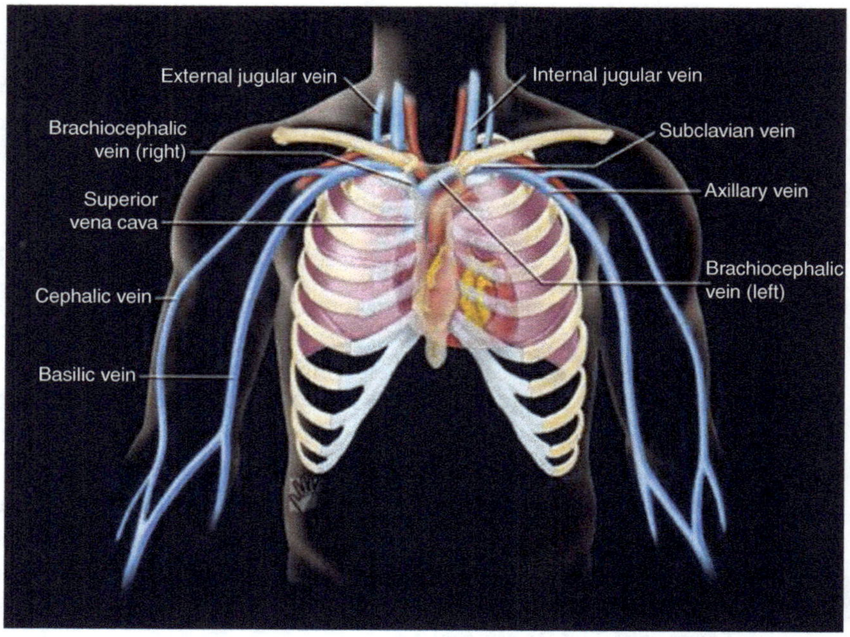

Fig. 7.1 Anatomy of the arm and chest (used with permission of N. Moureau, PICC Excellence)

eral X-ray film, the catheter can be distinguished as it changes course from the vertical SVC and may turn abruptly moving posteriorly and inferiorly. Smaller vessels such as the superior intercostal veins are important as a catheter may migrate into these during the insertion of upper thoracic CVADs. VADs inserted via the femoral veins should have their tips placed in the inferior vena cava (IVC) above the level of the diaphragm (Gorski et al. 2016a). During femoral insertion, the catheter may migrate into smaller veins during insertion including lumbar, iliolumbar renal, suprarenal, common iliac, hepatic and inferior phrenic veins (Gorski et al. 2016a; Tortora and Derrickson 2006). The IVC drains blood from the lower part of the body, ascends along the anterior vertebral column and is around 2.5 cm wide (Gibson and Bodenham 2013).

Arm anatomy—Moving away from the larger more central veins, there are the axillary, brachial, cephalic and basilic veins of the upper arm. Moving distally, the veins start to become smaller in diameter, and blood flow is reduced. When considering veins of the upper arm for PICC and midline placement, the main vessels include basilic, brachial and cephalic veins. Moving distally to around the antecubital area, the median cubital and cephalic are often prominent veins; smaller vessels include the accessory cephalic, brachial and intermediate antebrachial. Within the forearm, there are the branches of the basilic, cephalic and median veins together with radial, posterior/anterior ulna and accessory cephalic veins. The dorsum of the hand includes metacarpal veins and the dorsal venous arch (DVA) which has many tributaries; the medial aspect of the DVA leads the flow to the cephalic veins, and the lateral aspect flows to the basilic veins (Fig. 7.2). Anatomy is not universal, and variations exist from person to person. Assessment is the key to identifying anatomical variations and optimal vein and VAD site. Ultrasound is an excellent visualization and enhances assessment of veins, arteries and nerves.

Cannulation—Insertion of a short PIV has been described as the most frequent invasive procedure in acute care, with the most common complications being dislodgement and phlebitis (2.3–67%) but has a particularly low incidence of infection relative to other vascular devices (0.5/1000 catheter days) (Bertoglio et al. 2017). Catheter sizes from 20G to 22G are recommended for adult patients if possible (Gorski et al. 2016a). The forearm is strongly recommended (Bertoglio

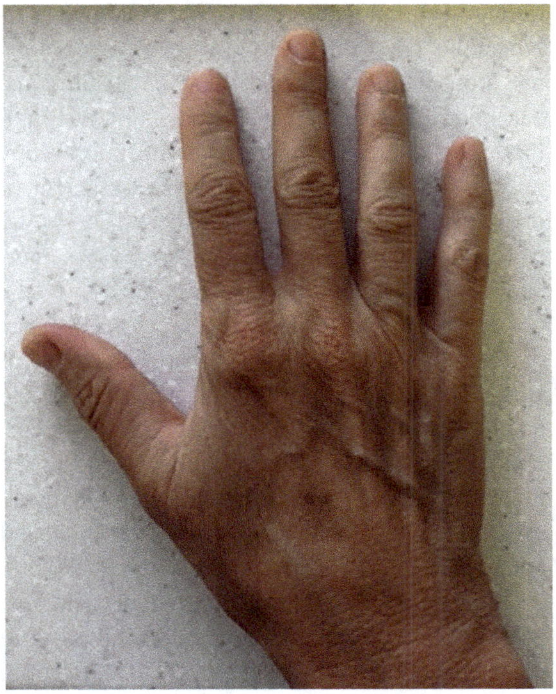

Fig. 7.2 Hand and dorsal venous arch (used with permission of N. Moureau, PICC Excellence)

et al. 2017). Selecting the optimal site for placement of PIV impacts upon the functional lifespan of the device, Wallis et al. (2014) identified that the forearm is the optimal position for the longest dwell time; this area is also associated with decreased pain (Gorski et al. 2016a). Risk factors for patients receiving chemotherapy include placement of the catheter in the hand and antecubital fossa and upper arm when compared to the forearm (Gorski et al. 2016a). A thorough assessment is necessary, not only of the suitability of the vessels but to the length of the PIV related to the depth of the vein. INS recommends two-thirds of the catheter be placed in the vein to establish safety (Gorski et al. 2016a). Consider the use of longer PIV lengths or midlines if a safe amount of catheter cannot be established within the vessel. An ultrasound-guided cannula placed in the upper arm is at increased risk of extravasation and infiltration (Gorski et al. 2016a). PIV sites such as the wrist and antecubital should be avoided, as areas of flexion they have increased rates of complications (Gorski et al. 2016a). Furthermore, patients planned for future mastectomy surgery or dialysis fistula should not have PIVs placed over joints, forearm is preferred (Bertoglio et al. 2017). Due to the relatively short length of most PIVs, site selection becomes an important determinant of tip position, as the insertion site and tip are within a short distance of each other.

Lower limbs should be avoided for insertion of intravenous devices unless absolutely necessary as they are at increased risk of tissue damage (Gorski et al. 2016a), alternative sites should be explored preferably. PIV position should ideally be in the non-dominant arm, and ventral surfaces of the wrist may increase pain and risk of nerve damage and thrombosis (Gorski et al. 2016a; RCN 2016). For many years, first attempt PIVs have been made on the dorsal aspect of the hand, but with advent of infrared and ultrasound technology, non-visible or difficult to palpate veins are now easier to assess and access. Veins of the forearm can lie slightly deeper than veins on the dorsum of the hand and overlying the antecubital area and enhanced by aids such as visualisation technology. In situations where intravenous access is needed, more urgently peripheral catheters may be inserted into the external jugular (Gorski et al. 2016a) or leg veins by a suitably trained clinician and when treatment is less than 4 days (Chopra et al. 2015).

Midline catheters are used for appropriate peripheral solutions; the Michigan appropriateness guide for intravenous catheters (Moureau and Chopra 2016) suggests that they are preferred for solutions up to 14 days but may be used in a manner consistent with the clinically indicated removal of peripheral catheters. Midline catheters come in a variety of length and diameters; INS principles should be followed when selecting a VAD with the smallest outer diameter (Gorski et al. 2016a). The midline is placed into the basilic, cephalic or brachial veins, by way of sterile procedure similar to PICC placement, with the exception of need to verify terminal tip since the midline remains in the peripheral veins (Gorski et al. 2016a). Adults and older children should have the tip of the midline placed at the level of the axilla and distal to the shoulder (Gorski et al. 2016a).

The axillary vein by definition is:

> the continuation of the basilic and brachial veins running from the lower border of the teres major muscle to the outer border of the first rib where it becomes the subclavian vein. (Farlex Medical Dictionary 2012)

The teres major muscle is attached to the scapula and to the humerus and is the most inferior positioned muscle of the muscles connected to the scapula; its function is to aid adduction of the arm.

One of the advantages of the midline compared to CVADs is that chest X-ray or ECG confirmation is not required. When the midline is appropriate, it may be more time efficient for the vascular access clinician and a more cost-effective solution, as midlines are often a comparably cheaper option versus other CVADs. Like all devices, it must be inserted according to the manufacturer's instructions; if there are concerns during insertion, impaired blood return or resistance to flushing an X-ray or replacement device should be considered (Alexandrou et al. 2011). As the tip position of a midline is placed at the level of the axilla where extravasation could be a risk, thus placing other anatomical structures at risk such as arteries and nerves, if fluid escapes into the tissues, it may be harder to detect than in the forearm or hand (Hadaway 2000).

Central venous catheter tip location—CVAD tip position for many years has been confirmed by the means of a radiograph or chest X-ray (CXR). In recent years, electrocardiograph (ECG)-based systems have been developed to confirm catheter tip position, some of which also have additional navigational elements. In this section we will discuss traditional radiographic techniques, the evolution of current practice and the adoption of tip confirmation technology.

Undertaking CVAD insertions under direct X-ray screening/fluoroscopy offers real-time visualisation of elements of the insertion, such as position of the guidewire tip deep in the thorax, migration and immediate confirmation of tip position. This has been, and is still for many institutions, the mainstay for CVAD insertions because of the advantages offered and because in many hospitals CVAD insertions still fall within the remit of interventional radiologists. Undertaking a post-procedure chest X-ray following a fluoroscopic insertion should be decided on an institutional basis; this is mainly for exclusion of pneumothorax as assessment is limited with fluoroscopy only; ultrasound sliding lung and assessment of pneumothorax may also be considered. A similar technique, but not radiographically robust as interventional suites, is for a CVAD insertion to take place in theatre or procedural area with assistance of a portable X-ray system or C-arm image intensifier. The technology has advanced, and image quality has improved; however portable systems remain inferior to fluoroscopy imaging. Both the fluoroscopy and C-arm approach are relatively expensive models of practice due to the capital and maintenance costs related to the systems.

Other models of insertion practice involve insertion in a designated area, or a multipurpose room that is suitable also for CVAD insertion. Using this, tip location can be confirmed during insertion using ECG confirmation system or by sending the patient to X-ray. The latter X-ray approach is prone to increased risk malposition as confirmation of tip position is sought following insertion. Lastly, many services place PICCs by the bedside, but this approach too is prone to higher insertion-related malposition unless using tip confirmation technology versus post-procedure X-ray confirmation. As we continue to see the adoption of ECG guidance systems, fluoroscopy remains inextricably linked to vascular access services for patients with complex congenital or disease-related anatomy, stenosis, etc., where more advanced insertion techniques are required. However, cost associated with fluoroscopy and the need to schedule and transport patients makes bedside PICC with ECG guidance more attractive and reasonable given the level of precision and accuracy associated with ECG.

7.4 ECG Tech Development

The concept of confirming catheter tip position by alternative means to X-ray is not a new one. As the knowledge and skills of identifying cardiac electrical impulses have evolved over the last century, this has given us the fundamental principles of ECG that we use in clinical practice today. Using this knowledge and transferring it into clinical applications allow us in today's clinical practice to confirm tip position of a CVAD using ECG technology.

Carlo Matteucci a professor of physics in Florence initially identified electrical impulses relating to cardiac pulsation (Matteucci 1842). Marey (1876) used an electrometer to record cardiac electrical activity from an exposed frog heart. Soon after Sanderson and Fredrick identified the two phases of cardiac electrical activity (Burdon-Sanderson and Page 1878) and at the turn of the century, Arthur Cushny at University College London reported the first case of auricular fibrillation (atrial fibrillation), making the connection between an irregular pulse and atrial fibrillation (Cushny and Edmonds 1906). Augustus Waller published the first human electrocardiogram, using a capillary electrometer, where the surface electrodes were strapped to the front of the chest and back and used saline jars where the limbs were immersed in saline solution. He identified that 'each beat of the heart is seen to be accompanied by an electrical variation' (Bestman and Creese 1979; Waller 1887).

Much of Waller's work was overshadowed by his colleague Willem Einthoven (1895) who developed the electrical waveforms we know today as P-, Q-, R-, S- and T-waves and eventually received a Nobel Prize for his work in the discovery of the mechanism of the electrocardiogram. The prize was awarded in 1924; sadly Waller could not be considered for the prize as he died in 1922.

Hellerstein continued the practical application of electrocardiography and in 1949 monitored the heart's electrical action at the distal catheter tip using saline within the catheter lumen, as an agent to conduct the cardiac electrical signals, using an adapter on the proximal end of catheter and an ECG monitor. He noted a pronounced increase in the P-wave as the catheter tip entered the right atrium (Hellerstein et al. 1949). Several years have elapsed since these early experimental technologies gave birth to commercially dedicated systems.

Today there are a number of systems commercially available that confirm catheter tip position, and there is an increasing trend to include or have optional navigational functionality.

The catheter tip confirmation systems available today are fundamentally based around the principles of ECG developed by the pioneers and predecessors such as Augustus Waller, who paved the way for our practice today. Focusing upon the cardiac impulses, the current systems are reliant upon the sinoatrial (SA) node and atrial electrical impulses. As the SA node fires, it triggers depolarisation of the atria and contraction of the two chambers, which on an ECG is represented by the P-wave of the normal P-, Q-, R-, S- and T-wave ECG complexes (Fig. 7.3).

In a sinus rhythm, where conduction is following the normal electrical pathway through the heart, the P-wave can be easily distinguished. Certain heart rhythms affect the atrial conduction pathway and so affect the transmitted P-wave on the ECG. Atrial flutter and atrial fibrillation are conditions where the atrial electrical conduction is disrupted; this is represented on the ECG in P-wave distortion. When the P-wave is not discernible, then other means of catheter tip confirmation is required such as a CXR. It is important that in patients with extreme tachycardia or with a pace-

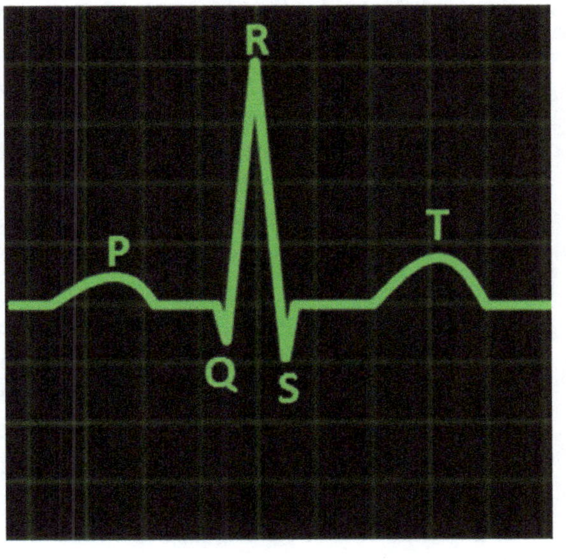

Fig. 7.3 Electrocardiogram normal sinus rhythm (used with permission of N. Moureau, PICC Excellence)

maker in situ, where the P-wave may not be discernible, an alternative method of tip confirmation is used. The instructions for use on most systems will require X-ray confirmation in these clinical instances. In some of these situations, changes in P-waves can be identified, aiding the clinician to achieve satisfactory tip position. However, X-ray confirmation is still required according to many systems' instructions. Technological advancements will soon develop systems that can provide tip confirmation, even when the clinician cannot readily identify the P-wave, such as when the heart is in atrial fibrillation.

The consoles are connected to the catheter via a sterile component that facilitates impulse conduction. ECG-alone systems detect the electrical impulses at the distal tip of the catheter during placement; the impulses are then processed by the console and presented in a graphical display for the operator to interpret. On the consular display screen, there are usually two ECG waveforms, one will be the standard ECG detecting cardiac electrical activity from the skin surface, and the other is an ECG detecting cardiac impulses from the internal catheter at the distal tip, the intracavity ECG.

The electrical impulses can be detected via the saline column in the lumen of the catheter or via a stylet/wire; both ways conduct the impulses from the distal tip of the catheter. The stylet system usually requires a crocodile clip, or an alternate means, to enable conduction from the stylet to the console or to a monitoring unit.

During a successful tip placement, the changes in ECG signal will firstly show a slight elevation in the P-wave as the catheter enters the SVC and moves towards the heart.

The P-wave continues to increase in size as it progresses towards the atria, which reaches its maximum amplitude at the cavoatrial junction.

As the catheter crosses the threshold of the cavoatrial junction, a portion of the atria and the SA node is now slightly superior to the tip of the catheter. This results in a reduction in the P-wave height and a portion of the P-wave becoming negative; a biphasic P-wave can be observed.

If the catheter is advanced, a further reduction of the P-wave height is observed together with an increasing biphasic signal.

The action of placing a catheter tip using ECG catheter tip confirmation system is a process, not just a matter of obtaining a particular waveform and leaving the catheter tip at that point. The process must include certain steps and acknowledgements of different waveforms to ensure that the catheter is indeed in the correct position. Once the catheter tip starts its journey down the SVC, the P-wave of the waveform starts to rise; at this time the catheter should be advanced slowly, allowing time for the system to translate the information received at the distal tip of the catheter into a graphical representation on the screen for the clinician to interpret. Cautious advancement of the catheter will see the P-wave begin to rise as the tip moves down the SVC to the cavoatrial junction.

Initial systems only offered ECG to provide tip confirmation, but evolution of this technology has seen the development of tracking and navigational options to provide added insight to the inserter of the position and direction the catheter during insertion and not just tip confirmation. Tip tracking technology may use magnetic or electromagnetic methods to track the movement of the catheter tip. Not all systems can be used with all different catheter types; some manufacturers limit the use of their systems to be used solely with their own products. PICCs have a longer venous pathway to arrive to their destination and have a greater opportunity to become misplaced compared to a non-tunnelled CVC being placed into the RIJ, where the pathway to the SVC and CAJ is a much straighter course and allows the passage of the catheter without guidance easier (AAGIB 2016). ECG only may be more suited for routine RIJ central venous insertions and navigation for other CVAD insertions.

Some tip tracking systems work by placing a T-piece sensor upon the chest of the patient, and then as the PICC is passing from the arm through the axilla towards the central veins, the tip can be tracked and displayed on the screen.

One system which uses alternative technology approach is VPS G4™, which uses Doppler signal to support the navigation. The Doppler signal is derived from transmitting bursts of fixed high-frequency energy from the stylet (illustrated by the grey wave fronts above) and then listening for the reflected sound from the blood particles. Blood particles flowing towards the stylet will generally reflect a slightly higher frequency (illustrated by the blue reflected wavelets above Fig. 7.4), whilst particles moving away from the stylet will reflect a slightly lower frequency back to the stylet sensor (shown by the magenta reflected waves (Fig. 7.5)).

The system can detect if the catheter is progressing with the flow of the venous blood, or if the catheter has migrated into the wrong vein, i.e. internal jugular, contralateral brachiocephalic or subclavian, by sensing retrograde blood flow and by displaying this on the console for the inserter see.

ECG—Walker et al. (2015) undertook a systematic review of RCTs (729 patients), looking at ECG only versus landmark/anatomical insertions with post-procedure CXR (Walker et al. 2015). It was identified that slightly higher complications occurred in the ECG arm in two of the studies reviewed; however these were mainly arterial punctures or haematoma. The authors point out that these complications pertain more towards insertion technique and use of ultrasound rather than related to the use of ECG. The review identified that ECG-based method was eighth times more effective than anatomy guided. The authors concluded that ECG confirmation appears a suitable replacement for post-procedural CXR confirmation (Walker et al. 2015).

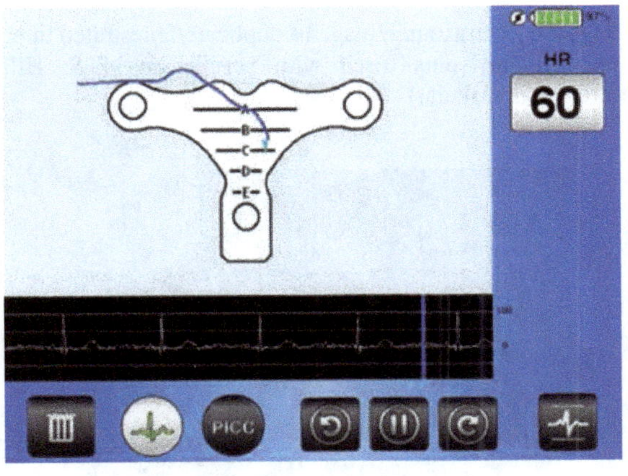

Fig. 7.4 Tip tracking and navigation technology (used with permission of Teleflex)

Yan Jin Liu (2015) studied two groups of patients using conventional PICC placement versus ECG-guided PICC placement, followed up then with CXR (Yan et al. 2017). In this randomised controlled study of 1007 patients, first attempt success was 89.2% in the ECG group versus 77.4% in the anatomical landmark group. The study also showed increased accuracy with ECG with right-sided placements versus left-arm approach.

The UK Royal College of Nursing Standards advises that tip position can be confirmed radiographically or with ECG guidance (RCN 2016). INS (2016) suggests post-procedure radiograph imaging is not necessary if alternative tip location technology confirms tip placement (Gorski et al. 2016a).

Ultrasound—In recent years there has been increasing interest in the role of ultrasound during tip placement; clinicians have examined its efficacy of confirmation of CVAD tip position. Duran-Gehing and colleagues (2015) describe the method of identifying CVC tip position using transthoracic ultrasound, a saline flush injected via the distal lumen of the CVC whilst visualising the right atrium with the ultrasound.

Fig. 7.5 Sound waves projecting image (used with permission of S. Hill, Precision Vascular)

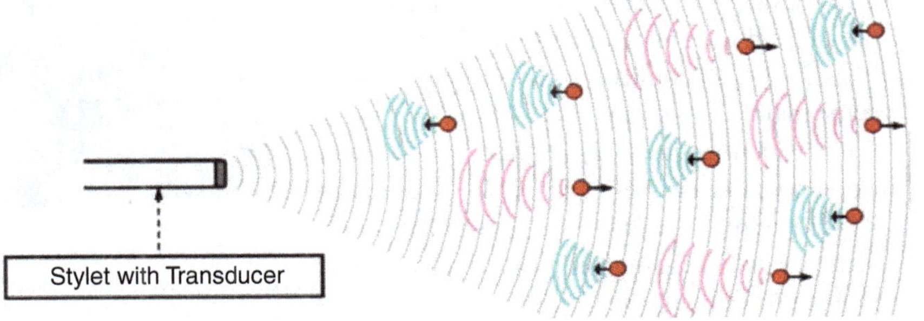

If microbubbles/turbulence of the saline can be observed within the RA in 2 s of the flush confirms satisfactory tip position, the authors suggest this method has 96% sensitivity. Marano et al. (2014) used transthoracic ultrasound to confirm PICC tip position in 53 patients; ultrasound was undertaken by a non-cardiologist and controlled by chest radiography. Catheter tip position was identified using this method successfully in 94.3% of cases, and 3 cases were malpositioned into the Mid-SVC; the authors suggested larger cohorts of patient to increase the validity of this method and noted that a limitation to this method is body habitus.

Weekes et al. (2016) prospectively inserted non-tunnelled catheters placed in emergency settings comparing ultrasound versus CXR for 151 patients. Four suboptimal catheter positions were detected by CXR; ultrasound identified three of these; again this study showed a shorter time to when the catheter could be used in the ultrasound arm. The authors concluded no significant difference in the accuracy between ultrasound and CXR for confirming tip position. Raman et al. (2017) compared non-tunnelled CVC tip position using transthoracic ultrasound versus CXR, monitoring the length of time before the tip position was confirmed and the catheter could be used, and identified that ultrasound confirmation allowed the catheter to be used in half of the time it took to gain CXR confirmation. This is a promising area of development regarding tip position ultrasound technology advances, as bedside ultrasound is becoming increasingly more capable and is no longer exclusively the realm of radiologists. Though limited by body habitus and patients with increased BMI, high accuracy of this approach provides another option for the experienced user, but further research and data is needed. INS (2016) reaffirms this point and suggests caution with ultrasound for CVAD tip location as its use to confirm tip location in all ages due to small sample sizes (Fig. 7.6).

However, the guidewire would not advance lower down the vessel (Fig. 7.7). The needle and guidewire were then removed. The lower vessel was then cannulated, and the guidewire was passed routinely without resistance; a fluoroscopic image then showed the guidewire has passed into the ipsilateral subclavian vein.

After removing the needle over the wire, the wire was then manipulated into satisfactory position (Fig. 7.8).

The guidewire continued into a satisfactory position, and the procedure continued routinely until the catheter was placed, and the catheter

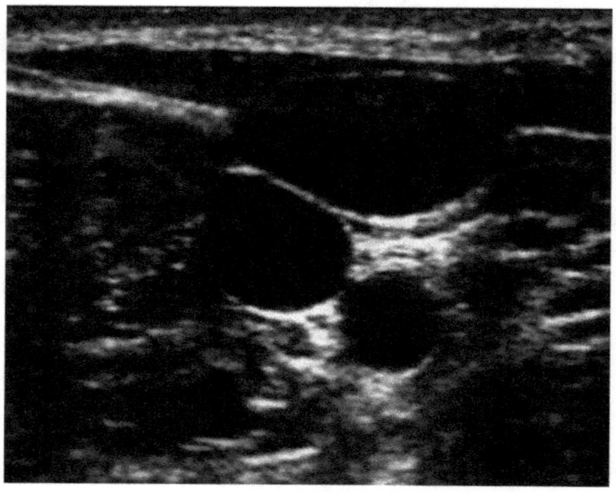

Fig. 7.6 Ultrasound image of duplicate/fenestrated internal jugular veins (used with permission of S. Hill, Precision Vascular)

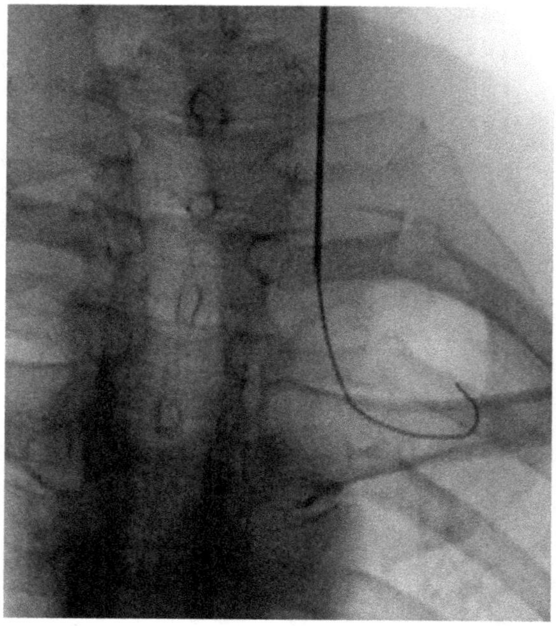

Fig. 7.7 Fluoroscopic image of guidewire advancement to left subclavian (used with permission of S. Hill, Precision Vascular)

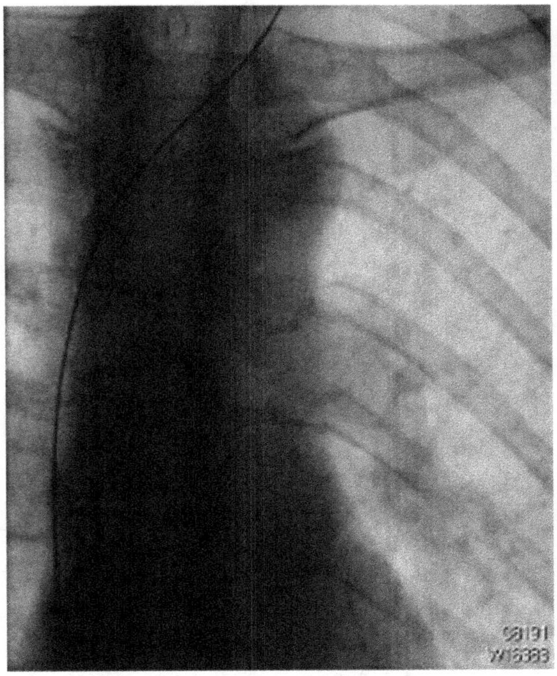

Fig. 7.8 Guidewire in satisfactory position (used with permission of S. Hill, Precision Vascular)

then doubled back on itself at the brachiocephalic junction with the SVC (Fig. 7.9).

The catheter was pulled back and readvanced through the peel-away sheath, and this time it passed into the contralateral veins. An angled hydrophilic guidewire was then used to facilitate passage of the catheter into the correct position.

Though many thousands of catheters are placed routinely without problems, some patients' anatomy present challenges. Having the necessary resources including skills and capacity within radiology is a fundamental necessity and is an inextricable element of vascular access services.

For many years X-ray has been the mainstay and viewed as the gold standard, but now viable alternatives to this are available. The reliability of X-ray is far from absolute. The suggested level of error for clinically significant or major error in radiology ranges from 2 to 20% (Goddard et al. 2001; Holt and Godard 2012), and a 'real-time' error rate among radiologists of daily practice averages between 3 and 5% (Brady et al. 2012). Where alternative systems exist that avoid the prescription of ionising radiation, then these systems must unequivocally be considered.

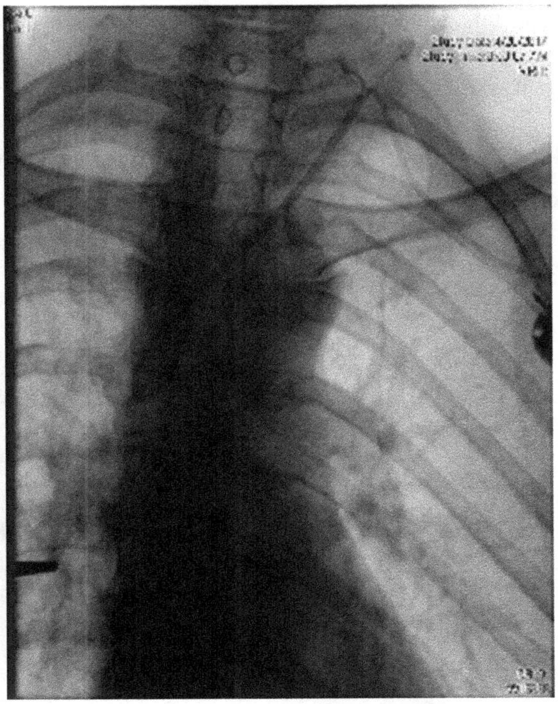

Fig. 7.9 Catheter doubling back into brachiocephalic junction with SVC (used with permission of S. Hill, Precision Vascular)

CVAD performance is directly related to the position of the terminal tip of the catheter (Sansivero 2012). CVAD safety and vein preservation are greatly impacted by tip positioning with device insertion and impacts the ability of the patient to receive prescribed therapy (Moureau et al. 2010). Insertions that are difficult with multiple threading manipulations may result in malpositioned catheters (Fig. 7.10). Suboptimal catheter tip position contributes to catheter dysfunction, thrombosis, vein erosion or continued malposition of the catheter (Eastridge and Lefor 1995; Moureau 2017; Petersen et al. 1999). For optimal upper extremity positioning, the terminal tip should terminate in the lower one-third of the superior vena cava (SVC) near the junction of the SVC and right atrium, where haemodilution rates are highest (Caers et al. 2005; Wuerz et al. 2016). Caers et al. (2005) found that catheter tip locations of CVADs positioned high in the SVC resulted in significant malfunctions. Malpositioned catheters, positioned in a suboptimal location in the SVC or in the adjacent areas, are much more likely to develop thrombosis and catheter dysfunction in the form of occlusion (Massmann et al. 2015; Petersen et al. 1999). The conclusions of the research indicated that the terminal tip of CVADs should be positioned as close to the SVC/right atrial junction as possible or slightly inside the right atrium. Multiple factors are involved with correct placement of the CVAD such as skill of the inserter, type of insertion, site selected for insertion and the patients' anatomy (Sansivero 2012).

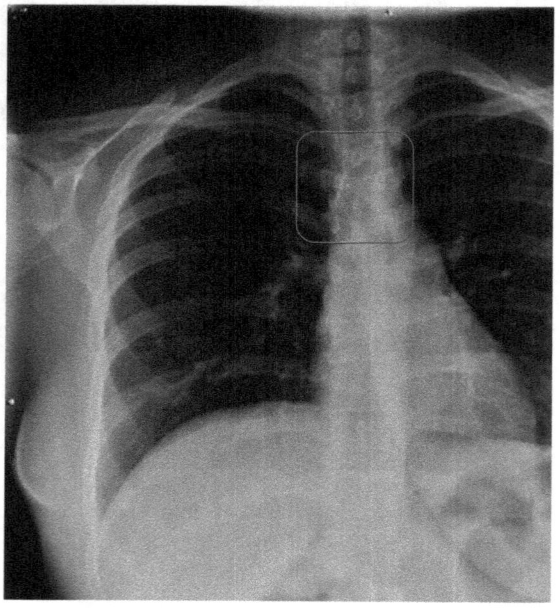

Fig. 7.10 PICC looped in the region of the mediastinum with P-wave elevation. Not distal SVC and no biphasic rhythm (used with permission of S. Hill, Precision Vascular)

Correct positioning of a CVAD is verified following the insertion procedure with radiologic confirmation or intraprocedural as with ECG or ultrasound verification. Radiological confirmation, by either chest X-ray or fluoroscopy, expose the patient to radiation and require interpretation on the part of the clinician. Interpretation is based on the anatomical landmarks and the knowledge of the clinician interpreting the results. Landmark determination of CVAD terminal tip precise location is controversial and may be influenced by patient positioning with oblique adjustments, by anatomical variation, complications of pneumothorax or other lung conditions which may impact ability to visualise the catheter tip. Often X-ray views are posterior/anterior and may not capture depth associated with azygous vein malpositioning or accidental arterial insertion (Fig. 7.11). Transoesophageal echocardiogram tip determination is a costly and invasive procedure that is very accurate, but not practical for CVAD insertion position verification.

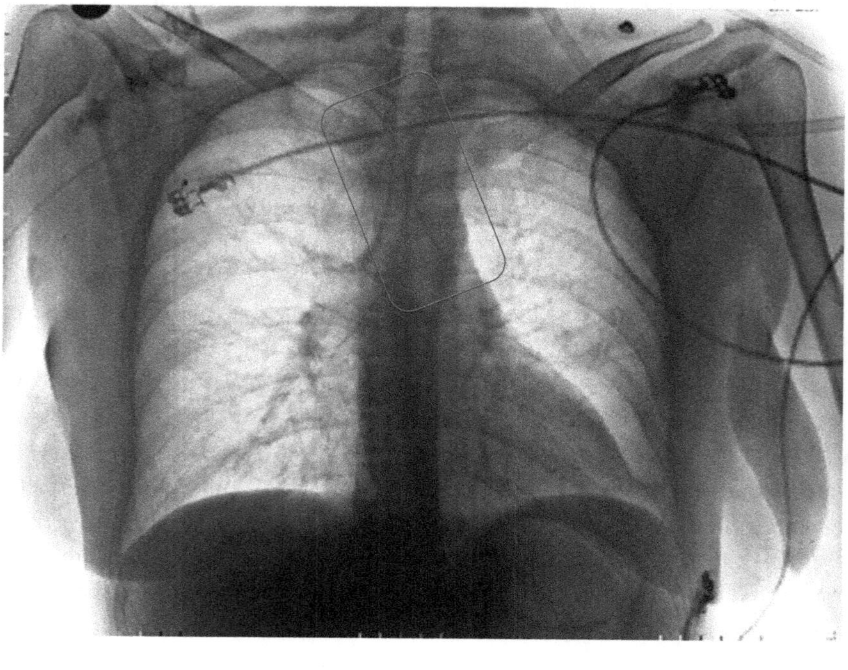

Fig. 7.11 Accidental arterial PICC insertion (used with permission of S. Hill, Precision Vascular)

Electrocardiographic intraprocedural positioning and tip confirmation has many advantages. Evidence supports the ECG method as accurate, precise and cost-effective for CVAD terminal tip positioning (Oliver and Jones 2014; Pittiruti et al. 2012; Rossetti et al. 2015; Schummer et al. 2004; Sette et al. 2010; Smith et al. 2010; Wolters et al. 2009). Precise positioning reduces the incidence of thrombotic malfunctions, vessel damage leading to venous thrombosis, arrhythmias, valve damage or other areas of malposition that impact the circulation or cardiac function (Fig. 7.12) (Pittiruti et al. 2011). ECG tip confirmation is performed during insertion using the real-time baseline rhythm connected to a lead on the patient, whilst the wire within the catheter functions as a separate lead (Fig. 7.13). Full description of the technique is included in multiple references (Moureau et al. 2010; Pittiruti et al. 2008, 2011, 2012; Rossetti et al. 2015).

The process for ECG positioning uses impulses from the sinoatrial (SA) node to demonstrate location in respect to the internal catheter. As the catheter advances through the venous system and approaches the SA node, the P-wave, as the first impulse of the pQRS complex, begins to elevate. Maximum intensity is reached as the catheter reaches the cavoatrial junction (CAJ) near the SA node, becoming diphasic with a negative deflection as the catheter passes the node (See Fig. 7.14). Limiting factors of intraprocedural ECG catheter positioning are the absence of a P-wave, as represented in atrial fibrillation and other cardiac rhythms where the P-wave may be indiscernible. Some clinicians have effectively

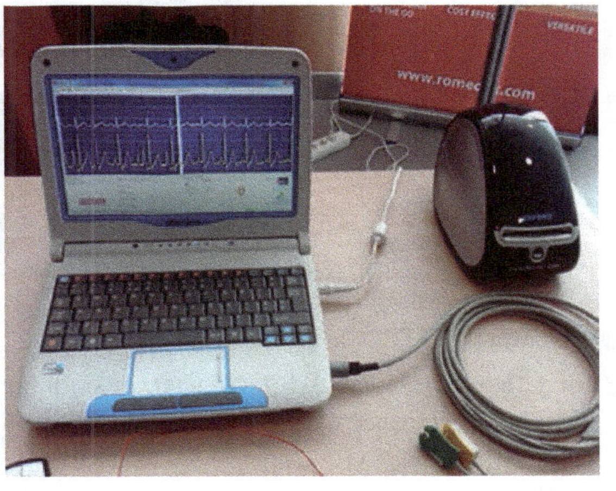

Fig. 7.13 Nautilus system ECG tip positioning system (used with permission of Romedex, Bucharest, Romania)

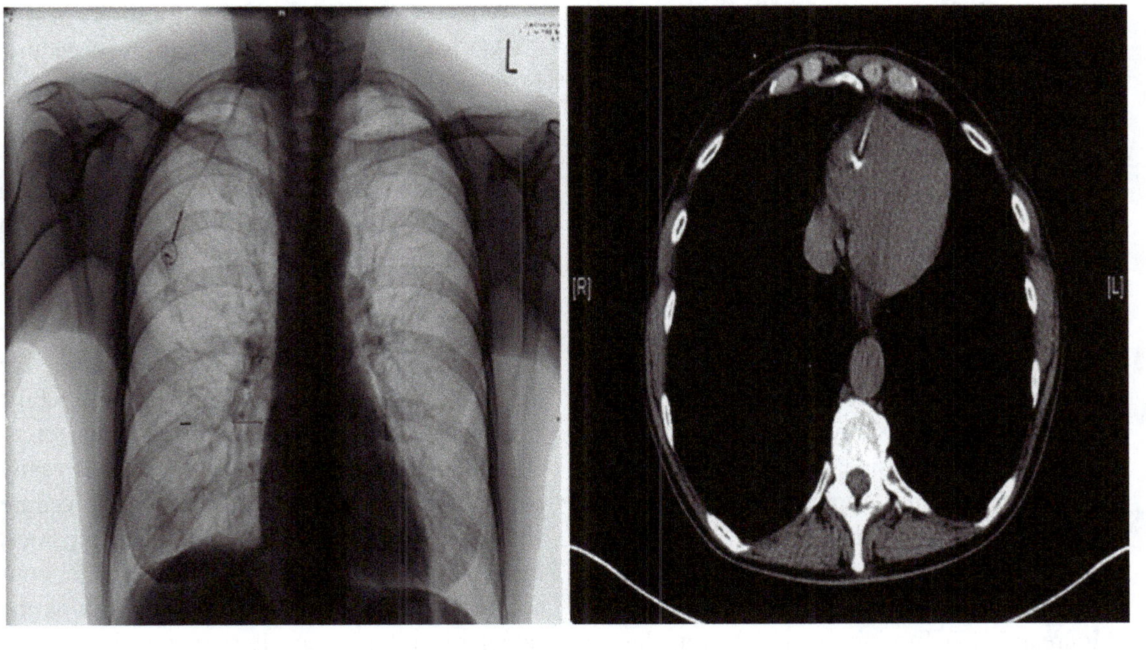

Fig. 7.12 Insertion of port at cavoatrial junction. Computer tomography scan at 20 months within the heart (used with permission of S. Hill, Precision Vascular)

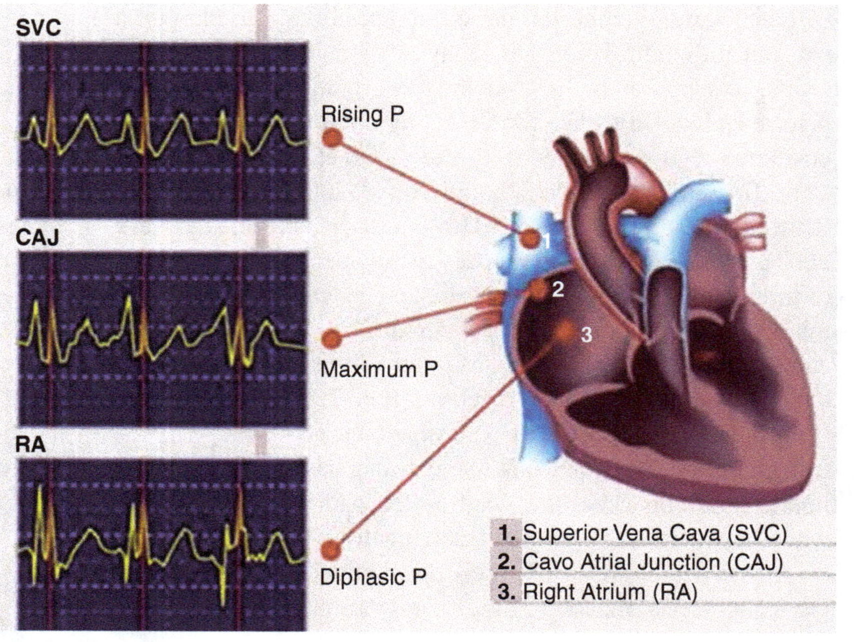

Fig. 7.14 Elevation of P-wave (used with permission of Romedex, Bucharest, Romania)

used the ECG system for catheter positioning even in the presence of atrial fibrillation (Pittiruti et al. 2014).

Chest X-ray provides confirmation of the catheter terminal tip position for CVADs whilst facilitating the evaluation of the lungs to rule out pneumothorax. Chest X-ray for CVAD tip verification is based on a one-dimensional view interpreted by the physician (Schuster et al. 2000; Verhey et al. 2008). Interpretation position can be inconsistent with variation from physician to physician; the junction of the SVC and the CAJ junction are not clearly defined on the anterior-posterior chest X-ray (Baldinelli et al. 2015; Pittiruti 2015; Schuster et al. 2000). Chest X-ray is a means to verify tip location but is subject to interpretation and is not precise and is prone (Moureau 2017). Chest X-ray to verify PICC tip position is far from ideal. The time involved in waiting for a chest X-ray to be performed and reported can be extensive, taking 30 min to multiple hours to complete. Typically, if the location of the terminal tip is incorrect on the X-ray, the clinician returns to the bedside, removes the dressing and repositions the catheter using ANTT. (Moureau 2017). In addition to increasing the risk of contamination, this manipulation can require an additional X-ray to verify whether the repositioning exercise was successful (Gordon 2016). Verification of terminal tip position is a safety requirement which can be satisfied by ECG guidance during placement of the device without the need for X-ray (Moureau 2017).

With ECG guidance, the location of the CVAD is known during the insertion procedure. ECG positioning is both accurate and precise (Pittiruti et al. 2008). ECG positioning is typically not applicable for patients with no discernible P-wave in the QRS complex, with fibrillation or arrhythmias (Pittiruti et al. 2011, 2014). In these situations, a chest X-ray is recommended for verification of the catheter terminal tip.

ECG catheter tip verification is performed by physicians and nurses effectively reducing the time necessary to confirm proper location whilst still in the insertion procedure (Moureau et al. 2010; Pittiruti et al. 2011). The process is easily adapted to the catheter and insertion procedure with equipment provided by multiple companies. In addition, any cardiac monitor can be connected using the lead from the right arm as the catheter lead for intracavitary monitoring.

7.5 Steps for Placing ECG-Guided PICC with Guidewire Technique (Moureau et al. 2010)

1. Attach (three or five lead) monitor to patient (always apply all new leads); determine if the patient is in normal sinus rhythm (NSR) and atrial fibrillation or is dependently paced. If the patient is in NSR, proceed with ECG-guided CVAD insertion.
2. Detach the right arm lead from the patient, and attach it to the ECG device or cable. Prepare the cable for use in the sterile procedure (the cable will attach to the guidewire within the catheter).
3. Select the vein and location for CVAD insertion using ultrasound scanning.
4. Measure selected vein to estimated location of caval atrial junction (CAJ).
5. Set up sterile field; prep and drape patient.
6. Don personal protective equipment (PPE).
7. Determine catheter length based on external measurement. Adjust the guidewire to the very distal end of the CVAD but not extended outside the catheter. Flush CVAD with normal saline. Guidewire must be specific for the length of that catheter and marked in advance for intracavitary ECG.
8. Place the sterile ECG cable into the field.
9. Insert the CVAD using ultrasound-guided modified Seldinger technique (MST).
10. Insert CVAD to its intended goal of the distal SVC/CAJ; attach the ECG. Attach alligator cable to the guidewire in the CVAD.
11. Flush the CVAD again with normal saline. The guidewire is acting as an electric conductor of ECG activity.
12. A QRS complex should appear on the monitor with a clearly identifiable P-wave. The P-wave is normal size initially, increasing in amplitude as the CVAD is advanced (Fig. 7.2). Compare P-wave size from initial normal complex to peak level. (Note: Size may vary with QRS complex comparison with P-wave and be larger than QRS. The determinant is positive P-wave change measured to peak with biphasic notch.)
13. When the P-wave is about 3/4 of the full peaked level, approx. 3/4 the size of the QRS, the CVAD tip is in the lower or distal SVC (also known as proximal SVC in relation to the heart).
14. When the P-wave is fully peaked or at the highest amplitude (positive P-wave), it is at the caval atrial junction (SVC/RA).
15. When a small negative wave spike is seen in the P-wave, the tip is in the upper part of the right atrium.
16. When the P-wave becomes biphasic (negative and positive P-wave of the same size—expanding beyond the baseline up and down), the CVAD tip is in the middle right atrium. This is known as an atrial spike.
17. If no QRS pattern change is seen during advancement of the catheter, the CVAD has malpositioned in the internal jugular or contralateral in the opposite subclavian vein. Attempts to reposition can be made until the P-wave enlargement is seen on the monitor.
18. Print final strip with P-wave at the same amplitude as QRS to confirm location of the tip. Include this ECG strip as part of the patient's record. (Note: You may see some respiratory variation in the waveform.)

7.6 Steps for Placing ECG-Guided PICC with Saline-Filled Lumen (Moureau et al. 2010)

1. Attach (three or five lead) monitor to patient (always apply all new leads); determine if the patient is in normal sinus rhythm (NSR) and atrial fibrillation or is dependently paced. If the patient is in NSR, proceed with ECG-guided CVAD insertion.
2. Detach the right arm lead from the patient, and attach it to the ECG device or cable. Prepare the cable for use in the sterile procedure.
3. Select the vein and location for CVAD insertion using ultrasound scanning.
4. Measure selected vein to estimated location of CAJ.

5. Set up sterile field; prep, and drape patient. Drop ECG cable with saline adapter septum onto the sterile field.
6. Don personal protective equipment (PPE).
7. Determine catheter length based on external measurement. Adjust the guidewire to the very distal end of the CVAD but not extended outside the catheter. Flush CVAD with normal saline. Guidewire must be specific for the length of that catheter and marked in advance for intracavitary ECG.
8. Prefill 20 cm^3 syringe with saline and attach a steel needle.
9. Insert the CVAD using ultrasound-guided modified Seldinger technique (MST).
10. Insert CVAD to its intended goal of the distal SVC/CAJ; attach the ECG. Insert needle into ECG saline adapter. Attach alligator clamp to the needle in the CVAD.
11. Flush the CVAD again with normal saline. Saline is acting as an electric conductor of ECG activity.
12. A QRS complex should appear on the monitor with an identifiable P-wave. The P-wave is normal size initially, increasing in amplitude as the CVAD is advanced (Fig. 7.2). Compare P-wave size from initial normal complex to peak level. (Note: Size may vary with QRS complex comparison with P-wave and be larger than QRS. The determinant is positive P-wave change measured to peak with biphasic notch.)
13. When the P-wave is about 3/4 of the full peaked level, approx. 3/4 the size of the QRS, the CVAD tip is in the lower or distal SVC (also known as proximal SVC in relation to the heart).
14. When the P-wave is fully peaked or at the highest amplitude (positive P-wave), it is at the CAJ (SVC/RA).
15. When a small negative wave spike is seen in the P-wave, the tip is in the upper part of the right atrium.
16. When the P-wave becomes biphasic (negative and positive P-wave of the same size—expanding beyond the baseline up and down), the CVAD tip is in the middle right atrium. This is known as an atrial spike.
17. If no QRS pattern change is seen during advancement of the catheter, the CVAD has malpositioned in the internal jugular or contralateral in the opposite subclavian vein. Attempts to reposition can be made until the P-wave enlargement is seen on the monitor.
18. Print final strip with P-wave at the same amplitude as QRS to confirm location of the tip. Include this ECG strip as part of the patient's record. (Note: You may see some respiratory variation in the waveform.)
19. Print final strip with P-wave at peak amplitude as QRS to confirm location of the tip. Include this ECG strip as part of the patient's record. (Note: You may see some respiratory variation in the waveform.)

7.7 Tip Movement

The catheter tip is exposed to many mechanical forces, exerted by the internal mechanical functions of the human body that can affect and alter the internal position, namely, the expansion and deflation of the lungs during the respiratory cycle and the pulsation of the heart and arterial structures. Vesely (2003) confirms the continual movement of the catheter tip from cardiac pulsation can lead to thrombosis development (Vesely 2003). The position of the patient will also affect the position of the catheter tip whether sitting, standing, supine or when considering PICCs if the arm is abducted or adducted. Foaurer and Alonzo (2000) measured the effect of moving the arm from an abducted to adducted position in 61 patients and found that 43 patients move caudally (lower/towards the heart), 7 moved cephalad (higher or superiorly) and 3 did not change position; the authors summarised that 58% of PICCs move 2 cm or more (Foaurer and Alonzo 2000). Hostetter et al. (2010) confirm that movement of catheter tip position is reported to be 2–3 cm; a correctly CAJ placed catheter has the potential to retract into the SVC and advance into the RA. Considering such variation occurs when the arm is abducted, bringing the arm away from the 90% extended, abducted position prior

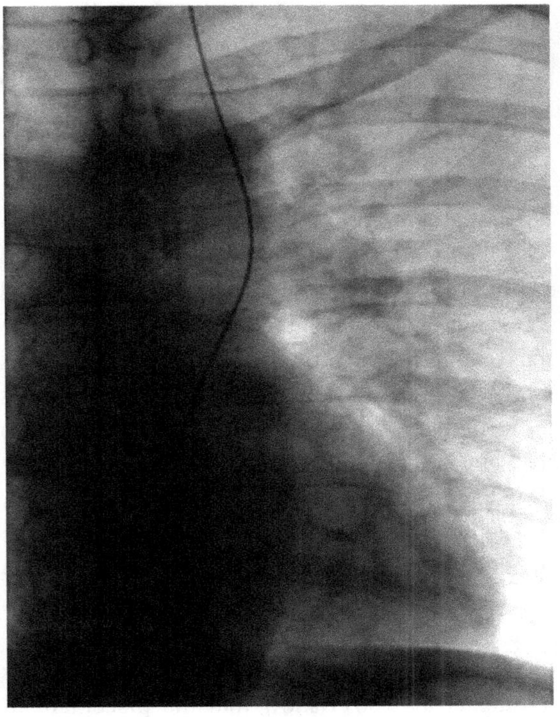

Fig. 7.15 Left internal jugular placement with incidental finding of left-sided SVC (used with permission of S. Hill, Precision Vascular)

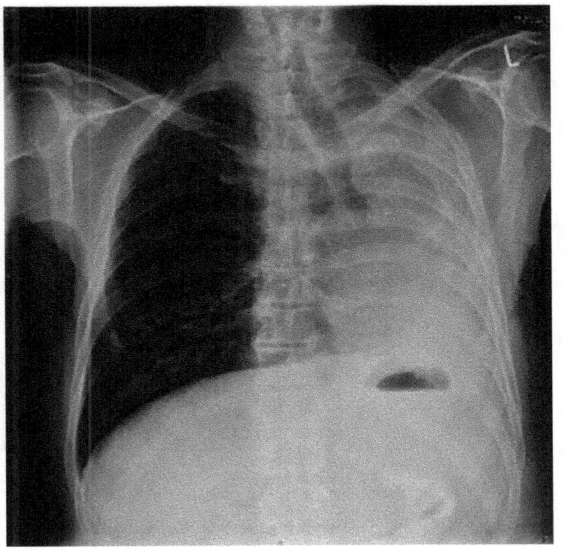

Fig. 7.16 Left pneumonectomy, right-sided PICC insertion; the PICC extended across the mediastinum to reach optimal position (used with permission of S. Hill, Precision Vascular)

to confirming tip position, more in line with the body's natural position may reduce migration associated with arm abduction.

Anatomical deviations may be present such as scoliosis, dextrocardia, left-sided SVC (Fig. 7.15) or iatrogenic abnormalities such as pneumonectomy (Fig. 7.16). Catheter tip position is not static like the snapshot image that an X-ray provides, which portrays a moment in time of the catheter tip position. Furthermore, this snapshot is often not a typical representation of the catheter tip position. It is standard practice to ask the patient to take a deep breath and hold the breath when the X-ray is being taken. The deep inhalation and breath holding force the diaphragm low, lowering the position of the heart within the thorax and altering the tip position of the catheter. Similarly, the position of the patient can affect the position of the catheter tip.

7.8 Thrombosis

The position of the catheter tip can influence the risk of VAD-related thrombosis. The actual position of the catheter tip can influence the likelihood of the catheter developing a thrombus. If the position of the catheter is too long and too short, abuts the wall of a vessel or is positioned optimally, all can influence the risk of thrombosis. An older study looking at right atrial thrombus on 48 patients with tunnelled CVC in situ, tip positions were in the superior vena cava and the right atrium (RA). Thrombus was found in 12.5% of cases by follow-up with transoesophageal echocardiograph, all of the thromboses were identified in the RA group, and all were asymptomatic (Gilon et al. 1998). Other studies have found higher incidence of thrombus in the SVC (Vesely 2003).

A larger randomised controlled study looked at this issue. Figure 7.17 is from a study looking at 428 CVC insertions, followed up with linograms, venograms and Doppler ultrasounds. What the study showed was that the relative position of

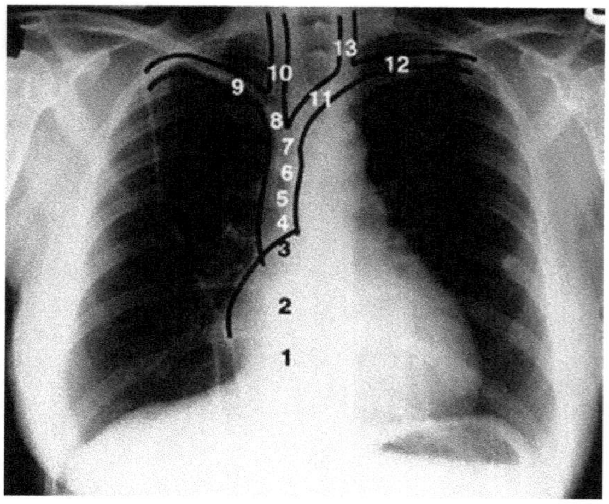

Fig. 7.17 Radiologic anatomy and tip position for CVADs (Cadman et al. 2004)

the catheter tip was directly proportional to the risk of thrombosis development. For instance, on the image, numbers 3 and 4 indicate distal SVC/ cavoatrial junction, and for the catheters with the tips positioned in this zone, the thrombosis rates were 2.6%; in the middle third of the SVC, 5.3%; and in the proximal position (proximal SVC or thoracic inlet veins), 41% resulted in thrombosis, an increase of 16 times the risk of those catheters placed in a distal position. The reason the authors gave for increased risk of short left-sided catheters was the catheter abutting the wall of the SVC, causing mechanical damage and also the potential for chemical damage from cytotoxic drugs inducing thrombotic changes (Cadman et al. 2004; Vesely 2003). Hallam et al. (2016) also include device selection based on nutritional solutions containing final concentrations exceeding 10% dextrose and/or 5% protein and explain that these also should be administered via a central venous catheter with tip placement in the superior vena cava. DeChicco et al. (2007) also identify that thrombosis is greater in the proximal SVC versus lower SVC and RA.

The study by Cadman and colleagues shows significant associations between thrombosis and females (twice the risk of males), left-sided insertions and proximal tip position. Catheter tip in the proximal third of the SVC and above was 16 times more likely to develop venous thrombosis. Women were twice more likely to develop thrombosis than men. Left-sided CVAD insertions may lead to damage as stiff dilators/introducers are passed through the brachiocephalic vein to the SVC (Vesely 2003).

Hostetter et al. (2010) points out that the presence of thrombosis may lead to infection. The apparent symbiotic relationship between thrombosis and infections has been avidly discussed within the field of vascular access. Theorists and clinicians suggest that the composites of a thrombus encourage the growth of pathogenic microbes and conversely the presence of infection releases coagulative processes that increase the patient to catheter-related thrombosis (Mehall et al. 2002; Raad and Bodey 1992; Ryder 2001).

Right atrial thrombus—Some studies have looked at the development of thrombosis in the heart. Vesely (2003) explains that catheters placed within the heart may lead to intracardiac thrombosis but points out that some studies (Kung et al. 2001) show that the placement of the catheter tip in the SVC did not prevent the formation of right atrial thrombus (RAT). Dreyer and Bingham (2005) investigating the right atrial thrombosis related to haemodialysis catheters reporting from 22 cases of RAT report that a 33% mortality exists if RAT is associated with infection versus 14% without infection (Dreyer and Bingham 2005). In terms of management of RAT, the authors suggest that thrombectomy has been associated with lower mortality than conservative management with anticoagulants and antibiotics. A strategy adopted by some includes a thrombosis less than 2 cm being managed conservatively (anticoagulants for 6 months) with repeated transoesophageal echocardiograph and catheter removal, larger than 2 cm, especially if infected, thrombectomy with antibiotics and anticoagulants (Dreyer and Bingham 2005). However, the authors concede that the optimal management of haemodialysis RAT is unknown.

Current practice in many institutions is still for a post-procedural chest X-ray to be used to verify the tip position of the catheters following insertion, for services inserting by the bedside, or in a designated procedure room without ECG guidance or X-ray screening. This can result in patient delays until the X-ray has been undertaken and verified. The limitations of this approach are that there is limited intraprocedural awareness of catheter tip position from the point of insertion to the landing zone.

Rates of malposition vary depending upon experience and type of insertion. Ibrahim (2012) identifies a bedside malposition rate for non-tunnelled CVCs of 14%, with 55% of these tips being misplaced into the RA and 14% into the left brachiocephalic vein. Other studies have shown that CVCs have 6.7% malposition rate (Roldan and Paniagua 2015) and PICC malposition rates of 9.3% both without guidance technology, confirmed by Hill (2012) whose combined PICC and CVC non-guided malposition rates were reported at 8%. Some studies show much higher malposition rates, up to 41% for central placements, including tips placed in the proximal third of SVC, including thoracic inlets, and PICC malposition rates up to 63% (Johnston et al. 2013). In cases of malposition, the catheter may require manipulation under fluoroscopy, retracting if too long or removing and replacement (Fig. 7.18). Manipulation of a catheter depends upon the availability of the fluoroscopy suite and radiologist or suitably trained clinician. If fluoroscopy is in high demand, immediate access may not be possible, increasing patient treatment delay and increasing costs attributed to the use of fluoroscopy. The additional interventions required to rectify misplaced catheters cause increased patient anxiety/distress and increase the risk of infective and mechanical complications. The additional interventions also decrease the efficacy and cost efficiency of the vascular access (VA) team.

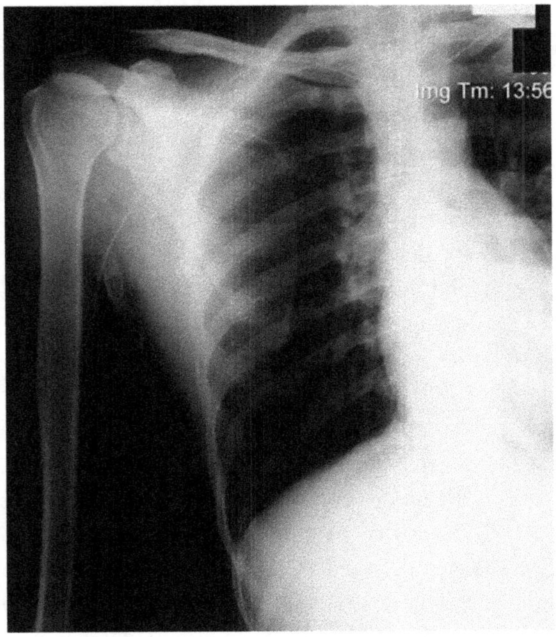

Fig. 7.18 Contralateral malposition with oblique (used with permission of N. Moureau, PICC Excellence)

Dialysis—Tal et al. (2013) explain dialysis catheter guidelines recommend the catheter to be placed into the RA. The authors also advocate that not only the tip of the catheter but the 'functional tip' of the catheter should be placed in the RA whilst ensuring that the catheter does not touch the atrial floor as to avoid mural thrombus, arrhythmias and erosion. The authors describe the function tip as the portion of the catheter from the most proximal side hole to the catheter tip. SVC placement of dialysis catheters can lead to higher recirculation rates, damage to the vessel wall, stenosis and catheter occlusion (Tal et al. 2013). Mandolfo et al. (2002) identifies that dialysis catheter tips placed at the cavoatrial junction benefit from higher blood flow. Equally Vesely (2003) suggests that stagnation of blood within the RA may lead to thrombus formation.

The national kidney foundation clinical guidelines advocate:

> The catheter tip should be adjusted to the level of the caval atrial junction or into the right atrium to ensure optimal blood flow. (Atrial positioning is only recommended for catheters composed of soft compliant material, such as silicone) (Opinion) NKF-K/DOQI (2001)

The CAJ cannot be definitively identified on an X-ray; rather the position of the CAJ is inferred by looking at other visible anatomical structures.

CXR—X-ray images are also subject to an element of magnification; here is an example in practice. The magnification associated with fluoroscopy is illustrated by placing two identical-sized coins, one on the anterior chest wall and the second coin level with the patient's back/spine. The extent to which magnification affects the image is dependent upon the distance the inten-

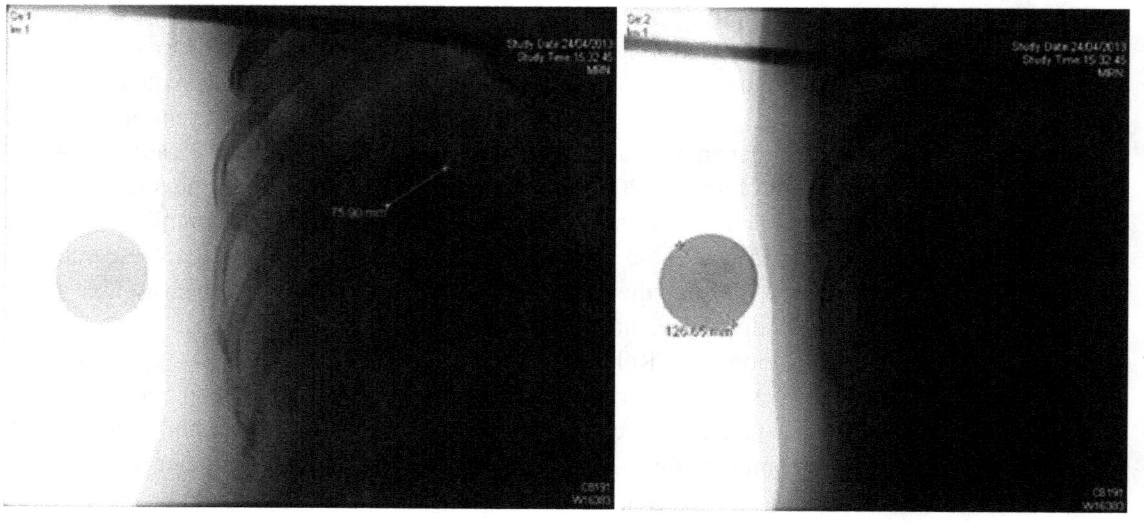

Figs. 7.19 and 7.20 Lateral view with magnification of the chest using coin perspective (used with permission of S. Hill, Precision Vascular)

sifier is from the patient. The patient's physical size can affect this, i.e. an increase in patient size results in increased distance from intensifier to plate resulting in more magnification. This is illustrated in Figs. 7.19 and 7.20 using the same size coins, one placed level with the anterior surface of the chest and the second with the patient's back. The coin placed posteriorly appears significantly larger (126.65 mm) versus the anteriorly placed coin measuring 75.90, which illustrates the increasing magnification of internal anatomy the closer it is to the image receptor.

Parallax—Vesely (2003) describes that the phenomenon of parallax can be an influential in determining catheter tip position.

Parallax is defined as:

> the position of the image on each emulsion of dual emulsion film; it is accentuated by tube-angled x-ray techniques.
>
> Miller-Keane (2003)

The objects in the lateral view are affected depending upon their relative position to each other and the angle at which they are viewed. Place a finger in front of you and view it with one eye closed then alternate by closing that eye and opening the other, the differing visual perspectives is an example of how the parallax effect works.

Considering the effects in practice, when viewing tip position on X-ray, it is important to select an anatomical structure closest to the catheter tip position to help to determine its position. Parallax may have more effect the further away the structure is from the point of interest; for instance, determining tip position by looking at the ribs and selecting anatomy in different anatomical planes can lead to error (Aslamy et al. 1998). Ryu et al. (2007) points out that parallax is greater and more variable with portable anterior-posterior CXR, such as in intensive care and operating theatres (Ryu et al. 2007).

Aslamy et al. (1998) suggested the tracheobronchial angle was the best radiographic landmark to determine the upper margin of the SVC. The authors determined these conclusions by studying 42 patients who had undergone magnetic resonance imaging scans (Aslamy et al. 1998). Hostetter et al. (2010) explain the carina later replaced this landmark because the structure can be identified more clearly. Baskin and colleagues confirmed this by examining 100 CT scans of patients from the ages of 12 to 28 years and found no association between age and any other parameters. The authors go on to explain that the cavoatrial junction lies lower than commonly believed and suggest that two vertebral bodies below the carina (with the intervertebral disc included) is a reliable estimate of the position of the cavoatrial junction (Baskin et al. 2008). Aslamy et al. (1998) importantly identified that the right superior heart border that is commonly used to determine catheter tip location, in 38% of cases, was formed by the left atrium.

Movement of tip position—Catheter tips are prone to movement; the still image of a radiographic X-ray detracts from this notion. The catheter tip is subjected to a range of dynamic movements from cardiac pulsation and lungs/diaphragmatic movement, which all contribute to the perpetual motion of the catheter tip (Mandolfo et al. 2002). The position of the patient can affect tip, whether standing, holding their breath for an X-ray, abducting or adducting their arm position (Fig. 7.21). The catheter with the most potential for internal catheter movement is a PICC. If the arm is abducted away from the body, this can cause downward internal movement of the PICC towards the heart of up to 2 cm; right-sided PICCs have higher rates of this type of movement vs the left (Aslamy et al. 1998).

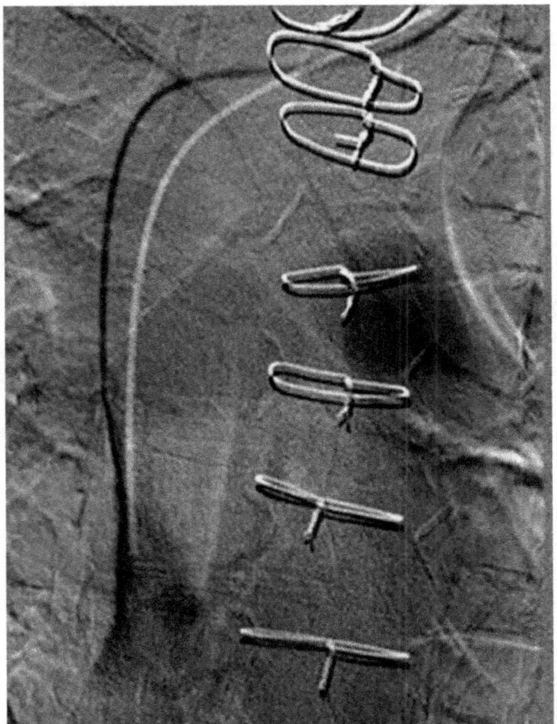

Fig. 7.21 PICC tip movement during high-pressure injection (used with permission of S. Hill, Precision Vascular)

Tunnelled CVCs and implanted ports can have different anatomical sites where they can be situated. Typically, they are placed on the anterior chest wall, which has an immediate benefit over PICCs in the stakes of internal movement, as they are not influenced to the same extent by the arm movement as the peripherally inserted counterparts. However, what is commonly appreciated by vascular access clinicians, especially those working in fluoroscopy, is that significant catheter tip movement is associated with patient position changing from supine to standing. Gibson and Bodenham (2013) point out that this movement is due to gravity, and as the abdominal contents move downwards, so do the diaphragm and the mediastinum, inadvertently causing an upward movement of the catheter tip. The authors also point that this is exacerbated in obese patients. I would add that the most profound movement observed of long-term catheters is in ladies who have an increased body mass index, who have large breasts and where the CVADs are being placed on the left. The movement for left-sided long-term devices appears to be more significant compared with those on the right, one way of counteracting this is to stabilise the chest wall in a position that simulates a supine position. This can be done by placing downward traction of the upper chest wall with adhesive drapes or using sensitive tapes; this simulation of supine chest wall/breast position limits, but does not eradicate, the tip movement from the patient moving from supine to the standing position. Large breast tissue has been documented in several studies as an influential factor in catheter tip placement (Gibson and Bodenham 2013; Cadman et al. 2004; Vesely 2003).

X-ray outcomes are also subject to the skill of the radiographer and the presentation of the patient, obesity, patient position, if the patient needs a mobile X-ray, or there may be other factor such as Harrington rods used for spinal support that may obscure the view of the catheter tip. The objective of a normal posterior (PA) anterior X-ray is to provide a balanced field of view to enable examination of the skeletal structures, organs and tissues. The objective of an X-ray post-CVAD insertion is to primarily identify the tip position, but at the same time, the clinician will ensure there are no kinks or loops in the catheter. There may be occasion that the purpose of the X-ray is dual fold, for the identification of tip position and to view the thoracic anatomical structures. The radiation prescription for a standard X-ray film may not necessarily be the dose needed to adequately view the tip position of a smaller-sized vascular device such as a PICC. Obtaining adequate exposure to identify the catheter tip is essential, or repeated X-rays may be needed. If a repeat CXR is required, a lateral view may provide an alternative angle if the tip is obscured on a PA or X-ray can be coned in to focus on the mediastinal area, which will reduce the radiation dose to the surrounding thoracic anatomy.

7.9 Conclusion

Tip position continues to be an emotive and controvertial subject. Clinicians must be aware of the range of movements a CVAD catheter tip is subjected to when the patient changes positions, from supine to standing the abdominal contents drop causing upward movement of the catheter tip (Vesely 2003), and the movement of PICCs particularly with abduction of the arm, and consider these potential movements when finalising catheter tip position. The revolution in catheter tip navigation and confirmation is now in full flow; the paradigm shift from radiological confirmation to ECG-based technology is now being reflected practice across the globe. The accuracy, safety benefits, elimination of radiation exposure, improved patient experience and vascular access service efficiency no longer allow X-ray confirmation to be the 'gold standard'.

Case Study

The patient was a 60-year-old female with a diagnosis of colonic adenocarcinoma, who had received a previous tunnelled CVC via the right internal jugular side that had been removed due to infection during a previous cycle of intravenous anticancer therapy. The patient attended for a pre-assessment for an implanted port and underwent all the necessary checks, including a review of the patient history, assessment of the right anterolateral upper chest wall (intended port implantation site), blood tests and ultrasound review of the relevant vasculature, taking time to talk through the procedure with the patient and provide the supportive literature about the procedure. The assessment was completed, and no concerns were noted about venous or other anatomy, and blood tests were obtained as per hospital protocol. During the procedure, ultrasound-guided cannulation was performed routinely, but the clinician could not pass guidewire; a more experienced operator attended who experienced same issue. As the procedure was undertaken in a dedicated procedure room intended to be placed under ECG guidance, it was decided that the procedure should be undertaken in the X-ray department under fluoroscopy and was rescheduled for another day, as not available that day. A left-sided internal jugular approach was planned. The ultrasound assessment showed an interesting image of duplicated left internal jugular veins. Passing the ultrasound from higher up the neck to the base, superiorly to inferiorly, the veins were one vessel (higher in the neck) which then split into two as they both then led separately to form part of the brachiocephalic vein. The vein positioned more anteriorly was cannulated under ultrasound, being more superficial and the larger of the two vessels (Fig. 7.6).

Case Study

A call was received from a radiologist to the vascular access team. The radiologist explained there was a patient who had undergone a CT scan and noticed that the catheter tip was in the ventricle. With great concern, the team evaluated the terminal tip position. The patient had also had a CXR that showed the catheter tip well into the heart. This implanted port had been in for 20 months. What had gone wrong, and how had this been missed? The port chamber was in its original position and had not slipped out of position; the catheter was still securely attached to the injectable reservoir and had not fractured and migrated. Upon closer investigation of this case, it became apparent that the port position hadn't changed but rather the internal anatomy. Unfortunately, over the 20 months from insertion, the patient had slowly developed bulky abdominal disease leading to upward movement of the diaphragm, resulting in the downward displacement of the catheter tip. Position was corrected by port revision with tip placed in the distal SVC rather than at the CAJ to avoid continued deterioration of the patient. Documentation was established in the medical record to alert medical providers of the changes in anatomy and impact on the port if the abdominal mass is removed.

Case Study

A patient required 6 weeks of antibiotic treatment for osteomyelitis. It was determined that a PICC would be the best device for the treatment duration and medication. The patient was positioned and measured for a placement length estimate. The PICC was placed by a trained specialist. The PICC was inserted with maximum sterile barriers, ultrasound guidance and ECG. The monitor and leads were prepared in advance and connected in a sterile fashion during the procedure. Prior to the procedure, the baseline EKG was established. During the procedure, the internal EKG rhythm demonstrated advancement of the PICC as the catheter entered the SVC. The P-wave continued to increase in amplitude as the catheter approached the cavoatrial junction (CAJ) reaching maximum. No biphasic or downward deflection of the P-wave noted. PICC was aspirated to confirm blood return, flushed with normal saline, secured and the procedure completed.

Summary of Key Points

1. The aim for vascular access clinicians is to place the catheter tip in the optimal location.
2. The implications of catheter malposition can contribute to increased morbidity.
3. The evolution of radiation-based methods to confirm catheter tip position can no longer claim the title of the 'gold standard' in practice.

References

Alexandrou E, Ramjan L, Spencer T, Frost S, Salamonson Y, Davidson P, Hillman K. The use of midline catheters in the adult acute care setting—clinical implications and recommendations for practice. J Assoc Vasc Access. 2011;16(1):35–41.

Aslamy Z, Dewald CL, Heffner JE. MRI of central venous anatomy. Implications for central venous catheter insertion. Chest. 1998;114:820–6.

anatomy: implications for central venous catheter insertion. Chest. 1998;114(3):820–6.

Baldinelli F, Capozzoli G, Pedrazzoli R, Marzano N. Evaluation of the correct position of peripherally inserted central catheters: anatomical landmark vs. electrocardiographic technique. J Vasc Access. 2015;16(5):394–8. https://doi.org/10.5301/jva.5000431.

Baskin KM, Jimenez RM, Cahill AM, Jawad AF, Towbin RB. Cavoatrial junction and central venous anatomy:

implications for central venous access tip position. J Vasc Interv Radiol. 2008;19(3):359–65.

Bertoglio S, Van Boxtel T, Goossens GA, Dougherty L, Furtwangler R, Lennan E, Pittiruti M, Sjovall K, Stas M. Improving outcomes of short peripheral vascular access in oncology and chemotherapy administration. London: SAGE Publications; 2017.

Bestman E, Creese R. Waller-pioneer of electrocardiography. Br Heart J. 1979;42(1):61–4.

Brady A, Laoide RÓ, McCarthy P, McDermott R. Discrepancy and error in radiology: concepts, causes and consequences. Ulster Med J. 2012; 81(1):3.

Burdon-Sanderson JS, Page FJM. II. Experimental results relating to the rhythmical and excitatory motions of the ventricle of the heart of the frog, and of the electrical phenomena which accompany them. Proc R Soc Lond. 1878;27(185–189):410–4.

Cadman A, Lawrance J, Fitzsimmons L, Spencer-Shaw A, Swindell R. To clot or not to clot? That is the question in central venous catheters. Clin Radiol. 2004;59(4):349–55.

Caers J, Fontaine C, Vinh-Hung V, De Mey J, Ponnet G, Oost C, et al. Catheter tip position as a risk factor for thrombosis associated with the use of subcutaneous infusion ports. Support Care Cancer. 2005;13(5):325–31.

Campisi C, Biffi R, Pittiruti M. Catheter-related central venous thrombosis: the development of a nationwide consensus paper in Italy. J Assoc Vasc Access. 2007;12(1):38–46.

Chopra V, Flanders SA, Saint S, Woller SC, O'Grady NP, Safdar N, Trerotola SO, Saran R, Moureau N, Wiseman S, Pittiruti M, Akl EA, Lee AY, Courey A, Swaminathan L, Ledonne J, Becker C, Krein SL, Bernstein SJ, Michigan Appropriateness Guide for Intravenouse Catheters Panel. The Michigan Appropriateness Guide for Intravenous Catheters (MAGIC): results from a multispecialty panel using the RAND/UCLA appropriateness method. Ann Intern Med. 2015;163:S1–40.

Cushny AR, Edmunds CW. Paroxysmal irregularity of the heart and auricular fibrillation. In: Bulloch W, editor. Studies in pathology. Written by alumni to celebrate the quatercentenary of the University of Aberdeen and the quarter-centenary of the chair of pathology therein. Aberdeen: Aberdeen University; 1906. p. 95.

DeChicco R, Seinder D, Brun C, Steiger E, Stafford J, Lopez R. Tip position of long-term central venous access devices used for parenteral nutrition. J Parenter Enter Nutr. 2007;31(5):382–7.

Dreyer G, Bingham C. Right atrial thrombus as a complication of a temporary haemodialysis catheter—a potentially avoidable complication. Nephrol Dial Transplant. 2005;20(2):474–5.

Duran-Gehring PE, Guirgis FW, McKee KC, Goggans S, Tran H, Kalynych CJ, Wears RL. The bubble study: ultrasound confirmation of central venous catheter placement. Am J Emerg Med. 2015;33(3):315–9.

Eastridge B, Lefor A. Complications of indwelling venous access devices in cancer patients. J Clin Oncol. 1995;13(1):233–8.

Einthoven W. Ueber die Form des menschlichen Electrocardiogramms (Using an improved electrometer and a correction formula developed independently of Burch, distinguishes five deflections which he names P, Q, R, S and T). Pflügers Arch Eur J Physiol. 1895;60(3):101–23.

Farlex. Farlex Partner Medical Dictionary. Splinting; 2012.

Foaurer AR, Alonzo M. Change in peripherally inserted central catheter tip position with abduction and adduction of the upper extremity. J Vasc Radiol. 2000;11(10):1325–8.

Gibson F, Bodenham A. Misplaced central venous catheters: applied anatomy and practical management. Br J Anaesth. 2013;110(3):333–46.

Gilon D, Schechter D, Rein AJ, Gimmon Z, Or R, Rozenman Y, Slavin S, Gotsman MS, Nagler A. Right atrial thrombi are related to indwelling central venous catheter position: insights into time course and possible mechanism of formation. Am Heart J. 1998;135(3):457–62.

Goddard P, Leslie A, Jones A, Wakeley C, Kabala J. Error in radiology. Br J Radiol. 2001;74(886):949–51.

Gordon S. Bedside chest radiographs and how ambiguous peripherally inserted central catheter tips happen: a case report. J Assoc Vasc Access. 2016;21(4): 237–41.

Gorski L, Hadaway L, Hagle M, McGoldrick M, Orr M, Doellman D. Infusion therapy: standards of practice. J Infus Nurs. 2016a;39(Suppl 1):S1–S159.

Gorski L, Hadaway L, Hagle M, McGoldrick M, Orr M, Doellman D. INS infusion therapy: standards of practice (supplement 1). J Infus Nurs. 2016b;39:S1–S159.

Hadaway LC. I. V. infiltration: not just a peripheral problem. Nurs Manag. 2000;31(11):25–32.

Hallam C, Weston V, Denton A, Hill S, Bodenham A, Dunn H, Jackson T. Development of the UK Vessel Health and Preservation (VHP) framework: a multi-organisational collaborative. J Infect Prev. 2016;17:65–72.

Hellerstein HK, Pritchard WH, Lewis RL. Recording of intracavity potentials through a single lumen, saline filled cardiac catheter. Proc Soc Exp Biol Med. 1949;71(1):58–61.

Hill S. VasoNova Arrow VPS™ technology evaluation. Hospital Pharmacy Europe; 2012.

Holt J, Godard P. Discrepancy and error in diagnostic radiology. WEMJ. 2012;111(2):4.

Hostetter R, Nakazawa N, Tompkins K, Hill B. Precision in central venous catheter tip placement: a review of the literature. J Assoc Vasc Access. 2010;15(3):112–25.

Ibrahim G. Central venous placement: where is the tip? Am J Crit Care. 2012;21(5):370–1.

Johnston AJ, Bishop SM, Martin L, See TC, Streater CT. Defining peripherally inserted central catheter tip position and an evaluation of insertions in one unit. Anaesthesia. 2013;68(5):484–91.

Kung SC, Aravind B, Morse S, Jacobs LE, Raja R. Tunneled catheter–associated atrial thrombi: successful treatment with chronic anticoagulation. Hemodial Int. 2001;5(1):32–6.

Liu Y-J, Dong L, Lou X-P, Miao J-H, Li X-X, Li X-J, Li J, Liu Q-Q, Chang Z-W. Evaluating ECG-aided tip localization of peripherally inserted central catheter in patients with cancer. Int J Clin Exp Med. 2015;8(8):14127–9.

Mandolfo S, Piazza W, Galli F. Catheter tip position and haemodialysis patient; a difficult symbiosis. J Vasc Access. 2002;3(2):64–73.

Marano L, Izzo G, Esposito G, Petrillo M, Cosenza A, Marano M, et al. Peripherally inserted central catheter tip position: a novel empirical-ultrasonographical index in a modern surgical oncology department. Ann Surg Oncol. 2014;21(2):656–61.

Marey EJ. Des variations électriques des muscles et du coeur en particulier, étudiées au moyen de l'électromètre de M. Lippmann. CR Acad Sci. 1876;82:975–7.

Massmann A, Jagoda P, Kranzhoefer N, Buecker A. Local low-dose thrombolysis for safe and effective treatment of venous port-catheter thrombosis. Ann Surg Oncol. 2015;22(5):1593–7.

Matteucci C. Sur un phenomene physiologique produit par les muscles en contraction. Ann Chim Phys. 1842;6:339–41.

Mehall J, Saltzman D, Jackson R, Smith S. Fibrin sheath enhances central venous catheter infection. Crit Care Med. 2002;30(4):908–12.

Miller-Keane. Encyclopedia and dictionary of medicine, nursing, and allied health. 7th ed. 2003. http://medical-dictionary.thefreedictionary.com/parallax+effect. Accessed 24 May 2017.

Moureau NL. Vessel health and preservation: vascular access assessment, selection, insertion, management, evaluation and clinical education. Doctor of Philosophy by Publication (PhD) Thesis and Exegesis (PhD Doctorate), Griffith University. 2017. https://www120.secure.griffith.edu.au/rch/items/e6aea329-fae8-4c41-aa3f-6b4f80298977/1/. https://www120.secure.griffith.edu.au/rch/items/e6aea329-fae8-4c41-aa3f-6b4f80298977/1/ (gu1507011216006).

Moureau N, Chopra V. Indications for peripheral, midline, and central catheters: summary of the michigan appropriateness guide for intravenous catheters recommendations. J Assoc Vasc Access. 2016;21:140–8.

Moureau N, Dennis G, Ames E, Severe R. Electrocardiogram (EKG) guided peripherally inserted central placement and tip position: results of a trial to replace radiological confirmation. J Assoc Vasc Access. 2010;15(1):9–15. https://doi.org/10.2309/java.15-1-3.

National Association of Vascular Access Networks. NAVAN position statement on terminal tip placement. J Vasc Access Devices. 1998;3:8–10.

NKF-K/DOQI. Clinical practice guidelines for vascular access. Am J Kidney Dis. 2001;37(1):S137–S18. https://doi.org/10.1016/S0272-6386(01)70007-8.

Oliver G, Jones M. ECG or X-ray as the 'gold standard' for establishing PICC-tip location? Br J Nurs. 2014;23(Suppl 19):S10–6. https://doi.org/10.12968/bjon.2014.23.Sup19.S10.

Petersen J, Delaney J, Brakstad M, Rowbotham R, Bagley C. Silicone venous access devices positioned with their tips high in the superior vena Caba are more likely to malfunction. Am J Surg. 1999;178(1):38–41.

Pittiruti M. Sweet Spot' vs. Carina: two criteria for verifying tip location by chest X-ray. J Assoc Vasc Access. 2015;20(4):240–1.

Pittiruti M, Scoppettuolo G, LaGreca A, Emoli A, Brutti A, Migliorini I, et al. The EKG method for positioning the tip of PICCs: results from two preliminary studies. J Assoc Vasc Access. 2008;13(4):179–86. https://doi.org/10.2309/ava.13-4-4.

Pittiruti M, Hamilton H, Biffi R, MacFie J, Pertkiewicz M. ESPEN guidelines on parenteral nutrition: central venous catheters (access, care, diagnosis and therapy of complications). Clin Nutr. 2009;28(4):365–77. https://doi.org/10.1016/j.clnu.2009.03.015.

Pittiruti M, La Greca A, Scoppettuolo G. The electrocardiographic method for positioning the tip of central venous catheters. J Vasc Access. 2011;12(4):280–91. https://doi.org/10.5301/JVA.2011.8381.

Pittiruti M, Bertollo D, Briglia E, Buononato M, Capozzoli G, De Simone L, et al. The intracavitary ECG method for positioning the tip of central venous catheters: results of an Italian Multicenter study. J Vasc Access. 2012;13(3):357–65.

Pittiruti M, LaGreca A, Emoli A, Calabrese M, Biasucci DG, Scoppettuolo G. Tip location of central venous access in patients with atrial fibrillation and pacemakers: an algorithm minimizing X-RAY exposure. J Assoc Vasc Access. 2014;19(4):210–1.

Raad I, Bodey G. Infectious complications of indwelling vascular catheters. Clin Infect Dis. 1992;15(2):197–208.

Raman D, Sharma M, Moghekar A, Wang X, Hatipoğlu U. Utilization of thoracic ultrasound for confirmation of central venous catheter placement and exclusion of pneumothorax: a novel technique in real-time application. J Intensive Care Med. 2017;0885066617705839.

RCN. Standards for infusion therapy. 4th ed. Royal College of Nursing; 2016. p. 1–94.

Roldan C, Paniagua L. Central venous catheter intravascular malpositioning: causes, prevention, diagnosis, and correction. West J Emerg Med. 2015;16(5):658–64.

Rossetti F, Pittiruti M, Lamperti M, Graziano U, Celentano D, Capozzoli G. The intracavitary ECG method for positioning the tip of central venous access devices in pediatric patients: results of an Italian multicenter study. J Vasc Access. 2015;16(2):137–43. https://doi.org/10.5301/jva.5000281.

Ryder M. The role of biofilm in vascular catheter-related infections. N Dev Vasc Dis. 2001;2:15–25.

Ryu HG, Bahk JH, Kim JT, Lee JH. Bedside prediction of central venous catheter insertion depth. Br J Anaesth. 2007;98(2):225–7.

Sansivero GE. What's new in vascular access devices and technology? Br J Nurs. 2012;21(Suppl 1):S16–20.

Schummer W, Schummer C, Schelenz C, Brandes H, Stock U, Muller T, et al. Central venous catheters—the inability of intra-atrial ECG to prove adequate positioning. Br J Anaesth. 2004;93(2):193–8.

Schuster M, Nave H, Piepenbrock S, Pabst R, Panning B. The Carina as a landmark in central venous catheter placement. Br J Anaesth. 2000;85(2):192–4.

Scott W. Central venous catheters. An overview of Food and Drug Administration activities. Surg Oncol Clin N Am. 1995;4(3):377–93.

Sette P, Azzini AM, Dorizzi RM, Castellano G. Serendipitous ECG guided PICC insertion using the guidewire as intra-cardiac electrode. J Vasc Access. 2010;11(1):72.

Smith B, Neuharth RM, Hendrix MA, McDonnall D, Michaels AD. Intravenous electrocardiographic guidance for placement of peripherally inserted central catheters. J Electrocardiol. 2010;43(3):274–8. https://doi.org/10.1016/j.jelectrocard.2010.02.003.

Tal M, Friedman T, MojiBian H. The Function tip: a different look at a contentious topic. Endovasc Today. 2013;73–5.

Tortora G, Derrickson B. Principles of anatomy and physiology. 11th ed. Wiley; 2006.

Verhey P, Gosselin M, Primack S, Blackburn P, Kraemer A. The right mediastinal border and central venous anatomy on frontal chest radiograph—direct CT correlation. J Assoc Vasc Access. 2008;13(1):32–5.

Vesely T. Central venous catheter tip position: a continuing controversy. J Vasc Interv Radiol. 2003;14(5):527–34.

Walker G, Alexandrou E, Rickard CM, Chan RJ, Webster J. Effectiveness of electrocardiographic guidance in CVAD tip placement. Br J Nurs. 2015;24(Suppl 14):S4–S12.

Waller AD. A demonstration on man of electromotive changes accompanying the heart's beat. J Physiol. 1887;8(5):229–34.

Wallis M, McGrail M, Webster J, Marsh N, Gowardman J, Playford E, Rickard C. Risk factors for peripheral intravenous catheter failure: a multivariate analysis of data from a randomized controlled trial. Infection Control Hospital Epidemiology. 2014;35(1):63–8. https://doi.org/10.1086/674398.

Weekes AJ, Keller SM, Efune B, Runyon M. Prospective comparison of ultrasound and CXR for confirmation of central venous catheter placement. Emerg Med J. 2016;33(3):176–80.

Wolters, Kluwer, Lippincott. ECG interpretation: an incredibly easy pocket guide. Published Book; 2009.

Wuerz L, Cooke J, Hentel K, Ince-Barnes J, Dawson R. Successful implementation of electrocardiogram-placed peripherally inserted central catheters at a major academic medical teaching organization. J Assoc Vasc Access. 2016;21(4):223–9.

8

Insertion-Related Complications

Steve Hill

Abstract

The reduction of complications is an integral theme of VHP; complications can occur during or post insertion. This chapter examines insertion-related complications including arterial puncture, nerve damage, and air embolus. The relationship between catheter complications and insertion site is explored including peripheral vein, internal jugular, axillary, and femoral-placed CVADs. Methods for clinicians to reduce insertion-related complications are discussed, including thorough patient assessment with pre-assessment of vasculature using ultrasound, visualization aids, and real-time imaging during the insertion.

Keywords

Adverse events · Accidental arterial access Nerve injury · Air emboli · Complications Central venous catheter · Femoral catheter Axillary catheter · Jugular catheter Ultrasound

S. Hill (✉)
The Christie NHS Foundation Trust, Manchester, UK

Precision Vascular and Surgical Services Ltd, Manchester, UK
e-mail: info@precisionvascular.co.uk; steve.hill@christie.nhs.uk

8.1 Introduction

There are several complications and injuries that can occur during insertion of a VAD including arterial puncture, nerve injury, air embolism, and infection. Arterial puncture of the insertion needle occurs in 3.7–12%; more significant injury with advancement of dilator occurs in 0.1–1.0% (Kornbau et al. 2015). Nerve impingement or injury occurs in a small percentage of VAD access and is characterized by intense pain reported by the patient, electric-type shooting pain, and numbness not unlike arterial access. The arterial and nerve access must be differentiated, and when unintended, the access attempt should be immediately aborted. Air embolism is a complication that may occur during insertion or post insertion when any access point to a central vein is left open to air. Other complications of infection, phlebitis, and thrombosis are post insertional complications where signs and symptoms will occur days, weeks, or months after placement of the device.

8.2 Arterial Access

Arterial access may be accidental, as in the case of intended venous access, or intentional for arterial blood sampling or hemodynamic monitoring. Accidental arterial puncture is often easy to spot secondary to pulsatile blood flow but may be less easy to identify in the arteries in extremities or on a hypotensive critically ill patient (Kornbau et al. 2015). Signs and symptoms include:

1. Forceful or pulsatile flow
2. Pain expressed by the patient when applicable
3. Pallor if in an extremity occurring below the site of access
4. Paresthesia/numbness/tingling reported by the patient
5. Color difference in blood, lighter than venous blood

If there is uncertainty of arterial punctured vessel, a pressure transducer can be used to assess for venous/arterial waveform or arterial blood gas sample analyzed (Kornbau et al. 2015). Training, supervision, and demonstrated ability to identify and manage accidental arterial access are a requirement of inserters.

Following identification of arterial access, a determination must be made for management based on peripheral or central vein access and the ability to compress. Arterial access in the periphery is easily managed with digital compression-promoting coagulation. Depending on the patient's medical condition and use of anticoagulating medications, pressure is continuously applied for five or more minutes. Application of a tourniquet for subsequent cannulation may result in harm, loss of coagulation to the area, and additional bleeding/hematoma formation impacting nerves and structures in the region. Arterial access in the regions of the neck or chest should result in consultation by a vascular surgeon to safely ligate and mitigate any future bleeding.

Complications from arterial puncture include compromised airway from hematoma, cerebral ischemia, excessive bleeding, arteriovenous fistula, hemothorax, pseudoaneurysm, thrombus formation, and death (Dixon et al. 2017). Dixon et al. (2017) undertook a systematic review of the literature related to inadvertent arterial puncture and reviewed 80 cases to identify optimal management. Eight out of 44 cases that were managed by removal and compression at the site of injury were complicated by stroke or thrombus. The authors found that fewer complications occurred if the device was left in situ while preparations were being made for endovascular or surgical intervention. Serious complications can still occur with needle or guidewire—the authors suggest that the lack of case study reporting was due to patients potentially being managed by removal and pressure. Reflected in the cases reviewed as only 4 of the 80 cases included placement of needle or guidewire puncture only. Surgical intervention was considered optimal intervention for those patients who are fit for general anesthesia; endovascular repair was only marginally less successful and may be more appropriate in medial subclavian injury due to restricted surgical access.

There may be several reasons for arterial placement of catheters while using ultrasound. During cannulation of the vein using ultrasound, visualization of the needle tip may be confused with visualization of the needle shaft (Bowdle 2014). This may provide false reassurance as the clinician is watching the needle tip on the ultrasound screen, but the ultrasound beam is over a section of the needle shaft, and the needle tip is actually placed in the artery. Alternatively, the needle may be within the vein while being inserted under ultrasound but then inadvertently placed into the artery when placing the guidewire as at this point ultrasound is not being used (Bowdle 2014). Learning practitioners may be more prone to needle movement at this stage until their skills are polished. Holding the needle with the non-dominant arm while resting the arm on the patient may increase stability and reduces movement of the needle tip and the risk of it moving out of the vein.

8.3 Vein Wall Injury

Damage to the vein wall can occur during VAD insertion; significant injury can lead to venous tears. Bodenham et al. (2016) suggest that the longitudinal cell structure of a vein makes it more prone to linear tears (Bodenham 2006). Kornbau et al. (2015) notes another mechanism for this injury is that the guidewire becomes trapped against the vessel wall, and subsequent passage of the dilator causes the wire to bow and push up against the vessel wall, potentially resulting in a linear tear (Kornbau et al. 2015). In addition, the risk of perforation increases if a catheter lies against the wall of the vein at an angle of greater than 40°, and major intrathoracic injuries may even require cardiopulmonary bypass to achieve cardiovascular stability while the injuries are repaired (Kornbau et al. 2015).

8.4 Nerve Injury

Nerve injury can be insertion-related, such as a needle being advanced into a nerve branch during insertion, or post insertion such as hematoma causing neuropathic symptoms. The incidence of nerve injury is estimated to be 1.6%, and resolution of neuropathic symptoms related to CVAD placement may take up to 6–12 months (Kornbau et al. 2015). Reports of phrenic nerve palsy following the insertion of an internal jugular CVC have been recorded; effects can be transient or may require surgical intervention (Ahn et al. 2012). Other sites include Brachial plexus, phrenic nerve, and median nerve or other upper arm nerves. Howes and Dell (2006) describe nerve injury that occurred following the insertion of a catheter for hemofiltration via the femoral vein. The patient was free from motor or sensory symptoms but complained of pain, which became severe. Limb perfusion was not affected, and peripheral pulses were intact. Nerve compression from the catheter was suspected; it was removed and replaced with an internal jugular catheter. The symptoms resolved almost immediately, and the patient did not suffer any lasting neurological deficits (Hows and Dell 2006). Zhao and Wang (2014) report an incidence of PICC-related nerve injury of 0.8% from a review of 739 cases; all of the injuries were related to brachial vein approach.

8.5 Air Embolism

Air embolism can occur when negative intrathoracic pressure draws air into the vein (Kornbau et al. 2015). This can occur at cannulation when disconnecting the syringe to insert the guidewire, when the dilator is removed from the Peel-Away sheath prior to advancing the catheter, by not priming the catheter according to manufacturer instructions, or leaving catheter clamps open. If air embolism does occur, the patient should be placed in the left decubitus position, localizing air in the right atrium and right lung and preventing emboli from entering the pulmonary arterial system, suggests Kornbau et al. (2015); the author adds that this maneuver is not effective in patients with abnormal anatomy. Case study option here.

8.6 Different Veins and Associated Risks

The axillary vein drains the cephalic, basilic, and brachial veins; it is closely accompanied by the axillary artery. Bodenham et al. (2004) look in detail at this approach, recording 200 cases and measuring various elements of the insertion and anatomical structures. The authors identified that moving more laterally, the axillary vein reduces in size and the depth of the vein increases. The mean length of right axillary catheters was 21.4 cm and 24.6 for catheters inserted on the left; axillary insertions were successfully inserted in 96% of cases. Complications included axillary arterial puncture in three cases (1.5%) and transient neuralgia in two cases (1%). Limitations of the technique were patients with increased BMI, due to decreased image quality, and difficulty passing guidewires and dilators was experienced with higher BMI patients because of the angle caused by deeper veins. Another limitation of this approach is misplacement of the guidewire, and the catheter occurred 15.5% and 12.9%, respectively, illustrating that the insertion technique would benefit from fluoroscopy or ECG/navigation technology (Fig. 8.1).

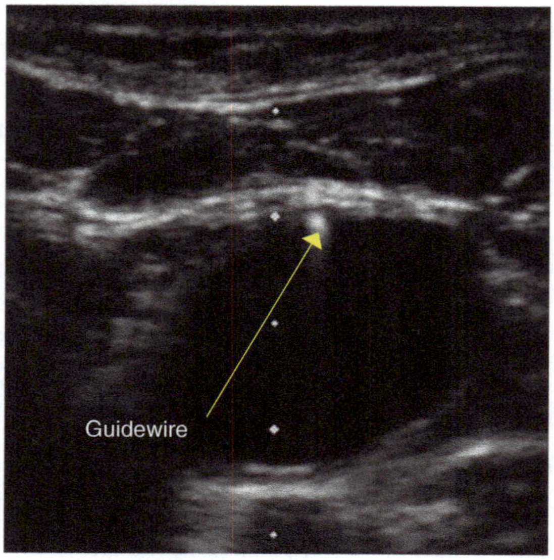

Fig. 8.1 Right internal jugular showing hyper-echogenic guidewire in position (used with permission of S. Hill)

Table 8.1 Incidence of complications for CVADs (Plumhans et al. 2011)

Complication	Axillary/subclavian	Internal jugular
Thrombosis	3%	0%
Arterial puncture	4 cases	1 case
Dislocation device	1 case	0

8.7 Axillary (Subclavian) Versus Jugular

Plumhans et al. (2011) compared internal jugular versus axillary and subclavian vein insertions on 138 oncology patients and found that pain perception, radiation dose, tip migration, thrombosis, risk of arterial puncture, and dislocation of the device were all lower in the patients that received devices via the internal jugular vein (Plumhans et al. 2011). Plumhans et al. noted as follows: thrombosis, arterial puncture, and device dislocation rates for IJ and subclavian insertions. Conclusions from this publication were that IJ complications were less frequent (Table 8.1).

8.8 Internal Jugular

In a review of 123 consecutive patients who had a CT, the right internal jugular (RIJ) had an average diameter of 15.6 mm versus 11.7 left internal jugular, the overlap with the carotid artery was not significantly different comparing right to left, and depth of the skin to vein was also similar (Ozbek et al. 2013). The authors also examine the incidence of veins less than 7 mm, which was 4.4% for RIJs and 21.9% for left internal jugular veins. Anatomy that presented outside of the expected landmarks occurred in 5.5% of cases, illustrating the importance of ultrasound and the limitation of landmark approach; human anatomy is not universal, and anatomical variations occur necessitating thorough ultrasound assessment, prior to the procedure and guidance during insertion (Lamperti et al. 2012; National Institute for Clinical Excellence 2002). Trendelenburg significantly increases the size of the internal jugular vein, increasing the safety of the procedure (Lewin et al. 2007). Parry (2004) assessed the influence of patient position upon the internal jugular approach and identified that the ideal position for the majority of patients was a 15% Trendelenburg position, with a small pillow

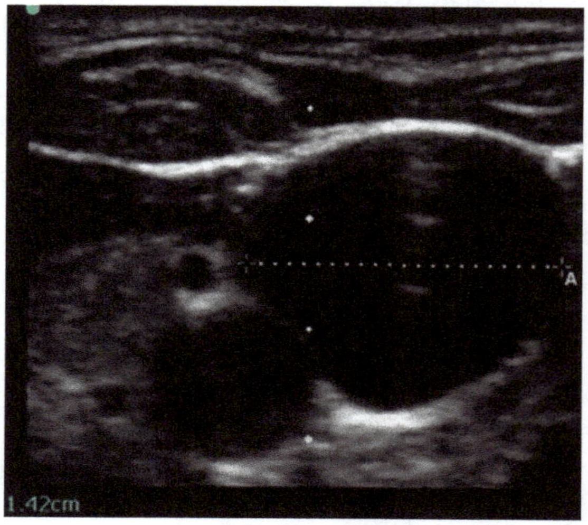

Fig. 8.2 Right internal jugular without Valsalva (used with permission of S. Hill)

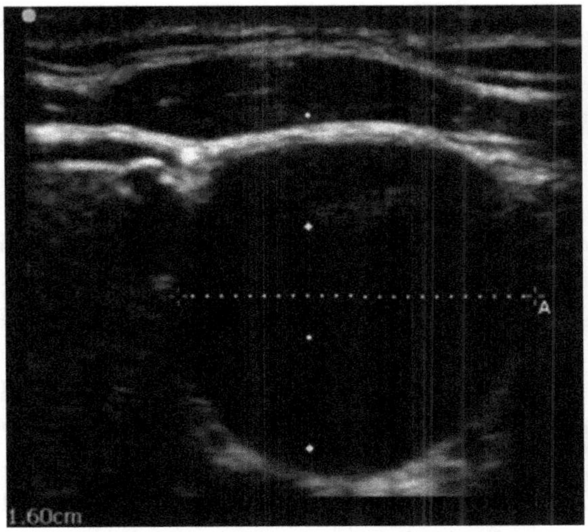

Fig. 8.3 Right internal jugular with Valsalva increase of 12.6% (used with permission of S. Hill)

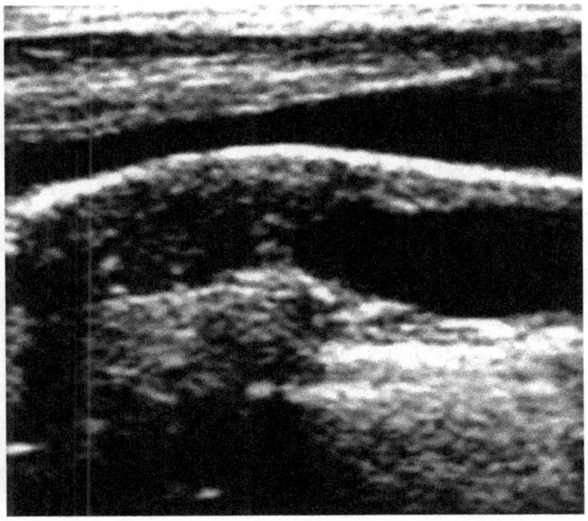

Fig. 8.4 Stenosis of the vein (used with permission of N. Moureau, PICC Excellence)

under the head and with the head positioned close to the midline; however, positioning of the head close to the midline would be balanced against ease of access to the insertion site and effect on sterility of the procedure (Parry 2004).

The internal jugular was associated with the lowest mechanical complications compared with subclavian and femoral approaches using ultrasound (Tsotsolis et al. 2015).

Figures 8.2 and 8.3 show changes in the diameter of the RIJ with and without a Valsalva maneuver.

8.9 Stenosis

Once a catheter is placed, it can still have longer-term detrimental effects on the vein, inflammation, microthrombi, intimal hyperplasia, fibrotic changes, and stenosis (Agarwal 2009). Stenosis is not an immediate or always obvious complication of vascular access; patients may not always present with symptoms. It may only be identified when a further VAD is needed and either identified on ultrasound, a guidewire not passing, or by subtle enhancement of collateral vasculature. Yevzlin (2008) reviewed rates of stenosis in hemodialysis catheters and found from subclavian-placed catheters that stenosis rates varied from 40 to 50% and that comparative studies comparing 50 internal jugular-placed hemodialysis catheters to 50 subclavian-placed catheters saw 42% stenosis in the subclavian group versus 10% in those receiving internal jugular access (Fig. 8.4) (Yevzlin 2008). Gonsalves et al. (2003) looked at the 154 patients who underwent PICC insertions, and at the time of insertion, venography showed normal central veins (Gonsalves et al. 2003). Further evaluation showed that three patients developed central vein stenosis and that one patient developed central vein occlusion. From the 154 patients, 8 of the subsequent venograms showed vein occlusion and 10 patients had stenosis; a 7% incidence of stenosis or occlusion was found in patients with initial normal venograms. Patients in the study with longer dwell times were more likely to develop central vein anomalies. Related to the pathophysiological processes of PICC on vasculature, El Ters et al. (2012) looked at the associations between arteriovenous fistula function of 425 patients and found a strong independent association between PICC use and lack of functioning arteriovenous fistula (El Ters et al. 2012). Therefore, advice related to PICC for renal patients suggested by; the AV fistula first breakthrough initiative national coalition recommends NOT using PICC lines in patients at risk for, or with known mid-stage 3CKD, stage 4 and 5CKD or end-stage renal disease. A small-bore central catheter in the internal jugular vessels is recommended instead (Hoggard et al. 2008). Anatomical site and vein selection remain intrinsically linked to VHP and clinical outcomes, and it is essential to be aware of complications relevant to the selected site for CVAD insertion.

Wu et al. (2016) undertook a meta-analysis of percutaneous insertions internal jugular vs. subclavian vein implanted port placements and suggested that the internal jugular vein is a safer insertion site for implanted ports and is associated with lower risk mechanical complications (Wu et al. 2013).

To preserve patients' vasculature, INS standards (2016) include avoidance of placing PICCs in patients with chronic kidney disease due to the risk of central vein stenosis and occlusion (Gorski et al. 2016). The MAGIC recommendations quantify this and suggest PICCs should not be considered appropriate for patients with renal disease stage 3 or greater, with GFR of less than 44 mL/min, or for any patients receiving renal replacement therapy (Chopra et al. 2015). When considering the implication of stenosis from central venous catheterization, RCN guidelines recommend the internal jugular vein due to the lower relative risk of complication and suggest that the subclavian, external jugular, and femoral veins should be avoided due to the high risk of stenosis (RCN 2016).

8.10 Femoral Approach

Merrer et al. (2001) undertook an RCT that compared subclavian (144) vs. femoral site (145) insertions, mechanical complications differed, arterial puncture (AP) in the femoral group were higher, 13 in femoral versus 7 in the subclavian arm (Merrer et al. 2001). The APs in the femoral group led to two significant retroperitoneal hematomas that required blood transfusions or surgery. Ultrasound scans were undertaken to detect the presence of thrombosis; in the subclavian group, thrombosis occurred in 1.9% patients and in 21.5% patients in the femoral arm, similar to thrombosis rates identified by Trottier (1995). Thrombosis was significantly higher in the femoral group at 21.5% versus 1.2 for the subclavian approach, seven patients in the femoral thrombosis group had complete catheter-related thrombosis, and pulmonary embolus was documented in two of the cases. Within this study they added that three patients would need to be treated using subclavian rather than femoral approach to prevent one complication. The authors looked at associations related to mechanical complications of insertion and found that there was an increased risk of mechanical complications associated with insertions that took place during the night, if the clinician was less experienced and if duration of insertion was prolonged.

Uhl and Gillot (2010) assessed 336 limbs to assess anatomical variations in femoral vein and found 12% with anatomical variations. Fronek et al. (2001) found the average width of the femoral vein to be 11.84 mm and that from the age of 60 years, size declined and velocity at rest significantly decreased over the age of 50 years (Fronek et al. 2001). Trendelenburg did not significantly improve femoral vein size but Valsalva maneuver was found to increase size by up to 40% (Lewin et al. 2007). Though mechanical risks exist, AAGBI guidelines suggest that in coagulopathic patients, the femoral approach may be advantageous, in the hands of an experienced clinician, as it allows easy compression of the site.

8.11 Infection and Femoral Site

Merrer et al. (2001) identified an incidence of infection for femoral insertions at 20 per/1000 and subclavian at 3.7 per/1000 cases and sepsis at 4.4% versus 1.5% (Merrer et al. 2001). Marik et al. (2012) undertook a systematic review looking at CRBSI risk or femoral subclavian and internal jugular catheters (Marik et al. 2012). The authors concluded that there was no significant difference between the infection rates of internal jugular and femoral sites in more recent studies and no difference between the three sites in terms of BSI (Marik et al. 2012). Timsit et al. (2013) looked at infection risk of jugular (1.0 per 1000 catheter days) versus femoral catheter (1.1 per 1000 catheter days) and found that femoral and internal jugular access leads to similar risk of infection, echoed by INS (2016) (Gorski et al. 2016; Timsit et al. 2013). Other factors with insertion leading to advantages of including femoral placement are tunneling techniques, moving the insertion site away from the inguinal fold with positioning toward the mid-thigh (Pittiruti 2014).

8.12 Conclusion

Acute care patients present with increasing comorbidities and complexities of illnesses. Clinicians must be aware, recognize, and subsequently safely manage insertion of the most appropriate intravenous devices to deliver treatment while avoiding complications to promote the best patient outcomes (Kornbau et al. 2015). While complications cannot be eliminated completely, prevention should be the ultimate goal.

Case Study

A 48-year-old male presented at the emergency room with severe shortness of breath, diaphoresis, low blood pressure, and lethargy. Following application of oxygen to the patient, the emergency department physician placed a right internal jugular catheter without ultrasound or visualization technology. The difficult insertion required three attempts. As the patient's adult-onset respiratory distress syndrome improved, he began complaining of chest pain, shortness of breath only when lying flat, and cough. During a sniff test of the diaphragm, right phrenic nerve paralysis was confirmed related to the insertion of the internal jugular catheter.

Summary of Key Points

1. Insertion-related complications can lead to profound implications for patients receiving CVADs.
2. An understanding of anatomy, thorough patient assessment, knowledge of patient history, use of ultrasound to assess the patient, and real-time imaging results in reduced complications.
3. Inserting clinicians must be able to recognize and manage CVAD-related complications.
4. Optimal patient outcomes for CVAD insertion requires the inserting clinician to be a vigilant, knowledgeable, and skilled practitioner; increased insertion attempts and clinician experience are closely linked to complication risk.

References

Agarwal AK. Central vein stenosis: current concepts. Adv Chronic Kidney Dis. 2009;16:360–70.

Ahn EJ, Baek CW, Shin HY, Kang H, Jung YH. Phrenic nerve palsy after internal jugular venous catheter placement. Korean J Anesthesiol. 2012;63:183–4.

Bodenham A, R Sharma A, Mallick A. Ultrasound-guided infraclavicular axillary vein cannulation for central venous access. Br J Anaesth. 2004;93(2):188–92. Epub, Jun 25.

Bodenham A. Ultrasound imaging by anaesthetists: training and accreditation issues. Br J Anaesth. 2006;96:414–7.

Bodenham A, Babu S, Bennett J, et al. Association of Anaesthetists of Great Britain and Ireland: safe vascular access 2016. Anaesthesia. 2016;71(5):573–85.

Bowdle A. Vascular complications of central venous catheter placement: evidence-based methods for prevention and treatment. J Cardiothorac Vasc Anesth. 2014;28:358–68.

Chopra V, Flanders SA, Saint S, Woller SC, O'Grady NP, Safdar N, Trerotola SO, Saran R, Moureau N, Wiseman S, Pittiruti M, Akl EA, Lee AY, Courey A, Swaminathan L, Ledonne J, Becker C, Krein SL, Bernstein SJ. The Michigan Appropriateness Guide for Intravenous Catheters (MAGIC): results from a multispecialty panel using the RAND/UCLA appropriateness method. Ann Intern Med. 2015;163:S1–S40.

Dixon OG, Smith GE, Carradice D, Chetter IC. A systematic review of management of inadvertent arterial injury during central venous catheterisation. J Vasc Access. 2017;18:97–102.

El Ters M, Schears GJ, Taler SJ, Williams AW, Albright RC, Jenson BM, Mahon AL, Stockland AH, Misra S, Nyberg SL, Rule AD, Hogan MC. Association between prior peripherally inserted central catheters and lack of functioning arteriovenous fistulas: a case-control study in hemodialysis patients. Am J Kidney Dis. 2012;60:601–8.

Fronek A, Criqui MH, Denenberg J, Langer RD. Common femoral vein dimensions and hemodynamics including Valsalva response as a function of sex, age, and ethnicity in a population study. J Vasc Surg. 2001;33:1050–6.

Gonsalves C, Eschelman D, Sullivan K, Dubois N, Bonn J. Incidence of central vein stenosis and occlusion following upper extremity PICC and port placement. Cardiovasc Intervent Radiol. 2003;26:123–7.

Gorski L, Hadaway L, Hagle M, Mcgoldrick M, Orr M, Doellman D. Infusion therapy: standards of practice (supplement 1). J Infus Nurs. 2016;39:S1–S159.

Hoggard J, Saad T, Schon D, Vesely T, Royer T. Guideline for venous access in patients with chronic kidney disease: a position statement from the American Society of Diagnostic and Interventional Nephrology Clinical Practice Committee and the Association for Vascular Access. Semin Dial. 2008;21:186–91.

Howes B, Dell R. Risk of nerve damage from vascular access catheters, vol. 61. The Association Anaesthetists of Great Britain; 2006. p. 618.

Kornbau C, Lee KC, Hughes GD, Firstenberg MS. Central line complications. Int J Crit illn Inj Sci. 2015;5:170.

Lamperti M, Bodenham AR, Pittiruti M, Blaivas M, Augoustides JG, Elbarbary M, Pirotte T, Karakitsos D, Ledonne J, Doniger S. International evidence-based recommendations on ultrasound-guided vascular access. Intensive Care Med. 2012;38:1105–17.

Lewin MR, Stein J, Wang R, Lee MM, Kernberg M, Boukhman M, Hahn I-H, Lewiss RE. Humming is as effective as Valsalva's maneuver and Trendelenburg's position for ultrasonographic visualization of the jugular venous system and common femoral veins. Ann Emerg Med. 2007;50:73–7.

Marik PE, Flemmer M, Harrison W. The risk of catheter-related bloodstream infection with femoral venous catheters as compared to subclavian and internal jugular venous catheters: a systematic review of the literature and meta-analysis. Crit Care Med. 2012;40:2479–85.

Merrer J, De Jonghe B, Golliot F, Lefrant J, Raffy B, Barre E, Rigaud J, Casciani D, Misset B, Bosquet C, Outin H, Brun-Buisson C, Nitenenberg G, French Catheter Study Group in Intensive Care. Complications of femoral and subclavian venous catheterization in critically ill patients: a randomized controlled trial. JAMA. 2001;286:700–7.

National Institute for Clinical Excellence. NICE Technological Appraisal Guidance: guidance on the use of ultrasound locating devices for placing central venous catheters. NICE Technological Appraisal Guidance, 2002. p. 1–24.

Ozbek S, Apiliogullari S, Erol C, Kivrak AS, Kara I, Uysal E, Koplay M, Duman A. Optimal angle of needle entry for internal jugular vein catheterization with a neutral head position: a CT study. Ren Fail. 2013;35:492–6.

Parry G. Trendelenburg position, head elevation and a midline position optimize right internal jugular vein diameter. Can J Anesth. 2004;51:379.

Pittiruti M. The "off-label" use of PICCs. In: Sandrucci S, Mussa B, editors. Peripherally inserted central venous catheters. Milan: Springer; 2014.

Plumhans C, Mahnken AH, Ocklenburg C, Keil S, Behrendt FF, Günther RW, Schoth F. Jugular versus subclavian totally implantable access ports: catheter position, complications and intrainterventional pain perception. Eur J Radiol. 2011;79:338–42.

RCN. Standards for infusion therapy. 4th ed. London: Royal College of Nursing; 2016. p. 1–94.

Timsit J-F, Bouadma L, Mimoz O, Parienti J-J, Garrouste-Orgeas M, Alfandari S, Plantefeve G, Bronchard R, Troche G, Gauzit R. Jugular versus femoral short-term catheterization and risk of infection in intensive care unit patients. Causal analysis of two randomized trials. Am J Respir Crit Care Med. 2013;188:1232–9.

Trottier S, Veremakis C, O'Brien J, et al. Femoral deep vein thrombosis associated with central venous catheterization; results from a prospective randomised controlled trial. Crit Care Med. 1995;23:52–9.

Tsotsolis N, Tsirgogianni K, Kioumis I, Pitsiou G, Baka S, Papaiwannou A, Karavergou A, Rapti A, Trakada G, Katsikogiannis N. Pneumothorax as a complication of central venous catheter insertion. Ann Transl Med. 2015;3(3):40.

Uhl J, Gillot C. The foot venous pump: anatomy and physiology. Monaco: XVI World Congress of the Union Internationale de Phlebologie; 2009.

Uhl F, Gillot C. Anatomical variation of the femoral vein. J Vasc Surg. 2010;52(3):714–9.

Wu S, Ling Q, Cao L, Wang J, Xu M, Zeng W. Real-time two-dimensional ultrasound guidance for central venous cannulation: a meta-analysis. J Am Soc Anesthesiol. 2013;118:361–75.

Yevzlin AS. Hemodialysis catheter-associated central venous stenosis. Semin Dial. 2008;21(6):522–7.. Wiley Online Library

Zhao L, Wang Y. A descriptive study of nerve injury related to upper arm PICC placement. WoCoVa presentation. Zhejiang University School of Medicine; 2014.

9

Securement in CVAD Care

Steve Hill and Nancy L. Moureau

Abstract

This chapter considers the role of securement in CVAD care, providing an overview of the background and how knowledge and research has evolved in this area. The complications of inadequate securement such as infection, migration, pistoning, and medical adhesive-related skin injury (MARSI) are examined to understand contributing factors that lead to their development. Practices that enhance optimal securement and mitigate risks are discussed as part of the clinician's role in the prevention of complications in our endeavor to reach our ultimate goal of achieving zero CVAD complications.

Keywords

Securement · Intravenous catheter · Central catheter · Stabilization · Dislodgement · Catheter failure

S. Hill
The Christie NHS Foundation Trust, Manchester, UK

Precision Vascular and Surgical Services Ltd, Manchester, UK
e-mail: info@precisionvascular.co.uk; steve.hill@christie.nhs.uk

N. L. Moureau (✉)
PICC Excellence, Inc., Hartwell, GA, USA

Menzies Health Institute, Alliance for Vascular Access Teaching and Research (AVATAR) Group, Griffith University, Brisbane, QLD, Australia
e-mail: nancy@piccexcellence.com

9.1 Introduction

Following the insertion of a VAD, methods to secure the position and reduce movement of the catheter contribute to the longevity and functionality of the venous access device. Securement of a VAD plays a crucial role in the performance and the success of the device. The importance of securement is established by the rates of catheter failure, malposition, infection, and complications of dislodgment/pistoning. The impact of poor securement upon the patient can be significant, leading to delays or missed treatments and infection (Oliver and Jones 2014). Inadequate securement may also prolong hospital stays, and further interventions are needed or a replacement VAD is required. Accidental dislodgement incidence is estimated at 1.8–24% of all VADs (Dugger et al. 1994; Moureau et al. 2002). Use of manufactured securement is intended to reduce the incidence of catheter failure due to dislodgement (Marsh et al. 2015). VHP provides a context for application of standardized securement processes that address issues of sutures, dressings, and forms of securement that combine both the use of cyanoacrylate and dressings. Securement is designed to minimize or eliminate dislodgment and related complications.

In the literature catheter failure rates prior to completion of therapy reflect an incidence of up to 69% (Marsh et al. 2015; Ullman et al. 2015a, b). Estimates reflect that 40–70% of peripheral intravenous catheters (PIVC) are due to dislodgment, occlusion, infiltration, or phlebitis, all complications which may be impacted by securement practices (Rickard and Marsh 2017). Movement of catheters in and out of the insertion site may cause inflammation, swelling, phlebitis, and infection that contribute to the need to remove and replace the catheter. Both peripheral and central catheters require adequate securement to reduce the risk of catheter failure and complications that contribute to increased morbidity and mortality during treatment.

For clinicians providing vascular access, there are few situations more frustrating and exasperating than after struggling painstakingly over a difficult placement and then to hear that the device has accidentally been pulled out. There are potential service implications too for vascular access teams or individual clinicians. Unnecessary repeated VAD insertions increase costs and reduce efficiency and may even increase waiting lists together with reducing capacity to respond to new patients referred who require a VAD.

As with the growth and divergence in vascular access devices, we have seen an increase in the variety of different methods of securing and dressing VADs. Once the VAD has been placed, our aim is to maintain cleanliness of the site by reducing microbial access and thereby reducing the cutaneous route of infection at the point where the device enters the skin. Protection and securement of a VAD must be effective to allow the VAD to achieve its intended dwell time and minimize complications.

Various studies have demonstrated the effectiveness of the differing types of securement with manufactured securement as the most highly recommended (Gorski et al. 2016; Ullman et al. 2015a, b). Types of catheter securement include tape and gauze, transparent film dressings that hold the catheter in place either independently or in conjunction with other forms of securement, more advanced dressings with borders and adherent strips, manufactured adhesive sutureless securement where the catheter is mounted and held in place through adhesive, anchoring or locking devices, tissue adhesives, more invasive subcutaneous securement, and sutures.

9.2 Purpose of Securement

The role of securement for devices is to limit movement, reduce transmission of external skin bacteria into the insertion site, and reduce the occurrence of accidental dislodgement often resulting in VAD failure. Effective forms of securement with a dressing cover help to protect the catheter and insertion site for up to 7 days as established in INS Standards (Gorski et al. 2016). The Standards also specify VADs should be stabilized and secured to prevent complications and unintentional loss of access. The Centers for Disease Control (CDC) recommends the use of sutureless securement to reduce the risk of infection for VADs (O'Grady et al. 2011). Commonly used forms of securement are transparent dressings that provide some degree of stabilization, allow visualization and assessment through the dressing, and prevent contamination from water or dirt while releasing moisture from the skin with varying levels of vapor permeability within the transparent film. Engineered stabilization devices are designed to reduce accidental dislodgement and other complications associated with movement and lack of securement.

9.3 Types of Securement

Devices used for securement of VADs include transparent dressings, tape and gauze, advanced dressings with borders and adherent strips, manufactured adhesive sutureless securement, anchoring or locking devices, tissue adhesives, subcutaneous securement, and sutures. Each of these forms of securement may be used in combination and can have slightly different applications. Patients with edema, anasarca, and drainage at the insertion site may require gauze and tape (Fig. 9.1) with dressing changes every 24–48 h in addition to an adhesive sutureless securement or subcutaneous securement device attached to the catheter. Sterile tape or reinforced strips can be used to secure the VAD to the skin and are most effective if used in a consistent and systematic manner by all staff. Manufacturers caution against the use of tape directly on catheters as it

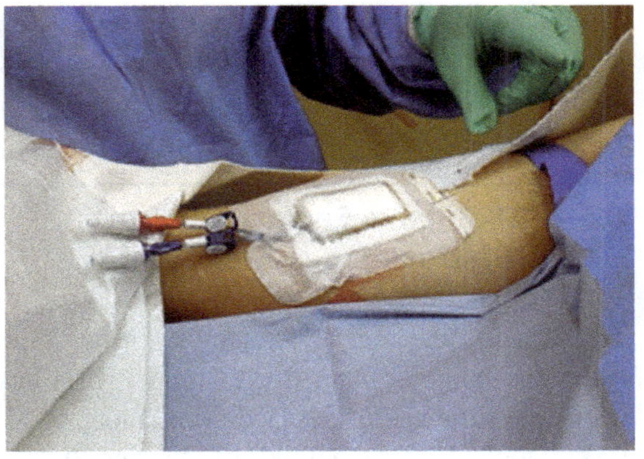

Fig. 9.1 Gauze dressing (used with permission of N. Moureau (PICC Excellence 2018))

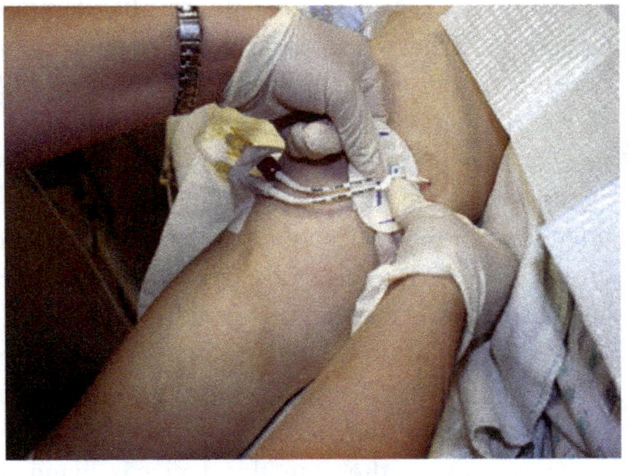

Fig. 9.2 Adhesive Securement Platform. Used with permission of Nancy Moureau, PICC Excellence

has been known to damage catheters during removal. Accidental dislodgement of catheters remains a problem when tape or reinforced strips are the only source of securement. Regardless of which product is used to secure the catheter, a securement device is changed with each dressing change or if it becomes soiled, bloody, or loose and is placed so that nothing interferes with insertion site assessment.

INS states a catheter stabilization device is the preferred alternative to tape or sutures (Gorski et al. 2016). There are several types of manufactured devices designed specifically for central venous catheters. Some are adhesive devices that allow the wings on the catheter hub to snap into a platform (Fig. 9.2), providing a firm base of stabilization. There are securement devices that have adhesive applied to skin and adhesive to hold the hub, and still others use a Velcro-strap material to cross over the hub to hold the lumens of the catheter and stabilize the device. Add-on plastic snap-on holders for the catheter create a place of securement around the catheter to lock onto a securement platform. Manufactured securement devices reduce dislodgement and are safer than sutures, tape, or strips. The manufactured devices are effective by maintaining a secure hold and preventing the catheter from pistoning in and out of the site. This reduction of movement of the catheter with adequate stabilization at the insertion site reduces movement of the catheter and may also reduce the introduction of microorganisms and catheter-related infection (Jeanes and Martinez-Garcia 2016).

9.4 Gauze and Tape Securement

In the early stages of VAD dressing development, Shivnan et al. (1991) compared the sterile gauze dressing with transparent adherent dressings for high-risk patients ($n = 96$) who were undergoing bone marrow transplants (Shivnan et al. 1991). In this study no significant difference was found in terms of infection, but transparent dressings were found to be less irritable than gauze and tape. Dressing types were evaluated for tunneled central venous catheters. Keeler et al. (2015) looked at the impact of three approaches and monitored rates of catheter-related infection and cost: no dressing, a gauze dressing, and a transparent dressing (Keeler et al. 2015). A total number of 432 patients were included in a single site comparison; no difference in infection rates, number of organisms, or days until the onset of an infection was noted between the groups. Gauze was found to have the highest cost of the three methods.

9.5 Transparent Dressings

Transparent dressings, as a type of securement, either alone or in conjunction with other forms of securement, include flat films or those with cloth borders. Bordered dressings may promote improved adherence of the edges with less lifting and reduce catheter dislodgement. According to INS, transparent dressings should not be relied upon to act as the single source of securement indicating the lack of supportive evidence (Gorski et al. 2016). Results of the study by Rickard et al. (2018) demonstrated similar dislodgement outcomes (7–10%) for transparent dressings, bordered transparent, adhesive sutureless securement, and transparent and tissue adhesive with transparent dressing (Rickard et al. 2018). While the tissue adhesive and transparent dressing had the lowest dislodgement (7%), the results were not statistically significant. This study, with single digit dislodgement rates reflected lower than average negative outcomes suggestive that initial securement by expert trained nurses (average of 87.7% of insertions) reduced complications. These results also emphasize the value of using a transparent dressing in combination with other forms of securement to reduce all complications. Dawn et al. (2010) undertook a prospective randomized study comparing adhesive sutureless securement with a transparent dressing with 302 subjects and found that the transparent dressing was non-inferior in respect of overall securement-related complications (Dawn et al. 2010).

Peripheral catheters are the most common form of VAD and have the highest failure rate, up to 69%, partially due to inadequate securement resulting in dislodgement (Rickard et al. 2010, 2012; Smith 2006). Evidence supports the use of two options for catheter stabilization of PIVCs (Fig. 9.3), one for the hub and one as a dressing (Bausone-Gazda et al. 2010; Gorski et al. 2016; Jackson 2012).

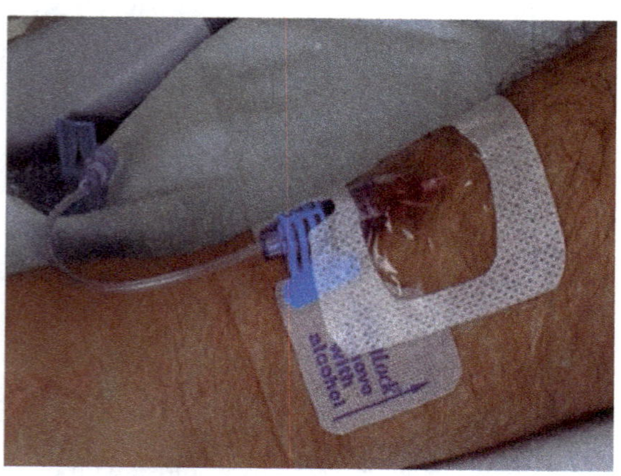

Fig. 9.3 Adhesive securement with PIVC dressing (used with permission of N. Moureau, PICC Excellence)

9.6 Adhesive Securement Platforms

Traditionally the mechanism for securing some catheters for non-tunneled CVC and PICCs has been to suture them in place. Yamamoto et al. (2002) looked at two methods of securing PICCs, traditional suturing and adhesive sutureless securement looking at rates of dislodgement, occlusion, leakage, infection, and thrombosis (Yamamoto et al. 2002). The results demonstrated the adhesive sutureless securement complications were lower than the sutures group (42 vs. 61), though the difference did not reach statistical significance. There was, however, a significantly lower rate of catheter-related bloodstream infections in the adhesive sutureless securement group (2 vs. 10). The study also identified one needlestick injury which occurred during suturing. Adhesive sutureless securement is used with PIVC, midline, PICCs, and some chest, neck, and femoral CVADs (Fig. 9.3). Used in conjunction with a transparent dressing, this device is changed every 7 days or when the dressing is changed.

9.7 Tissue Adhesive Securement

For many years surgical glue has been used successfully in healthcare for a variety of applications, from traumatic lacerations to trocar port incisions (Regalado and Funaki 2008). In more recent times, medical grade surgical glue has attracted the attention from clinicians within the specialty of vascular access. Tissue adhesives or glue are now used with VADs with one drop on the insertion site and an optional drop under the hub of the catheter to provide stabilization and also have evidence to suggest a level of microbial protection (Pittiruti and Scoppettuolo 2017; Rickard et al. 2018; Simonova et al. 2012). Scoppettuolo et al. (2015) found that cyanoacrylate glue can be used as an alternative to suturing and helps to reduce site bleeding for VADs (Scoppettuolo et al. 2015). The authors suggest a 40% reduction in PICC related bleeding at the insertion site with 0% bleeding observed at 1 h and at 24 h in 45 patients. In a study at the same hospital, using cyanoacrylate glue on 348 PICCs (pediatric and adult) with 165 non-tunneled CVADs including high-risk coagulopathic patients, the study showed that the glue was 100% effective at preventing post-insertion bleeding at the exit site (Pittiruti et al. 2016). In PICCs glue was effective in preventing extraluminal bacterial contamination of the catheter (Pittiruti et al. 2016). Furthermore, the authors used an insertion bundle, which included glue in pediatric CVADs which resulted in a tenfold decrease in infection. Other advantages include increasing the speed of skin closure, for instance, when closing the wounds for implanted ports versus tradition time-consuming suture closure. The ability to close the port sites more quickly may reduce the risk the site is exposed to infection and reduce the risk of needlestick injury (Regalado and Funaki 2008). As with any adhesive, MARSI or skin irritation may occur making it prudent for the clinician to perform a skin test prior to use of any of the tissue adhesive formulations. Tissue adhesives are typically used in conjunction with a transparent dressing cover providing added securement of the catheter even if the dressing becomes non-adherent.

9.8 Subcutaneous Securement

Another type of engineered securement is the subcutaneous snap-on stabilization device with tungsten flanges that anchor the device around the catheter and in the subcutaneous tissue of the patient (Egan et al. 2013). This type of securement has been successful with CVADs resulting in favorable clinician and patient satisfaction (Bugden et al. 2016; Gorski et al. 2016; Jeanes and Martinez-Garcia 2016; Zerla et al. 2017). Subcutaneous securement applied to a catheter is left in place for the entire life of the catheter without replacement, unless complication or device dislodgement occurs, providing an excellent option for securement similar to suturing without the added concerns of puncture site infection.

9.9 Sutures

Sutures are often used for internal jugular or subclavian acute care catheters and designed for short-term. The process of inserting sutures as a form of securement requires multiple punctures through the skin creating an added risk of secondary local infection for the patient (Frey and Schears 2006). INS recommends avoidance of sutures or tape noting they are not as effective as securement devices and that sutures are associated with needlestick injuries, biofilm growth, and an increased risk of infection (Gorski et al. 2016). Research has shown manufactured devices such as adhesive securement to be equal to or better than sutures for stabilizing catheters. Rickard and colleagues (2016) performed a four-way randomized controlled trial looking at CVAD securement for 221 cardiac surgical patients (Rickard et al. 2016). The study looked at dressings/securement combinations:

- Suture + bordered polyurethane (BPU), the control = 2 (4%).
- Suture + gauze absorbent dressing = 1 (2%).
- Adhesive sutureless securement + simple polyurethane dressing (SPU) = 4 (7%).
- Tissue adhesive + SPD = 4 (17%) – stopped mid-trial.
- Suture + tissue adhesive + SPU = 0 (0%).

After CVAD dislodgement in the tissue adhesive + SPU arm, the researchers decided to cease randomization to this arm of the study and created a fifth arm for the remaining 30 patients that included suture + tissue adhesive + SPU. The results demonstrated combination approach to securement, and dressing had the best outcomes for those with sutures and dressing or adhesive securement and dressing.

The authors concluded that tissue adhesive and SPU were ineffective for CVAD securement in challenging post-cardiac patients, suture + tissue adhesive + SPU appeared promising with zero CVAD failure, and further research was required. Infection rates were not measured. The study illustrates the limitations a number of approaches to secure VADs and that perhaps the solutions for successful securement/dressings outcomes are as a result of using a number of methods, which when combined, provide more favorable outcomes.

9.10 Add-On Securement Devices

Safety release valves, as disposable tubing stop-check valves, can contribute to the reduction of catheter failure from dislodgement and provide increased patient safety by blocking blood or fluid flow whenever disconnection of the catheter occurs. Disconnection of tubing and dislodgement of catheters often occurs with normal patient activity. Add-on devices in the form of quick release valves may reduce catheter failure and provide a novel option for securement.

9.11 Impact of Inadequate Securement

Regardless of the type of vascular access device, a PIVC, midline, PICC, and non-tunneled or tunneled CVAD, dislodgement and premature removal can occur. Dislodgement or accidental removal can disrupt patient therapy, perhaps even contributing to exacerbation of medical conditions through treatment delays, this can create anxiety for patients who may need a replacement of a VAD and increase healthcare cost. Rickard et al. (2015) estimate that up to 69% of PIVC fail prior to treatment completion (Rickard et al. 2015). The most common reason for PIVC failure is due to infiltration or dislodgement (Royer 2003), and it is estimated that 10% simply fall out (Rickard et al. 2015). Ventura et al. (2016) quote dislodgement rates from 10.2 per 1000 cases in pretrial data and 0 per 1000 when trialing different methods of securement for midline catheters. Hughes et al. (2014) identified a PICC post-insertion misplacement rate was approximately 4.5%, based on 460 PICC insertions and an actual replacement rate of 21 PICCs using wound closure strips, adhesive sutureless securement device, and a semipermeable dressing (Hughes 2014). Lorente et al. (2004) reviewed accidental catheter removal including the rate of accidental catheter removal of non-tunneled CVADs, 2.02/100 catheter-days (Lorente et al. 2004). In a retrospective study looking at tunneled CVAD and PICC complications, Wong et al. (2015) identified a dislodgement/migration rate of 3 out of 29 PICCs (10.3%) versus the tunneled CVAD group of 4 out of 161 patients (2.4%) (Wong et al. 2015).

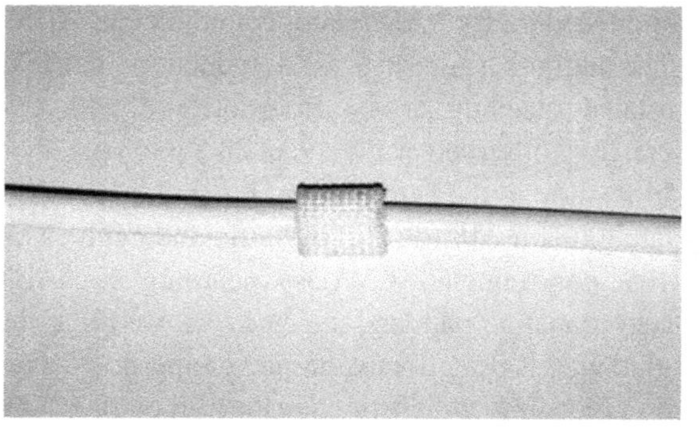

Fig. 9.4 Tunneled Dacron cuffed catheter (used with permission of S. Hill, Precision Vascular)

Even cuffed tunneled CVADs, where the patients' tissues engraft onto the cuff, are not completely resistant to dislodgement. The cuff, positioned approximately 1 cm within the insertion tract, becomes embedded into the tissues within weeks following insertion (Fig. 9.4). Until the cuff is fully secured, surgical glue or sutures and dressings may be used to aid securement and prevent infection. During those early weeks, before tissues have grafted onto the cuff, the catheter is as vulnerable to dislodgement as other non-cuffed devices. The catheter may be positioned under a dressing in a curved configuration that resists accidental pull of the catheter; the tension may be displaced by the curled catheter, thereby protecting the catheter cuff external migration. However, if the cuff is pulled out of the tissues and exposed (Simcock 2008), the catheter is no longer secured and resulting in distal CVAD tip migration.

Pistoning is the mechanical motion of the catheter in and out of the skin, which can lead to irritation of the intima of the vessel and over time potentially contribute to thrombotic changes (Macklin and Blackburn 2015). Macklin and

Blackburn (2015) elaborate particularly in respect to PICCs that "pistons" in the vein increase the possibility of phlebitis or infection. Rickard et al. (2018) explains the micro-motion is a phenomenon seen in PIVCs causing inflammation presenting with pain, swelling, occlusion, and infiltration and may increase infection (Rickard et al. 2018).

Ullman et al. (2015a, b) describe earlier methods to secure CVADs was to use simple tape or gauze. In the 1980s and 1990s, transparent dressings gained more prominence. When simple tape and gauze are used as a form of securement, the clinician's ability to inspect the site may be limited and visualization of the VAD site impaired until the dressing is changed. Next generation dressings that were transparent facilitated easier inspection of the site. Frasca et al. (2010) explains: "Because occlusive dressings trap moisture on the skin and provide an ideal environment for quick local microflora growth, these dressings for insertion sites must be permeable to water vapor" (Frasca et al. 2010). Webster et al. (2011) confirm this point in their Cochrane review; initial concerns were present that surface humidity may lead to infection. Dressings with vapor-permeable film are now used allowing moisture to pass through the dressing away from the skin while maintaining a water and contaminant barrier.

Dressing and securement devices are not free from adverse effects. Cutting (2008) suggests the repeated application and removal of adhesive tapes and dressings from the same site can cause damage to the skin by "skin stripping," namely, the removal of superficial stratum corneum, which can cause inflammation, skin reactions, edema, and soreness. Repeated dressing change within a short period of time may lead to changes in skin integrity, potentially causing damage, pain, increased costs, and incidence of skin colonization (Webster et al. 2011). Understanding and managing the effects of dressings/securement devices is multifaceted and can involve a multitude of single or combination of variables.

Ensuring adequate securement for VAD is a routine occurrence in many clinicians' everyday practice, but there are sometimes some unwanted side effects. Applying another layer upon the skin surface by using a dressing or securement occasionally leads to problematic skin reactions. The damage from reapplication and removal may not always be visible as superficial skin layers are damaged during this process. Skin injury is increased when the adhesive attachment to the skin is stronger than the cutaneous layers of the skin and their attachment to cells (McNichol et al. 2013).

A consensus summit was held of key opinion leaders in December 2012, specialists in dermatology, geriatrics, orthopedics, plastic surgery, and researchers in the panel providing guidance on the subject including assessment, prevention, and treatment of MARSI (McNichol et al. 2013). The specialist team defined MARSI as: "A medical adhesive–related skin injury is an occurrence in which erythema and/or other manifestation of cutaneous abnormality (including, but not limited to, vesicle, bulla, erosion, or tear) persists 30 minutes or more after removal of the adhesive."

Multiple factors that increase the likelihood of damage to the patient's skin when dressings and adhesive sutureless securement devices are applied to the skin are intrinsic or extrinsic (Fig. 9.5). The damage from reapplication and removal may not always be visible as superficial skin layers are damaged during this process. Intrinsic factors are patient-specific factors that influence the individual integrity of the skin such as topical infections, including eczema, dermatitis, or, for example, if the patient has been taking long-term steroidal therapy. Or there may be transient factors where the patient at particular point in time may be malnourished or dehydrated making their skin more fragile than in normal daily life. If the patient is receiving anticancer therapy and is immunosuppressed or has radiation treatment, these factors can lead to the fragility of the skin and its susceptibility to infections (McNichol et al. 2013). Increasing age is unfortunately not an ally to skin integrity, and an inverse relationship exists, as age increases, skin integrity eventually decreases. Mechanical changes also occur with age including reduced blood flow through reduced size of the vasculature, hydration is reduced, and inflammatory processes are enhanced (Cutting 2008). Aging

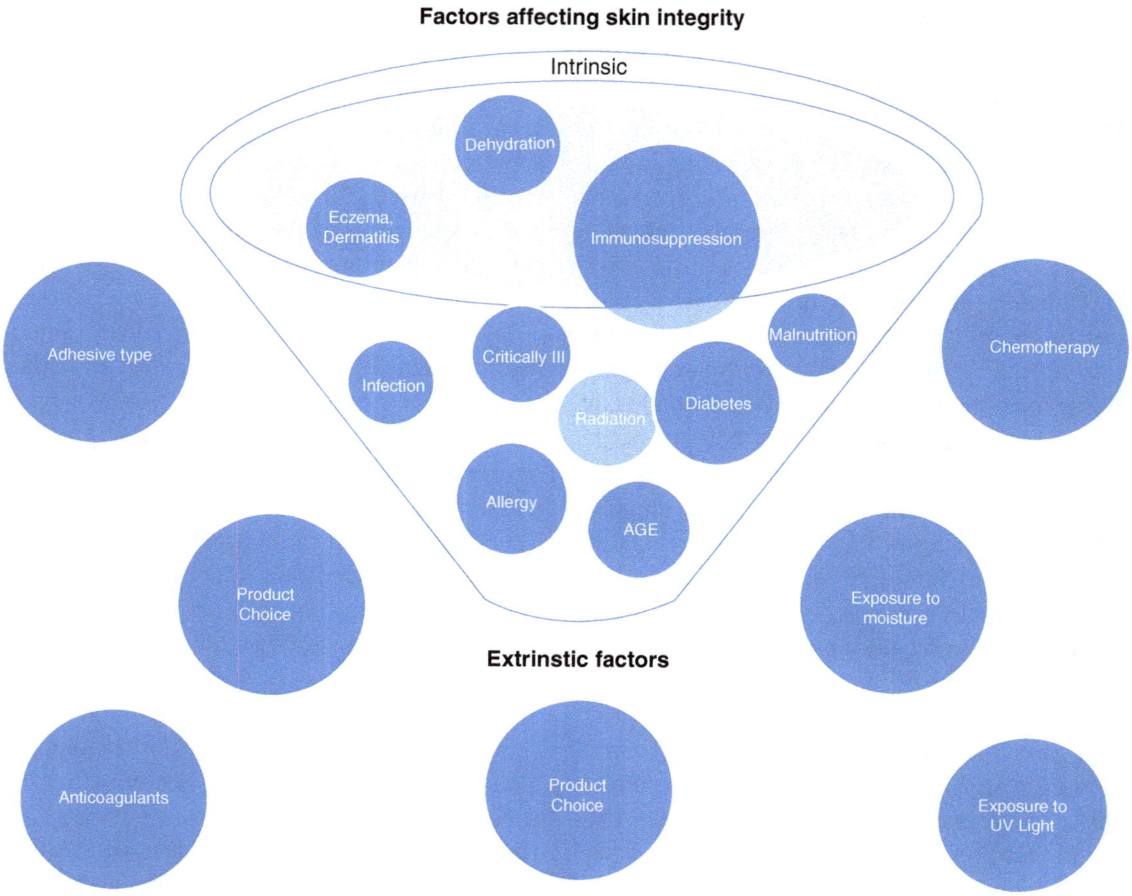

Fig. 9.5 Extrinsic factors for the skin and dressing securement. Modified from McNichol et al. (2013), understanding and guarding against medical adhesive-related skin injuries (MARSI) (Courtesy of 3M 2016)

affects the skin by loss of dermal matrix and subcutaneous tissue, reduced cohesion between dermal and epidermal layers and loss of elasticity (Thayer 2012). Enhanced inflammatory responses, reduction in cutaneous vessel size, and potentially neoplasms are increased the older we become; hydration and resiliency of skin are also intimately linked with age (Cutting 2008).

Extrinsic variables influence health of the skin, such as the prolonged exposure to moisture leading to maceration (Fig. 9.6) or application and removal technique (McNichol et al. 2013). The implications of using adhesive tapes and dressings on the skin can result in the superficial stratum corneum being removed with them, which Cutting (2008) describes as skin stripping. Medical adhesive can be pressure sensitive; increased application pressure increases the contact surface area that the dressing and adhesive has with the skin and may impact upon the superficial layers of skin when removal occurs. Thereby, increased pressure applied to the dressing increases the bond with the skin and may increase the damage to the skin upon removal.

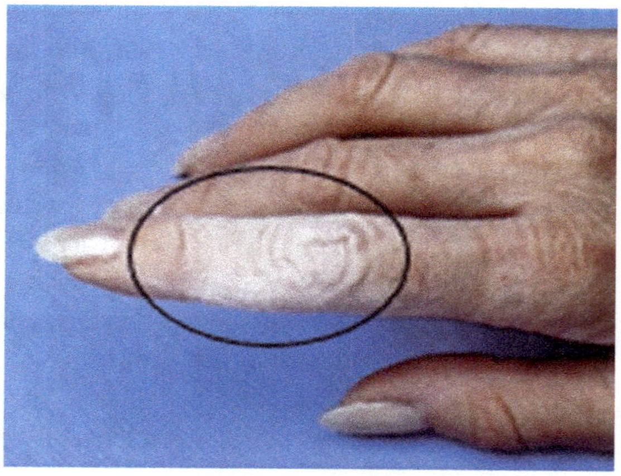

Fig. 9.6 Maceration from a saturated dressing (courtesy of 3M)

Skin assessment is an established part of healthcare, to check surgical site healing, avoiding dermatological conditions and by taking preventative measures such as the assessment of pressure related skin and tissue damage (Yue et al. 2014). Similarly, the assessment and monitoring of VAD sites is an integral part of many healthcare providers. Vascular access and infection prevention guidelines around the globe advocate the close monitoring of the vulnerable areas of the body where vascular devices break the protective barrier of the skin (Gorski et al. 2016; Loveday et al. 2014; Pittiruti et al. 2009; RCN 2016; RNAO 2008). The ongoing assessment and monitoring of the VAD insertion site is essential to detect any subtle changes that may indicate that the area has deteriorating skin integrity and could lead to infection or skin reactions. The VHP daily assessment tool (Fig. 9.7) advocates that the VAD site should be assessed regularly to ensure the device has not dislodged or is occluded and also to consider if the device is still appropriate and necessary. In some instances, changes in medical conditions or treatment therapy will indicate that an alternative VAD is appropriate (Hallam et al. 2016). VHP also promotes observation of the site for signs of leakage or infection and to assess this by using vascular access site scoring system, such as the VIP scoring system (Gorski et al. 2016; Jackson 1998). However, if we are to reduce and avoid incidence of MARSI, maceration, dermatitis, and other skin reactions, our assessment of VAD sites needs to be broader reaching in order to provide early detection of complications. Clinical practice should not solely focus upon signs of phlebitis and infection. We need to shift from practice being responsive and reactionary to problems related to dressings, securement, and VADs to a more proactive approach by employing a preventative approach. The aim should be to adopt a preventative healthcare culture with a holistic, comprehensive approach identifying patient-specific features and environmental and product-related factors that increase risk for patients while continuing to be vigilant monitoring, treating, and providing ongoing evaluation of VAD sight problems that may occur.

The success of a securement device can be judged on its durability and if it remains in place and supports the VAD and contributes to the device achieving its intended dwell time. Attention should also be given to how comfortable it is for the patient, how it affects the skin when applied and removed, and how user-friendly it is for the clinician to apply and remove (Ventura et al. 2016). A dressing should also provide protection against pathogens, allow visualization of the VAD site, be breathable, be comfortable for the patient, and be easy for the user to apply and remove.

Along with these desirable features we would choose for dressing and securement, selection should also be based upon its ability to reduce unwanted iatrogenic effects such as infection, skin irritation, and if the device achieves its intended dwell time.

Comprehensive patient assessment helps give the clinician insight into the individual vulnerabilities the patient may have and in turn inform the choice of dressing. Optimal dressing choice with consideration to the individual needs of the patient may increase the success of the dressing and/or securement and in turn minimize complications related the VAD being secured. Selection should be based upon the intended purpose, anatomical location, breathability, and flexibility, such as higher-risk areas like IJ (internal jugular) placement.

Consider high IJ placement of CVADs (Figs. 9.8 and 9.9), which is still common practice in many critical care settings. The weight of multiple IV infusions upon the catheter can pull and lift the dressing, releasing its contact from the skin and provide a route for pathogenic organisms to the CVAD site. There are alternative solutions to this problem, one is to avoid the high placement in the first instance by using a cannulation point at the lower aspect of the patient's neck or brachiocephalic access, allowing placement of the catheter upon the patient's clavicular/ upper pectoral area (discussed in Part III). Catheters in high IJ positions can lead to the problem of catheter drag, but there are alternate solutions. Not only is the appropriate dressing/ securement important but also the position of the patient, infusion pumps, tubing and that the tubing can move freely with the patient if conscious.

Daily Vessel Health Assessment Tool

Patient Medical ID #: ____________________ **Date:** ____ / ____ / ______
dd mm yyyy

Nursing Information

1. How comfortable is the patient with their vascular access device? (ask the patient)
   - ☐ 5 - Extremely comfortable
   - ☐ 4 - Somewhat comfortable
   - ☐ 3 - Comfortable
   - ☐ 2 - Somewhat uncomfortable
   - ☐ 1 - Very uncomfortable
   - ☐ N/A due to confusion /sedation or other ____________

   If #2 or #1 checked, please explain the reason for discomfort: ____________

2. What is the current device(s)? (check all that apply)

Type:	☐ PIV	☐ Midline	☐ PICC	☐ CVC	☐ Port	☐ Dialysis	
Number of Lumens	☐ 1	☐ 2	☐ 3	Which Device?		☐ PICC	☐ CVC
No. of Lumens in Use	☐ 1	☐ 2	☐ 3	Which Device?		☐ PICC	☐ CVC

3. What complications, if any occurred within the last 24 hours (PIV)? (check all that apply)
   - ☐ Infiltration ☐ Multiple restarts in 24 hrs
   - ☐ Phlebitis/thrombophlebitis ☐ Infection ☐ Other ____________

4. Did any complications occur within the last 24 hours with Central Venous Access Device(s)? ☐ Yes ☐ No
   If Yes, check all that apply. Which Device? ☐ PIV ☐ Midline ☐ PICC ☐ CVC ☐ Port ☐ Dialysis
   - ☐ Infection ☐ Phlebitis ☐ Occlusion
   - ☐ Partial Withdrawal Occlusion ☐ Thrombosis ☐ Other

5. Is this patient having any difficulty with eating and drinking? ☐ Yes ☐ No
6. Are there IV medications ordered other than PRN? ☐ Yes ☐ No
7. Is the VAD absolutely neccessary for blood draws with this patient? ☐ Yes ☐ No

Nursing Recommendation: **Print Name:** ____________ RN/NP/PA/IVRN (circle)

8. Referring to the VHP Right Line Tool is the Venous access device(s) most appropriate for the current treatment plan? ☐ Yes ☐ No
   If No, What device would apply based on Right Line Tool Selection? ____________
9. Is there any reason to maintain the current device(s)? ☐ Yes ☐ No
   If Yes, (other than the above reason) Why? ____________

RECOMMENDATIONS:
- ☐ Discontinue device(s) ☐ Maintain device(s)
- ☐ Consider new device(s) from VHP Assessment Trifold Recommended new device(s) ____________

Physician/Pharmacist Info: **Print Name:** ____________ MD/PharmD (circle)
(Information can be obtained by interview or by phone)

10. would switch to all oral medications be contraindicated at this time for this patient? ☐ Yes ☐ No
11. Is there an active blood stream infection? ☐ Yes ☐ No
12. Will access be required once the patient is released? ☐ Yes ☐ No
13. What is the current discharge plan? # of days left
14. Is the current IV device still necessary for this treatment plan and this patient? ☐ Yes ☐ No
    If Yes, please explain:
    - ☐ IV needed additional days Number of additional day(s) ____________
    - ☐ Critical condition ☐ Other ____________

MD Action Plan:
See nursing recommendation(s). If two or more NO answers, consider discontinuation of all IV devices to reduce risk to patient.

FINALACTION:
☐ Discontinue device(s) ☐ Maintain device(s) ________ # day(s)

For internal review: ☐ 25% ☐ 50% ☐ 75% ☐ 100%

Fig. 9.7 Daily assessment tool (used with permission of Teleflex)

As discussed, pathological/intrinsic factors and extrinsic factors (see Fig. 9.10) impact upon skin health can help mitigate the symptoms of MARSI, if we apply best practices and select the most appropriate dressings for the patient. INS guidelines suggest we should:

"Assess skin when the device is changed; anticipate potential risk for skin injury due to age, joint movement, and presence of edema" (Gorski et al. 2016) and that we should apply barrier solutions to skin exposed to the adhesive dressing to reduce the risk of MARSI (Gorski et al. 2016).

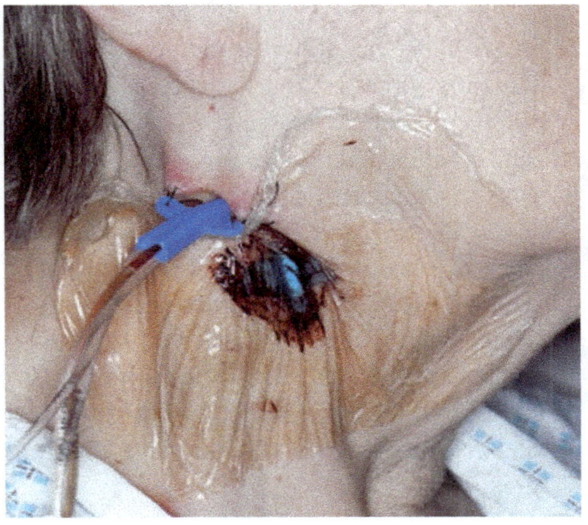

Fig. 9.8 Suture site with loose dressing and signs of infection (used with permission S. Hill, The Association for Safe Aseptic Practice (ASAP))

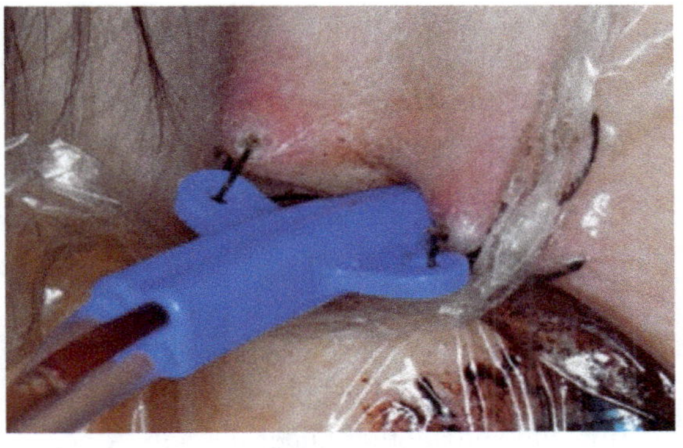

Fig. 9.9 Jugular Non-tunneled CVAD (used with permission S. Hill, The Association for Safe Aseptic Practice (ASAP))

Simply giving sufficient time for the skin to dry fully following cleaning prevents trapping moisture under the skin which can lead to dermatitis or maceration. Care should be taken not to overstretch the dressing and cause undue tension on the skin. Similarly, removal technique can result in unnecessary damage to the skin if done incorrectly. The skin must be supported as the dressing is being pulled back and continue to support the skin close to where it is being removed. Remove the dressing low and slow over itself in the direction of the hair growth and use medical adhesive remover if needed (McNichol et al. 2013) for vulnerable tissue and skin.

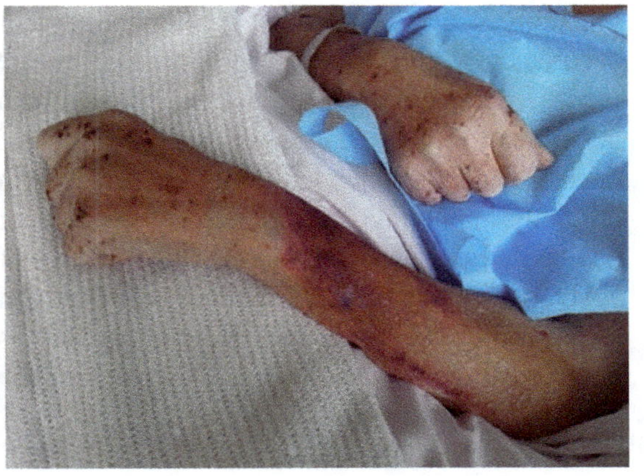

Fig. 9.10 Patient with aged skin and injury (used with permission S. Hill, The Association for Safe Aseptic Practice (ASAP))

When applying the dressing, ensure that undue pressure is not applied bearing in mind that many adhesives are pressure sensitive and increased adhesion occurs with increased pressure. Especially for the patient with a history of steroid medications and those with visibly thin, fragile skin special care should be given to application and removal. The pressure applied increases the skin surface area contact with the adhesive, and so greater pressure applied will increase the tension needed to remove the dressing and the stripping effect upon the patients' skin (McNichol et al. 2013). Optimal pressure must be applied to the individual needs of the patient, increased pressure may be appropriate for higher-risk areas such as IJ placements if skin integrity is sufficiently healthy, but a more sensitive application is required with patients with greater skin vulnerabilities. We cannot expect that we can exclude all risks of MARSI by solely focusing upon dressing choice, holistic assessment of the patient, and addressing risk factors by providing adequate nutrition, hydration, and balanced nutritional needs will all help to optimize patient outcomes.

9.12 Conclusion

Securement of VADs is a vital component to ensure patient safety through maximizing device dwell time and function while minimizing complications. Selecting the most appropriate form of securement with dressing type depends upon the device, the patient's previous experience with adhesives, the evidence supporting types of devices, and the knowledge of the clinician in correctly applying the selected securement device(s). Education is necessary in all phases of VAD management including the assessment and provision of dressings and securement and is essential to achieving the best outcomes in the VHP patient process.

Case Study

A young female patient in her 20s who was receiving chemotherapy for lymphoma. She was receiving this chemotherapy via a PICC secured with a standard polyurethane dressing with sutureless securement device plus sterile tapes. Some weeks into her treatment, she developed an allergy to the dressing. We discussed about dressing change frequency and general care and maintenance, to see if we could pick up anything from how it was being cared for that may have been contributing to the problems she was experiencing. However, she was being cared for by a very experienced team of hematology nurses who were seeing the patient once or twice a week, and the care being given was in line with hospital policy. We replaced the dressing with alternative polyurethane dressing and applied a sterile barrier film as to protect the skin from the adhesive and the dressing. We gave the patient the necessary information about looking out for increasing symptoms and to contact us at the earliest opportunity if there were any problems. The patient presented the next day with similar issues that she had experienced with the previous dressing and the medical/nursing team decided upon a pragmatic approach to identify the suitability of dressing for the patient and used small amounts of dressing from each of the available transparent, semipermeable dressings used in the hospital and placed them on the patient's forearm. The patient was monitored for an hour to see if there was any skin reaction and if the was one that did not cause a skin reaction. To the surprise of the team, all four came back having caused an allergic reaction to the skin. The team then decided to use sterile tape and gauze, supported with a tubular elasticated support; the patient had the PICC in for a further 2 months without infection or other complications and the reactions from the adhesive dressings resolved.

Case Study

A 75-year-old female was admitted to hospital for pneumonia and required an ultrasound-guided peripheral catheter (UGPIV) insertion due to difficult venous access and multiple failed attempts at PIVC placement. Following successful aseptic placement of the UGPIV, the clinician wanted to take special care to secure the catheter to prevent accidental dislodgement. The PIVC hub was secured with a small drop of tissue adhesive at the insertion site and another under the hub. A bordered transparent dressing applied on top of the insertion area with pressure applied to all edges to ensure proper adherence. Treatment with antibiotics continued for 5 days with no PIVC complications. Prior to discharge from hospital, the PIVC was inspected and removed. No skin irritation or other complications were noted.

Summary of Key Points

1. *Securement takes the form of a transparent dressing, tape, and gauze, advanced dressings with borders and adherent strips, manufactured adhesive securement platforms, anchoring or*

locking devices, tissue adhesives, subcutaneous securement, and sutures.

2. *Securement of VADs is a component necessary to promote complication free survival of a VAD.*
3. *Manufactured securement aids in reducing movement of the catheter stabilizing position and avoiding complications such as phlebitis, infection and dislodgement.*

References

Bausone-Gazda D, Lefaiver C, Walters S. A randomized controlled trial to compare the complications of 2 peripheral intravenous catheter-stabilization systems. J Infus Nurs. 2010;33:371–84.

Bugden S, Shean K, Scott M, Mihala G, Clark S, Johnstone C, Fraser JF, Rickard CM. Skin glue reduces the failure rate of emergency department–inserted peripheral intravenous catheters: a randomized controlled trial. Ann Emerg Med. 2016;68:196–201.

Cutting K. Impact of adhesive surgical tape and wound dressings on the skin, with reference to skin stripping. J Wound Care. 2008;17:157–62.

Dugger B, Macklin D, Rand B. Veni-gard (R) versus standard dressings on hemodynamic catheter sites. Dimens Crit Care Nurs. 1994;13:84–9.

Egan G, Siskin G, Weinmann R IV, Galloway M. A prospective postmarket study to evaluate the safety and efficacy of a new peripherally inserted central catheter stabilization system. J Infus Nurs. 2013;36:181–8.

Frasca D, Dahyot-Fizelier C, Mimoz O. Prevention of central venous catheter-related infection in the intensive care unit. Crit Care. 2010;14:212.

Frey A, Schears G. Why are we stuck on tape and suture? J Infus Nurs. 2006;29:34–8.

Gorski L, Hadaway L, Hagle M, Mcgoldrick M, Orr M, Doellman D. Infusion therapy: standards of practice (supplement 1). J Infus Nurs. 2016;39:S1–S159.

Hallam C, Weston V, Denton A, Hill S, Bodenham A, Dunn H, Jackson T. Development of the UK Vessel Health and Preservation (VHP) framework: a multi-organisational collaborative. J Infect Prev. 2016;17:65–72.

Hughes ME. Reducing PICC migrations and improving patient outcomes. Br J Nurs. 2014;23:S12–8.

Jackson A. Infection control—a battle in vein: infusion phlebitis. Nurs Times. 1998;94(68):71.

Jackson A. Retrospective comparative audit of two peripheral IV securement dressings. Br J Nurs. 2012;21:10–5.

Jeanes A, Martinez-Garcia G. Intravenous securement devices: an overview. Br J Healthcare Manag. 2016;22:488–92.

Keeler M, Haas BK, Northam S, Nieswiadomy M, McConnel C, Savoie L. Analysis of costs and benefits of transparent, gauze, or no dressing for a tunnelled central venous catheter in Canadian stem cell transplant recipients. Can Oncol Nurs J. 2015;25(3): 289–98.

Lorente L, Huidobro MS, Martín MM, Jiménez A, Mora ML. Accidental catheter removal in critically ill patients: a prospective and observational study. Crit Care. 2004;8:R229.

Loveday H, Wilson J, Pratt R, Golsorkhi M, Tingle A, Bak A, Browne J, Prieto J, Wilcox M. EPIC3: national evidence-based guidelines for preventing healthcare-associated infections in NHS Hospitals in England. J Hosp Infect. 2014;86:S1–70.

Macklin D, Blackburn P. Central venous catheter securement: using the Healthcare and Technology Synergy Model to take a close look. J Assoc Vasc Access. 2015;20:45–50.

Marsh N, Webster J, Flynn J, Mihala G, Hewer B, Fraser J, Rickard C. Securement methods for peripheral venous catheters to prevent failure: a randomized controlled pilot trial. J Vasc Access. 2015;16:237–44.

Mcnichol L, Lund C, Rosen T, Gray M. Medical adhesives and patient safety: state of the scienceconsensus statements for the assessment, prevention, and treatment of adhesive-related skin injuries. J Dermatol Nurs Assoc. 2013;5:323–38.

Moureau N, Poole S, Murdock M, Gray S, Semba C. Central venous catheters in home infusion care: outcomes analysis in 50,470 patients. J Vasc Interv Radiol. 2002;13:1009–16.

O'Grady N, Alexander M, Burns L, Dellinger E, Garland J, Heard S, Lipsett P, Masur H, Mermel L, Pearson M, Raad I, Randolph A, Rupp M, Saint S. Guidelines for the prevention of intravascular catheter-related infections. Center for Disease Control HICPAC Healthcare Infection Control Practices Advisory Committee: Guidelines for the prevention of intravascular catheter-related infections. Atlanta: Center for Disease Control and Prevention; 2011.

Oliver G, Jones M. ECG or X-ray as the 'Gold Standard' for establishing PICC-tip location? Br J Nurs. 2014;23(Suppl 19):S10–6. https://doi.org/10.12968/bjon.2014.23.Sup19.S10.

PICC Excellence. Online course manuals. In: Moureau N, editor. www.piccexcellence.com. Accessed Mar 2018.

Pittiruti M, Scoppettuolo G, Emoli A, Musarò A, Biasucci D. Cyanoacrylate glue and central venous access device insertion. J Assoc Vasc Access. 2016;21(4):249.

Pittiruti M, Scoppettuolo G. Gavecelt Manual of PICC and Midline: Indications, insertion, management, Italy, Edna S.p.A.; 2017.

Pittiruti M, Hamilton H, Biffi R, Macfie J, Pertkiewicz M. ESPEN guidelines on parenteral nutrition: central venous catheters (access, care, diagnosis and therapy of complications). Clin Nutr. 2009;28:365–77.

RCN. Standards for infusion therapy. 4th ed. London: Royal College of Nursing; 2016. p. 1–94.

Regalado S, Funaki B. Novel devices for wound closure in interventional radiology. Semin Intervent Radiol. 2008;25(01):058–64. © Thieme Medical Publishers.

Rickard CM, Marsh NM. Annals for hospitalists inpatient notes-the other catheter—the mighty peripheral IV. Ann Intern Med. 2017;167:HO2–3.

Rickard C, Mccann D, Munnings J, Mcgrail M. Routine resite of peripheral intravenous devices every 3 days did not reduce complications compared with clinically indicated resite: a randomised controlled trial. J BMC Med. 2010;8:53.

Rickard C, Webster J, Wallis M, Marsh N, Mcgrail M, French V, Foster L, Gallagher P, Gowardman J, Zhang L, Mcclymont A, Whitby M. Routine versus clinically indicated replacement of peripheral intravenous catheters: a randomised controlled equivalence trial. Lancet. 2012;380:1066–74.

Rickard CM, Marsh N, Webster J, Playford EG, Mcgrail MR, Larsen E, Keogh S, Mcmillan D, Whitty JA, Choudhury MA. Securing all intravenous devices effectively in hospitalised patients—the SAVE trial: study protocol for a multicentre randomised controlled trial. BMJ Open. 2015;5:e008689.

Rickard CM, Marsh N, Webster J, Runnegar N, Larsen E, Mcgrail MR, Fullerton F, Bettington E, Whitty JA, Choudhury MA. Dressings and securements for the prevention of peripheral intravenous catheter failure in adults (SAVE): a pragmatic, randomised controlled, superiority trial. Lancet. 2018;392(10145):419–30.

RNAO. Nursing Best Practice Guidelines: Assessment and Device Selection for Vascular Access. Nursing Best Practice Guidelines. Registered Nurses Association of Ontario; 2008.

Royer T. Improving short peripheral IV outcomes: a clinical trial of two securement methods. J Assoc Vasc Access. 2003;8:1–5.

Scoppettuolo G, Dolcetti L, Emoli A, La Greca A, Biasucci D, Pittiruti M. Further benefits of cyanoacrylate glue for central venous catheterisation. Anaesthesia. 2015;70:758.

Shivnan J, Mcguire D, Freedman S, Sharkazy E, Bosserman G, Larson E, Grouleff P. A comparison of transparent adherent and dry sterile gauze dressings for long-term central catheters in patients undergoing bone marrow transplant. Oncol Nurs Forum. 1991;18(8):1349–56.

Simcock L. No going back: advantages of ultrasound-guided upper arm PICC placement. J Assoc Vasc Access. 2008;13(4):191–7. https://doi.org/10.2309/java.13-4-6.

Simonova G, Rickard C, Dunster K, Smyth D, Mcmillan D, Fraser J. Cyanoacrylate tissue adhesives—effective securement technique for intravascular catheters: in vitro testing of safety and feasibility. Anaesth Intensive Care. 2012;40:460–6.

Smith B. Peripheral intravenous catheter dwell times: a comparison of securement methods for implementation of a 96-h scheduled change protocol. J Infus Nurs. 2006;29:14–7.

Thayer D. Skin damage associated with intravenous therapy: common problems and strategies for prevention. J Infus Nurs. 2012;35:390–401.

Ullman A, Cooke M, Mitchell M, Lin F, New K, Long D, Mihala G, Rickard C. Dressings and securement devices for central venous catheters (CVC). Cochrane Database Syst Rev. 2015a;(9):CD010367.

Ullman A, Cooke M, Rickard C. Examining the role of securement and dressing products to prevent central venous access device failure: a narrative review. J Assoc Vasc Access. 2015b;20:99–110.

Ventura R, O'Loughlin C, Vavrik B. Clinical evaluation of a securement device used on midline catheters. Br J Nurs. 2016;25:S16–22.

Webster J, Gillies D, O'Riordan E, Sherriff K, Rickard C. Gauze and tape and transparent polyurethane dressings for central venous catheters. Cochrane Database Syst Rev. 2011;(11):CD003827.

Wong W, Chan W, Ip S, Ng W, Chan C, Ho H, Siu K, Tan C. Infection rate of Hickman catheters versus peripherally inserted central venous catheters in oncology patients. Hong Kong J Radiol. 2015;18:197–204.

Yamamoto A, Solomon J, Soulen M, Tang J, Parkinson K, Lin R, Schears G. Sutureless securement device reduces complications of peripherally inserted central venous catheters. J Vasc Interv Radiol. 2002;13:77–81.

Yue J, Tabloski P, Dowal SL, Puelle MR, Nandan R, Inouye SK. NICE to HELP: operationalizing National Institute for Health and Clinical Excellence guidelines to improve clinical practice. J Am Geriatr Soc. 2014;62:754–61.

Zerla P, Canelli A, Cerne L, Caravella G, Gilardini A, De Luca G, Aricisteanu A, Venezia R. Evaluating safety, efficacy, and cost-effectiveness of PICC securement by subcutaneously anchored stabilization device. J Vasc Access. 2017;18(3):238–42.

Part IV

Prevention of Infections

10

Avoiding Infections Due to Insertion through Vascular Access Devices

Michelle DeVries

Abstract

The goal of vascular access devices is to provide for the administration of the therapies required to help the patient recover while causing the least amount of damage to the patient's vascular system. One of the ways to preserve patient vasculature is through the prevention of infections associated with these devices. The central line bundle, created by Peter Pronovost in a landmark study known as the keystone study in Michigan, consists of five components that, when strictly adhered to during the insertion of a central line catheter, are known to reduce the risk of catheter-related BSIs. The five components include hand hygiene, maximal barrier precautions during insertion, use of chlorhexidine as a skin antisepsis, optimal catheter site selection with avoidance of the femoral vein for central venous access in adult patients, and daily review of line necessity with prompt removal of unnecessary lines. These five components to prevent infection during the insertion of a central catheter are reviewed within this chapter. Care and maintenance considerations, equally important in the prevention of infection, are covered in detail throughout the rest of this book.

M. DeVries (✉)
Methodist Hospitals, Gary, IN, USA

Menzies Health Research Institute—Alliance for Vascular Access Teaching and Research (AVATAR) Group, Griffith University, Brisbane, QLD, Australia
e-mail: infectionprevention@comcast.net

Keywords

CVAD infection prevention · Central line bundle · Personal protective equipment · Site selection · Device necessity

10.1 Introduction

A monumental amount of attention has been devoted to preventing infections during the insertion phase of a vascular catheter's life cycle. The very act of breaking the skin barrier and inserting a medical device directly through the vein wall and into the blood stream deserves special attention, as the patient's natural infection prevention barriers have been disrupted. Defining key infection prevention elements during the insertion of a central catheter (known as the central line bundle) and monitoring adherence to these elements has resulted in tremendously positive results; knowledge of and adherence to these protocols has become a core expectation for all healthcare environments (APIC 2015; The Joint Commission 2012). Due to the positive impact sustained by adhering to the central line bundle, these core elements (hand hygiene, maximal barrier precautions during insertion, use of chlorhexidine as a skin antisepsis, optimal catheter site selection with avoidance of the femoral vein for central venous access in adult patients, daily review of line necessity with prompt removal of unnecessary lines) deserve further review and understanding.

10.2 Hand Hygiene

Since the days of Ignaz Semmelweis, hand hygiene has been a fundamental part of any infection prevention strategy (WHO 2009). Hand washing is the cornerstone to aseptic technique practiced by all medical professionals to decrease the risk of bacterial contamination and the transmission of microbes from patient to patient (PICC Excellence 2018).

The procedure for washing hands (Fig. 10.1) prior to insertion of a vascular access device or any invasive procedure as recommended by the World Health Organization is as follows (WHO 2015):

With Soap and Water:

1. Wet hands with water.
2. Apply enough soap to cover all hand surfaces.
3. Rub hands palm to palm.
4. Rub right palm over left dorsum with fingers interlaced. Repeat on other side.
5. Rub hands palm to palm with fingers interlaced.
6. Rub back of fingers to opposing palms with fingers interlocked.
7. Perform rotational rubbing of left thumb clasped in right palm and vice versa.
8. Perform rotational rubbing, backward and forward, with clasped fingers of right hand in left palm and vice versa.

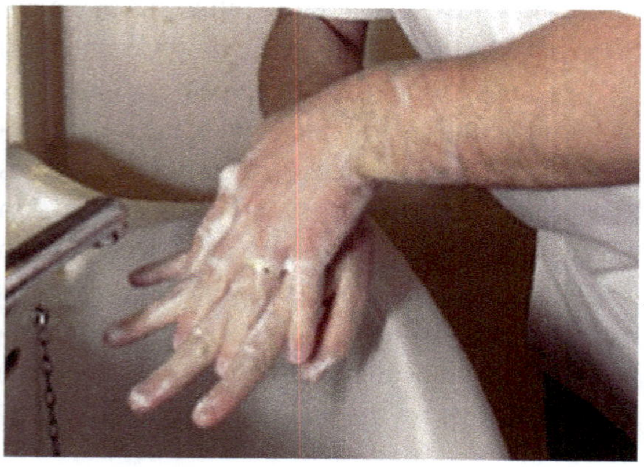

Fig. 10.1 Handwashing procedure. Used with permission N. Moureau PICC Excellence

9. Rinse hands thoroughly under running water.
10. Use clean paper towel to dry hands. Do not wave hands or blow on skin to dry.
11. Turn off faucet using same paper towel.

Alcohol-based waterless cleansing foam is extremely effective at reducing hand pathogens and can be used for intermittent hand cleansing in place of soap and water when hands are not visibly soiled (O'Grady et al. 2011b; Gorski et al. 2016).

Hand Rub Procedure (WHO 2015):

1. Apply a palm full of product in cupped hand and cover all surfaces.
2. Rub hands palm to palm.
3. Rub right palm over left dorsum with fingers interlaced and vice versa.
4. Rub hands palm to palm with fingers interlaced.
5. Rub backs of fingers to opposing palms with fingers interlocked.
6. Perform rotational rubbing of left thumb clasped in right palm and vice versa.
7. Perform rotational rubbing, backwards and forwards with clasped fingers of right hand in left palm and vice versa.
8. Allow to air-dry. Once dry, your hands are ready for your gloves.

Soap and water cleansing is still necessary after caring for patients who have *Clostridium difficile* as these spores are not susceptible to alcohol-based waterless cleansers (Gorski et al. 2016). Clostridium difficile has recently been renamed/reclassified as *Clostridiodes difficile.*

To protect the caregiver as well as the patient, gloves are used any time the hands will encounter blood or bodily fluids, or other potential pathogens, or when patients are on isolation precautions. Gloves are applied after hand hygiene has been performed, and hygiene is performed again following glove removal.

A summary of when handwashing/hand hygiene should occur and as well as hand hygiene requirements and recommendations according to each of the frequently referenced guidelines specific to vascular access is included

Table 10.1 Handwashing requirements and recommendations per guidance publications

SHEA Compendium (Marschall et al. 2014)	• Perform hand hygiene prior to catheter insertion or manipulation • Use an alcohol-based waterless product or antiseptic soap and water • Use of gloves does not obviate hand hygiene
Guidelines for the Prevention of Intravascular Catheter-Related Infections (O'Grady et al. 2011a)	• Perform hand hygiene procedures, either by washing hands with conventional soap and water or with alcohol-based hand rubs (ABHR) • Handwashing should be performed before and after palpating catheter insertion sites as well as before and after inserting, replacing, accessing, repairing, or dressing an intravascular catheter. Palpation of the insertion site should not be performed after the application of antiseptic, unless aseptic technique is maintained
EPIC3 (Loveday et al. 2014)	• Decontaminate hands and wear a new pair of clean non-sterile gloves before manipulating each patient's catheter. Decontaminate hands immediately following the removal of gloves • When decontaminating hands using an alcohol-based hand rub, hands should be free of dirt and organic material, and hand rub solution must come into contact with all surfaces of the hand; hands should be rubbed together vigorously, paying particular attention to the tips of the fingers, the thumbs, and the areas between the fingers, until the solution has evaporated, and the hands are dry
CDC Hand Hygiene Guidelines (2002) (Prevention 2002)	• When hands are visibly dirty or contaminated with proteinaceous material or are visibly soiled with blood or other body fluids, wash hands with either a non-antimicrobial soap and water or an antimicrobial soap and water • If hands are not visibly soiled, use an alcohol-based hand rub or an antimicrobial soap and water for routinely decontaminating hands in all other clinical situations • Decontaminate hands before donning sterile gloves when inserting a central intravascular catheter • Decontaminate hands before inserting indwelling urinary catheters, peripheral vascular catheters, or other invasive devices that do not require a surgical procedure • Decontaminate hands after removing gloves
INS Standards of Practice(Gorski et al. 2016)	• Perform hand hygiene with an alcohol-based hand rub or antimicrobial soap and water during patient care – Before having direct contact with the patient – Before donning sterile gloves when inserting a central intravascular catheter – Before inserting a peripheral vascular catheter – After contact with the patient's intact or non-intact skin – After contact with body fluids or excretions, mucous membranes, and wound dressings (if the hands are not visibly soiled) – After contact with inanimate objects (including medical equipment) in the immediate vicinity of the patient – After removing gloves • Use an alcohol-based hand rub routinely when performing hand hygiene unless the hands are visibly soiled, or there is an outbreak of a spore-forming pathogen or norovirus gastroenteritis
WHO Five Moments for Hand Hygiene (WHO 2009)	• Wash hands only when visibly soiled; otherwise hand rub • Hand rub before patient contact, before inserting catheters, after risk of exposure to bodily fluids, after patient contact, and after contact with patient surroundings

in Table 10.1. Regardless of which guideline is followed, handwashing compliance is essential for the prevention of infections during the insertion and manipulation of any vascular access device. A framework for monitoring and reporting handwashing compliance as it relates to vascular access insertions and manipulations is essential to patient safety and should be included in all infection control and vascular access programs.

10.3 Maximal Barrier Precautions

The purpose of maximal sterile barrier precautions is to establish an aseptic barrier minimizing the passage of microorganisms from non-sterile to sterile areas. Central venous catheter procedures are to be treated as surgical procedures, using maximum sterile full-body drapes, taking special care in the application of gloves and immediately managing any episodes of contamination. Maximal barriers include (Marschall et al. 2014):

- Non-sterile caps and masks
- Sterile gown
- Sterile gloves
- Sterile large full-body drapes

The clinician wears the gown, cap, gloves, and mask to protect the patient from the clinician's microorganisms, and the patient is covered in full-body drapes to protect the patient from having his own microorganisms or bed microorganisms move from non-treated areas into areas that have been cleaned in an aseptic manner.

10.3.1 Sterile Gown

The sterile gown is used as part of the insertion procedure to prevent the transfer of microbes from the clinician to the patient, reducing the risk of infection. The sterile gown, which should be donned prior to donning sterile gloves, is folded so that the clinician can don the gown in a manner that maintains sterility. The clinician slips hands through the armholes and moves the arms in an outward motion, being careful not to touch any non-sterile items in the area. The gown unfolds, covering the clinician's arms and shoulders. An assistant can then grasp the strings and tie the gown behind the clinician's neck. To avoid contamination of the sleeves, hands should not be put through the sleeves and out the open end of the gown; keep cuffs of gown well over hands. Once gown is on and tied, it is time to don the sterile gloves.

10.3.2 Gloves

Gloves are required for all intravascular insertion procedures. According to the CDC and INS, sterile gloves are to be worn for the insertion of all arterial, central venous and midline catheters (Gorski et al. 2016; O'Grady et al. 2011a). Requirement for the use of sterile versus non-sterile gloves for peripheral intravenous catheter (PIVC) insertions is in a period of evolution. The CDC recommendations indicate that clean gloves for the insertion of PIVC, but sterile gloves if the site is re-palpated (O'Grady et al. 2011a). INS standards specify the use of a new pair of disposable, non-sterile gloves for peripheral intravenous insertions if Standard-ANTT is being used (no re-palpation of the site after asepsis) throughout the insertion procedure but suggests increased attention to aseptic technique and consideration of sterile gloves, as well as contamination concerns with the use of clean versus sterile gloves (Gorski et al. 2016).

10.3.3 How to Don Sterile Gloves

Donning sterile gloves requires a specific technique and some preparation. The following procedure is recommended (PICC Excellence 2018):

1. Open the sterile pack prior to donning gown so that the gloves can be accessed easily. The gloves are folded and cuffed exposing the inner glove so that the outer glove is not touched by the hand.
2. Grasp the cuff of one glove with the fingertips of the opposite hand which is still covered by the sterile gown sleeve. This way, only the sterile gown touches the sterile glove.
3. Slip hand into glove and pull the cuff over to unroll glove and cover hand and sleeve cuff.
4. Using the gloved hand, open the second glove from underneath the cuff allowing the sterile glove to touch the sterile portion of the second glove; slide second hand into glove and unfold to cover hand and sleeve cuff.

Important tips (PICC Excellence 2018):

1. Always overlap sterile gown with glove cuffs.
2. It is essential to avoid touching non-sterile items once sterile gloves are applied; the hands and fingers may be kept interlaced and in front of you at or above waist level to avoid inadvertent contamination.

3. When clean gloves are used there is also potential for contamination by touching environmental surfaces prior to handling insertion supplies. Change clean gloves immediately before an invasive procedure such as VAD insertion.
4. Refrain from adjusting the mask or scratching the nose once sterile gloves are in place.
5. Any break or tear in the sterile gloves or touching the sterile glove to a non-sterile surface requires immediate removal with gown cuffs pulled down and application of new sterile gloves.

Audits may be performed to not only assess the appropriate application and use of gloves but also provide a more careful review of glove usage including considerations such as maintaining sterility and changing gloves when contaminated.

10.3.4 Sterile Drapes

A full-body sterile drape is placed on the patient to minimize the movement of microorganisms into the site selected for the catheter insertion procedure and to prevent contamination of the catheter prior to insertion into the bloodstream by allowing it to touch only the sterile surface of the full-body drape. Once the sterile drape is positioned, it is not moved or rearranged. Keep in mind that once a patient is draped, only the top surface of the draped area is considered sterile. Areas where skin is exposed, such as with a fenestration, should be skin adherent to avoid contamination from un-prepped skin. Exposed skin, regardless of prepping, remains a source of contamination. Do not touch skin with gloved hands or with the catheter.

10.4 Patient Skin Preparation

Skin preparation using chlorhexidine is another step in the central line bundle known to reduce the risk of infection. Two distinct steps must be performed prior to penetrating the skin barrier for the insertion of a vascular access device: the skin at and near the insertion site must be cleaned of any visible soil, and the insertion site must be prepared with an antiseptic agent (Gorski et al. 2016).

Many clinicians choose to cleanse the skin with soap and water or a skin cleansing wipe or other product formulation (Garland et al. 1995). This may help reduce the bioburden and the risk of inactivation of the antimicrobial solution if proteinaceous materials are present. However, a large French study failed to identify a difference in infection rates when a detergent cleansing was added prior to application of the antiseptic agent (Mimoz et al. 2015).

Chlorhexidine bathing is effective in reducing the bioload on the body especially when the chlorhexidine is applied without rinsing. Routine bathing of patients with chlorhexidine results in reduction of CLABSI. Randomized trials, meta-analyses, and guideline recommendations provide a strong basis for this practice (Timsit et al. 2018).

10.5 Appropriate Skin Decontamination

Once the skin is cleaned, it is ready to be prepared with an antiseptic. While alcohol and betadine offer some antimicrobial benefit, chlorhexidine gluconate (CHG) has become the standard for skin preparation prior to IV insertions for patients greater than 2 months old. According to the label, CHG must be used with caution in children less than 2 months of age. Commercially available preparations of CHG are combined with alcohol to achieve rapid kill as well as persistence. Early studies strongly supported the use of CHG over povidone-iodine for skin preparations (Maki et al. 1994). The CDC recommends >0.5% chlorhexidine (CHG) with 70% alcohol as the antiseptic of choice (O'Grady et al. 2011a). A recent study by McCann et al. did not find a statistically significant improvement in CLABSI rates when increasing CHG to 2% in alcohol over more routinely used concentrations (McCann et al. 2016). While no agent can completely rid the skin of every microorganism, CHG is proven to be effective over the most common infecting microbes. Chlorhexidine is recommended both for its broad-spectrum action on bacteria, viruses, and fungi and its residual effect. CHG provides continual residual killing action for 48–72 h after application. Label claims vary per formulation, but at least one product now has a label claim for a 7-day kill which may offer some benefits (Healthcare 2017).

With all products, understanding appropriate use requires careful reading of instructions prior to use. Each comes with specific instructions regarding appropriate application method, duration of scrub time and necessary dry time based on volume of product used and anatomical location. Ensuring that products are applied appropriately is a significant consideration that likely does not receive enough attention during process monitoring (Casey et al. 2017).

In general, the widely available skin disinfection products in the US market promote a frictional back and forth method of application using pressure as described below (Silva 2014):

Use the following technique to cleanse the catheter insertion site prior to catheter placement:

1. Apply antiseptic solution using a frictional back and forth motion until all applicator solution is used.
2. Allow antiseptic solution to air-dry (do not blow or blot dry).

Because chlorhexidine with alcohol dries much faster, it reduces the likelihood that the catheter will be inserted before bacteria have died. Regardless of the product selected, ensuring that the product has dried completely prior to application of the transparent dressing minimizes the risk of skin irritation.

10.6 Ultrasound

When ultrasound is used as part of the insertion process, the device's cleanliness and disinfection procedures need to be ascertained. For central and midline placement, the use of sterile gel and sterile probe cover during the insertion procedure is a standard practice. As with all medical equipment, cleaning and disinfection must follow manufacturer's recommendations and accepted infection control standards. Delicate transducers may require products that are not routinely used in the organization. If non-sterile gel is used during the initial assessment, ensure that single use sterile packets are available for use during the insertion procedure. Ensure that maintenance of non-sterile versus sterile gels is consistent with recommended practices to reduce inadvertent contamination (Oleszkowicz et al. 2015).

The Association for Vascular Access (AVA) published Guidance on Transducer Disinfection that established the need to develop processes for transducer (probe) cleaning in conjunction with patient use, validation of clinician training, and use of commercially manufactured sheath for all patient-based activities that involve contact with blood/body fluids or non-intact skin, evaluate outcomes, and document performance and training (Association for Vascular Access 2018). Programs should also review recommendations for frequency of probe cable and unit disinfection beyond just the transducer, as contamination of these surfaces is also noted as a significant concern.

For ultrasound-guided PIVC insertion, clinicians have found success with varying levels of ANTT. Be aware of facility policies which dictate the frequency of cleaning the entire surfaces of equipment (not just the probe) particularly when caring for patients in isolation precautions. For the infection control considerations of this chapter, ultrasound may also have additional impact by decreasing the number of attempts necessary to gain access.

10.7 Site Selection

The selected site for catheter placement is a result of many factors including (Gorski et al. 2016):

- Risk consideration based on knowledge of skin flora concentrations (arm veins versus femoral)
- Diagnosis (how long will the catheter be in use)
- Therapy (what kind of infusions are required)
- Vessel health and size (looking for straight, non-stenosed, bouncy, large veins)
- Age of patient (infant vs. adult)
- Length of time treatment required

Some areas of insertion, such as the neck or femoral area, are prone to higher infection rates than other sites (arm) due to high microbial counts, humidity, and difficulty in dressing adherence. These factors must be taken into consideration when selecting and disinfecting an insertion site. For example, the femoral site is generally avoided due to its heavy colonization; however, a more recent review article suggests that the risk of infection from this site may no longer be as disparate from other locations (Marik et al. 2012) as originally believed.

Tunneling a CVAD to an area of greater safety may improve outcomes as in the case of mid-thigh femoral vein insertion. Moving an insertion location from the groin, axilla, or neck onto the leg, mid-upper arm, or chest, respectively, improves the ability to maintain transparent dressing adherence, reduces contamination caused by dressing disruption, and moves the insertion location onto a more secure and stable platform.

When the internal jugular vein is selected, care must be given for optimal placement to allow for maintenance of an intact dressing, which may require updated insertion practices. An intact dressing provides an important barrier to microbial transmission. Understanding the importance of an intact dressing helps the inserter when considering various options for insertion site location.

The location of a PIVC can impact outcomes and failure rates. For peripheral devices, there has been much published in support of the use of the forearm as the preferred insertion site to promote longer dwell time; decrease pain, phlebitis, infiltration, and dislodgement; and facilitate patient self-care (Fields et al. 2012; Gorski et al. 2016; Wallis et al. 2014). Insertion in the forearm creates a stable location for securement and dressing. There are considerations for other locations and the ability to maintain an intact dressing such as present with devices located in the hand or antecubital fossa.

Careful assessment of specific anatomical characteristics along the vein path allows for planning of optimal needle insertion or exit site to minimize the risk related to ongoing care and maintenance of the device. This pre-insertion assessment should include an external visual inspection looking for optimal access sites (e.g., away from areas of flexion or skin irritation/compromise) and an internal inspection with use of ultrasound to determine vein path and health. The goal with any distal catheter tip placement is to maximize three factors.

10.8 Daily Review of Line Necessity

The most effective way to prevent catheter-related BSI is to simply not have a catheter. As basic as this sounds, it is paramount to infection prevention. As soon as the catheter is no longer medically necessary, it should be removed. While this is a recommendation by many healthcare groups and authors, establishing a policy and process with measured staff compliance for daily review is rare.

When performing daily assessment on a patient with a catheter, consider the following questions:

- Is the catheter still necessary for treatment of this patient or just convenient (don't retain for convenience such as periodic blood draws)?
- Can the patient be switched to a peripheral IV or to oral medications?
- Are there any catheter-related complications?
- Are there alternative therapies that could be used that would allow for the removal of the line?
- Is therapy completed or being discontinued?
- Is the patient satisfied and comfortable with the current delivery of medications?

The goal of vascular access devices is to provide for the administration of the therapies required to help the patient recover while causing the least amount of damage to the patient's vascular system. As soon as it is determined that the vascular access device is no longer medically necessary, it should be removed from the patient.

10.9 Use of Insertion Checklists and Observers

It is recommended that an observer be present during any central venous catheter (CVC) insertion procedure to ensure aseptic technique is maintained throughout the procedure (O'Grady et al. 2011a). The Society for Healthcare Epidemiology of America (SHEA) recommendations state, "CVC insertion should be observed by a nurse, physician or other healthcare personnel who has received appropriate education, is certified to perform the procedure and has received education in aseptic technique to ensure that aseptic technique is maintained" (Marschall et al. 2014). "This observer should be empowered to stop the procedure if breaches in aseptic technique are observed." Following a checklist during a central vascular insertion procedure has such a profound effect on patient safety that in 2013, the Agency for Healthcare Research and Quality named "bundles that include checklists to prevent central line-associated bloodstream infection (CLABSI)" one of the top 10 "strongly encouraged patient safety practices" (Chopra et al. 2013).

While specific procedures in aseptic technique have proven to reduce the risk of CLABSIs (central line bundle created by Peter Pronovost in the keystone study in Michigan (Pronovost et al. 2006)), without adherence to these practices, CLABSIs will continue to be a problem in healthcare facilities (Fig. 10.2). The purpose of an observer is not only to remind and affirm the use of ANTT through the use of a central line insertion procedure (CLIP) checklist (Fig. 10.3) but also to hold the inserter accountable to aseptic procedures during the insertion process (CDC and NHSN 2016). The observer follows a procedure checklist or CLIP form as established by the facility and is responsible to check off each step as the inserter performs each required protocol. Adherence to protocol is a must in the reduction of central line infections.

The use of CLIP was introduced with the expectation that it would be completed by a trained observer (ideally empowered to stop the procedure in the event of a breach in sterile technique). There is some concern with the nursing insertion teams at times being staffed without the ability to have a trained observer. Expert consensus is that it is not ideal to assess one's own compliance with Surgical-ANTT; expanding practice to allow a trained observer to be present is in the best interest of patient safety (of note, this need not be another vascular access nurse or even another registered nurse but can be accomplished by another staff member with adequate training). Work continues to be published evaluating the impact of care bundles and checklists as effective means to improve outcomes (Blot et al. 2014).

Although not as commonplace with peripheral devices, there are precedents for the use of PIVC insertion and maintenance bundles. In the United Kingdom, the Saving Lives campaign gave consideration to both aspects of PIVC insertion and management including the provision of audit tools to assess bundle compliance (Slyne et al. 2012). In Spain, researchers reported improved outcomes after establishing bundles focused on reducing phlebitis and infection related to peripheral devices (Mestre et al. 2013). In the United States, the concept of an insertion and maintenance bundle (Table 10.2) was successfully used when adopting a policy to allow longer dwell of short peripheral catheters (DeVries et al. 2016; Devries and Valentine 2016).

Checklist for Prevention of Central Line Associated Blood Stream Infections

Based on 2011 CDC guideline for prevention of intravascular catheter-associated bloodstream infections:
https://www.cdc.gov/infectioncontrol/guidelines/bsi/index.html
Strategies to Prevent Central Line–Associated Bloodstream Infections in Acute Care Hospitals: 2014 Update
http://www.jstor.org/stable/10.1086/676533

For Clinicians:

Follow proper insertion practices

☐ Perform hand hygiene before insertion.
☐ Adhere to aseptic technique.
☐ Use maximal sterile barrier precautions (i.e., mask, cap, gown, sterile gloves, and sterile full body drape).
☐ Choose the best insertion site to minimize infections and noninfectious complications based on individual patient characteristics.
- Avoid femoral site in obese adult patients.

☐ Prepare the insertion sitewith >0.5% chlorhexidine with alcohol.
☐ Place a sterile gauze dressing or a sterile, transparent, semipermeable dressing over the insertion site.
☐ For patients 18 years of age or older, use a chlorhexidine impregnated dressing with an FDA cleared label that specifies a clinical indication for reducing CLABSI for short term non-tunneled catheters unless the facility is demonstrating success at preventing CLABSI withbaseline prevention practices.

Handle and maintain central lines appropriately

☐ Comply with hand hygiene requirements.
☐ Bathe ICU patients over 2 months of age with a chlorhexidine preparation on a daily basis.
☐ Scrub the access port or hub with friction immediately prior to each use with an appropriate antiseptic (chlorhexidine, povidone iodine, an iodophor, or 70% alcohol).
☐ Use only sterile devices to access catheters.
☐ Immediately replace dressings that are wet, soiled, or dislodged.
☐ Perform routine dressing changes using aseptic technique with clean or sterile gloves.
- Change gauze dressings at least every two days or semipermeable dressings at least every seven days.
- For patients 18 yearsof age or older, use a chlorhexidine impregnated dressing with an FDA cleared label that specifies a clinical indication for reducing CLABSIfor short-term non-tunneled catheters unless the facility is demonstrating success at preventing CLABSI with baseline prevention practices.

☐ Change administrations sets for continuous infusions no more frequently than every 4 days, but at least every 7 days.
- If blood or blood products or fat emulsions are administered change tubing every 24 hours.
- If propofol is administered, change tubing every 6-12 hours or when the vial is changed.

Promptly remove unnecessary central lines

☐ Perform daily audits to assess whether each central line is still needed.

For Healthcare Organizations:

☐ Educate healthcare personnel about indications for central lines, proper procedures for insertion and maintenance, and appropriate infection prevention measures.
☐ Designate personnel who demonstrate competency for the insertion and maintenance of central lines.
☐ Periodically assess knowledge of and adherence to guidelines for all personnel involved in the insertion and maintenance of central lines.
☐ Provide a checklist to clinicians to ensure adherence to aseptic insertion practices.
☐ Reeducate personnel at regular intervals about central line insertion, handling and maintenance,and whenever related policies, procedures, supplies, or equipment changes.
☐ Empower staff to stop non-emergent insertion if proper procedures are not followed.
☐ Ensure efficient access to supplies for central line insertion and maintenance (i.e. create a bundle with all needed supplies).
☐ Use hospital-specific or collaborative-based performance measures to ensure compliance with recommended practices.

Supplemental strategies for consideration:

☐ Antimicrobial/Antiseptic impregnated catheters
☐ Antiseptic impregnated caps for access ports

Fig. 10.2 Checklist for prevention of central line-associated bloodstream infections (Center for Disease Control 2011) https://www.cdc.gov/HAI/pdfs/bsi/checklist-for-CLABSI.pdf

NHSN National Healthcare Safety Network

Form Approved
OMB No. 0920-0666
Exp. Date: 11/30/2021
www.cdc.gov/nhsn

Page 1 of 2
*required for saving

Central Line Insertion Practices Adherence Monitoring

Facility ID: ____________ Event #: ____________

*Patient ID: ____________ Social Security #: ___ ___ ___ - ___ ___ - ___ ___ ___ ___
Secondary ID: ____________ Medicare #: ____________
Patient Name, Last: ____________ First: ____________ Middle: ____________
*Gender: ☐ F ☐ M ☐ Other *Date of Birth: ___/___/_____ (mm/dd/yyyy)
Ethnicity (specify): ____________ Race (specify): ____________

*Event Type: CLIP *Location: ____________ *Date of Insertion: ___/___/_____ (mm/dd/yyyy)
*Person recording insertion practice data: ☐ Inserter ☐ Observer
Central line inserter ID: ________ Name, Last: ____________ First: ____________
*Occupation of inserter:

☐ Fellow ☐ Medical student ☐ Other student ☐ Other medical staff
☐ Physician assistant ☐ Attending physician ☐ Intern/resident ☐ Registered nurse
☐ Advanced practice nurse ☐ Other (specify): ____________

*Was inserter a member of PICC/IV Team? ☐ Y ☐ N
*Reason for insertion:

☐ New indication for central line (e.g., hemodynamic monitoring, fluid/medication administration, etc.)
☐ Replace malfunctioning central line
☐ Suspected central line-associated infection
☐ Other (specify): ____________

If Suspected central line-associated infection, was the central line exchanged over a guidewire? ☐ Y ☐ N
*Inserter performed hand hygiene prior tocentral line insertion: ☐ Y ☐ N (if not observed directly, ask inserter)
*Maximal sterile barriers used: Mask ☐ Y ☐ N Sterile gown ☐ Y ☐ N
Large sterile drape ☐ Y ☐ N Sterile gloves ☐ Y ☐ N Cap ☐ Y ☐ N
*Skin preparation (check all that apply) ☐ Chlorhexidine gluconate ☐ Povidone iodine ☐ Alcohol
☐ Other (specify): ____________
If skin prep choice was <u>not</u> chlorhexidine, was there a contraindication to chlorhexidine? ☐ Y ☐ N ☐ U
If there was a contraindication to chlorhexidine, indicate the type of contraindication:

☐ Patient is less than 2 months of age - chlorhexidine is to be used with caution in patients less than 2 months of age
☐ Patient has a documented/known allergy/reaction to CHG based products that would preclude its use
☐ Facility restrictions or safety concerns for CHG use in premature infants precludes its use

*Was skin prep agent completely dry at time of first skin puncture? ☐ Y ☐ N (if not observed directly, ask inserter)
*Insertion site: ☐ Femoral ☐ Jugular ☐ Lower extremity ☐ Scalp ☐ Subclavian ☐ Umbilical ☐ Upper extremity
Antimicrobial coated catheter used: ☐ Y ☐ N

Assurance of Confidentiality: The voluntarily provided information obtained in this surveillance system that would permit identification of any individual or institution is collected with a guarantee that it will be held in strict confidence, will be used only for the purposes stated, and will not otherwise be disclosed or released without the consent of the individual, or the institution in accordance with Sections 304, 306 and 308(d) of the Public Health Service Act (42 USC 242b, 242k, and 242m(d)).

Public reporting burden of this collection of information is estimated to average 25 minutes per response, including the time for reviewing instructions, searching existing data sources, gathering and maintaining the data needed, and completing and reviewing the collection of information. An agency may not conduct or sponsor, and a person is not required to respond to a collection of information unless it displays a currently valid OMB control number. Send comments regarding this burden estimate or any other aspect of this collection ofinformation, including suggestions for reducing this burden to CDC, Reports Clearance Officer, 1600 Clifton Rd., MS D-74, Atlanta, GA 30333, ATTN: PRA (0920-0666).
CDC 57.125 (Front) Rev 5, v8.8

Fig. 10.3 Central line insertion practices (CLIP) monitoring form (CDC and NHSN 2016) https://www.cdc.gov/nhsn/forms/57.125_CLIP_BLANK.pdf

Table 10.2 Clinical bundle modified (DeVries et al. 2016)

Components of protected clinical bundle	Rationale
Chlorhexidine and alcohol skin prep	Provide adequate skin disinfection of bacteria on skin
Sterile gloves if re-palpation of skin	Aseptic non touch technique
Intravenous catheter with integrated extension	Reduces manipulation consistent with INS standards
Chlorhexidine dressing	Indicated to reduce skin infections, skin colonization and bloodstream infection
Securement dressing	Securement is strong element in preventing catheter movement
Alcohol disinfection caps	Provide intraluminal protection

Case Study

A regional teaching hospital identified a rising rate of central line-associated bloodstream infections and wanted to verify the medical and nursing staff understood and applied the foundational principles of infection prevention to their insertion and maintenance practices with CVADs. Most of the infections were occurring in the early days following insertion, so the main emphasis was on insertion-related considerations.

A vascular access infection prevention committee was formed. The committee identified the foundational practices, standards, and guidelines from the Centers for Disease Control (CDC), Evidence-based Practices in Infection Control (EPIC), Society of Healthcare Epidemiology of America (SHEA), and others. They incorporated education on the central line bundle and checklist, evidence-based maintenance practices for aseptic technique, and prepared an evaluation tool for staff observation. A two-step process included education and observation to verify understanding of the foundational principles. Following the completion of the education, based on data collected during observation, it was decided that the central line bundle checklist required an independent observer to verify the steps. After analyzing the temporal association with this intervention with decreased early-onset infections, the committee determined the integration of the observer would provide a long-term solution for CVAD insertion infection prevention compliance in this teaching facility.

Due to the nature of changing medical staff and attrition among nursing staff, the committee was later deemed a permanent committee and went on to establish other methods to standardize infection prevention practices with all vascular access insertion and management at the hospital.

Summary of Key Points

1. The prevention of catheter-related BSIs is paramount to the preservation of vessel health.
2. Adhering to the components of the central line bundle during a central line insertion procedure has proven to be an effective way to prevent catheter-related BSIs.
3. The five components of the central line bundle include:
   (a) Hand hygiene
   (b) Maximal barrier precautions during insertion
   (c) Use of chlorhexidine as a skin antisepsis
   (d) Optimal catheter site selection with avoidance of the femoral vein for central venous access in adult patients
   (e) Daily review of catheter necessity with prompt removal of unnecessary catheters

4. As an infection prevention strategy, catheters should be removed as soon as they are deemed no longer medically necessary.
5. It is recommended that an observer be present during any central venous catheter (CVC) insertion procedure to ensure ANTT is maintained throughout the procedure.
6. The use of a checklist to prevent central line-associated bloodstream infection is one of the top 10 "strongly encouraged patient safety practices."

References

Apic. Guide to preventing central line-associated bloodstream infections, United States of America; 2015.

Association for Vascular Access. Guidance document transducer disinfection for assessment and insertion of peripheral and central catheters for vascular access teams and clinicians. In: Thompson J, Garrett JH, editors. www.avainfo.org; 2018.

Blot K, Bergs J, Vogelaers D, Blot S, Vandijck D. Prevention of central line-associated bloodstream infections through quality improvement interventions: a systematic review and meta-analysis. Clin Infect Dis. 2014;59:96–105.

Casey AL, Badia JM, Higgins A, Korndorffer J, Mantyh C, Mimoz O, Moro M. Skin antisepsis: it's not only what you use, it's the way that you use it. J Hosp Infect. 2017;96:221–2.

CDC, NHSN. National Healthcare Safety Network (NHSN) overview and Central Line Insertion Practices (CLIP); 2016.

Center for Disease Control. Checklist for prevention of central line associated blood stream infections [Online]. 2011. http://www.cdc.gov/HAI/pdfs/bsi/checklist-for-CLABSI.pdf.

Chopra V, Krein SL, Olmsted RN, Safdar N & Saint S. Prevention of central line-associated bloodstream infections: brief update review. Making health care safer II: an updated critical analysis of the evidence for patient safety practices. Rockville: Agency for Healthcare Research and Quality (US); 2013.

Devries M, Valentine M. Bloodstream infections from peripheral lines: an underrated risk. Am Nurse Today. 2016;11. https://www.americannursetoday.com/piv/.

Devries M, Valentine M, Mancos P. Protected clinical indication of peripheral intravenous lines: successful implementation. J Assoc Vasc Access. 2016;21:89–92.

Fields JM, Dean AJ, Todman RW, Au AK, Anderson KL, Ku BS, Pines JM, Panebianco NL. The effect of vessel depth, diameter, and location on ultrasound-guided peripheral intravenous catheter longevity. Am J Emerg Med. 2012;30:1134–40.

Garland J, Buck R, Maloney P, Durkin D, Toth-Lloyd S, Duffy M, Szocik P, Mcauliffe T, Goldmann D. Comparison of 10% povidone-iodine and 0.5% chlorhexidine gluconate for the prevention of peripheral intravenous catheter colonization in neonates: a prospect trial. Pediatr Infect Dis J. 1995;14:510–6.

Gorski L, Hadaway L, Hagle M, Mcgoldrick M, Orr M, Doellman D. Infusion therapy: standards of practice (supplement 1). J Inf Nurs. 2016;39(Suppl 1):S1–S159.

Healthcare P. Interventional care: prevantices [Online]. 2017. https://pdihc.com/all-products/prevantics. Accessed 4 Aug 2017

Loveday H, Wilson J, Pratt R, Golsorkhi M, Tingle A, Bak A, Browne J, Prieto J, Wilcox M. EPIC3: national evidence-based guidelines for preventing healthcare-associated infections in NHS Hospitals in England. J Hosp Infect. 2014;86:S1–70.

Maki DG, Ringer M, Alvarado CJ. Prospective randomized trial of povidone-iodine, alcohol, and chlorhexidine for prevention of infection associated with central venous and arterial catheters. Am J Infect Control. 1994;22:242.

Marik PE, Flemmer M, Harrison W. The risk of catheter-related bloodstream infection with femoral venous catheters as compared to subclavian and internal jugular venous catheters: a systematic review of the literature and meta-analysis. Crit Care Med. 2012;40:2479–85.

Marschall J, Mermel L, Fakih M, Hadaway L, Kallen A, O'Grady N, Pettis A, Rupp M, Sandora T, Maragakis L, Yokoe D. Strategies to prevent central line–associated bloodstream infections in acute care hospitals: 2014 update. Infect Control Hosp Epidemiol. 2014;35:753–71.

Mccann M, Fitzpatrick F, Mellotte G, Clarke M. Is 2% chlorhexidine gluconate in 70% isopropyl alcohol more effective at preventing central venous catheter–related infections than routinely used chlorhexidine gluconate solutions: a pilot multicenter randomized trial (ISRCTN2657745)? Am J Infect Control. 2016;44:948–9.

Mestre G, Berbel C, Tortajada P, Alarcia M, Coca R, Fernández MM, Gallemi G, García I, Aguilar MC, Rodríguez-Baño J, Martinez JA. Successful multifaceted intervention aimed to reduce short peripheral venous catheter-related adverse events: a quasiexperimental cohort study. Am J Infect Control. 2013;41:520–6.

Mimoz O, Lucet J-C, Kerforne T, Pascal J, Souweine B, Goudet V, Mercat A, Bouadma L, Lasocki S, Alfandari S, Friggeri A, Wallet F, Allou N, Ruckly S, Balayn D, Lepape A, Timsit J-F. Skin antisepsis with chlorhexidine–alcohol versus povidone iodine–alcohol, with and without skin scrubbing, for prevention of intravascular-catheter-related infection (CLEAN): an open-label, multicentre, randomised, controlled, two-by-two factorial trial. Lancet. 2015;386:2069–77.

O'Grady N, Alexander M, Burns L, Dellinger E, Garland J, Heard S, Lipsett P, Masur H, Mermel L, Pearson M, Raad I, Randolph A, Rupp M, Saint S, (Hicpac), H. I. C. P. a. C. Centers for Disease Control Guidelines for the prevention of intravascular catheter-related infections. Clin Infect Dis. 2011a;52:e162–93.

O'Grady N, Alexander M, Burns L, Dellinger E, Garland J, Heard S, Lipsett P, Masur H, Mermel L, Pearson M, Raad I, Randolph A, Rupp M, Saint S. Guidelines for the prevention of intravascular catheter-related infections. Center for Disease Control HICPAC Healthcare Infection Control Practices Advisory Committee: Guidelines for the prevention of intravascular catheterrelated infections. Center for Disease Control and Prevention; 2011b.

Oleszkowicz SC, Chittick P, Russo V, Keller P, Sims M, Band J. Infections associated with use of ultrasound transmission gel: proposed guidelines to minimize risk. Infect Control Hosp Epidemiol. 2015;33:1235–7.

Picc Excellence. Online course manuals. In: Moureau N, editor. 2018

Prevention CFDCA. Guideline for hand hygiene in healthcare settings: recommendations of the Healthcare Infection Control Practices Advisory Committee and the HICPAC/SHEA/APIC/IDSA Hand Hygiene Task Force. MMWR Recomm Rep. 2002;51(RR-16):1–45.

Pronovost P, Needham D, Berenholtz S, Sinopoli D, Chu H, Cosgrove S, Sexton B, Hyzy R, Welsh R, Roth G. An intervention to decrease catheter-related bloodstream infections in the ICU. N Engl J Med. 2006;355:2725–32.

Silva P. The right skin preparation technique: a literature review. J Perioper Pract. 2014;24:283–5.

Slyne H, Phillips C, Parkes J. Saving Lives audits: do they improve infection prevention and control practice? J Infect Prev. 2012;13:24–7.

The Joint Commission. Preventing central line–associated bloodstream infections: a global challenge, a global perspective [Online]. [Accessed] 2012.

Timsit J-F, Rupp M, Bouza E, Chopra V, Kärpänen T, Laupland K, Lisboa T, Mermel L, Mimoz O, Parienti J-J. A state of the art review on optimal practices to prevent, recognize, and manage complications associated with intravascular devices in the critically ill. Intensive Care Med. 2018;1–18.

Wallis M, Mcgrail M, Webster J, Marsh N, Gowardman J, Playford E, Rickard C. Risk factors for peripheral intravenous catheter failure: a multivariate analysis of data from a randomized controlled trial. Infect Control Hosp Epidemiol. 2014;35:63–8.

WHO. SAVE LIVES: clean your hands—WHO's global annual call to action for health workers [Online]. online: World Health Organization. 2015. http://www.who.int/gpsc/5may/en/. Accessed 9 Mar 2016, 2015.

World Health Organization. Historical perspective on hand hygiene in health care. WHO guidelines on hand hygiene in health care: First global patient safety challenge clean care is safer care. Genva; 2009.

11

Clinical Implementation of ANTT®

Stephen Rowley and Simon Clare

Abstract

Aseptic technique, which involves infection prevention actions designed to protect patients from infection when undergoing invasive clinical procedures, is universally prescribed by guideline makers as a critical competency in the prevention of infections. However, no meaningful explanation of what aseptic technique is or how it is to be applied to ensure patient safety is provided within any of the guidelines. The Aseptic Non Touch Technique (ANTT®), originated by Rowley in the late 1990s, was designed to help address variable aseptic technique standards of practice and provide a rationalized, contemporary, evidence-based framework to standardize this critical competency and help improve standards of practice. The ANTT® Clinical Practice Framework provides a comprehensive framework for aseptic technique for all invasive procedures based on an approach termed Key-Part and Key-Site Protection. During the insertion or manipulation of an intravascular device, the 'ANTT-Approach' provides a systematic method that supports the practitioner to include all the important elements of aseptic technique, with particular focus on the identification and protection of 'Key-Parts' and 'Key-Sites' throughout the preparation and the procedure. This chapter provides clinical examples of how the ANTT® is implemented in the healthcare setting, as well as, importantly, how to promote compliance of the technique.

Keywords

Aseptic technique · ANTT® · Sterile · Aseptic

S. Rowley (✉) · S. Clare
The Association for Safe Aseptic Practice (ASAP), London, UK
e-mail: Stephen.rowley@antt.org; simon.clare@antt.org

11.1 Which Aseptic Technique Is the 'Right' Aseptic Technique?

At its heart, aseptic technique involves a collection of infection prevention actions designed to protect patients from infection when undergoing invasive clinical procedures, including maintenance of indwelling medical devices. A combination of decontamination processes, sterilized equipment and handling technique is used to minimize potential transmission of pathogenic microorganisms (Clare and Rowley 2017). In terms of protecting patients from infection, aseptic technique is one of the most important and commonly used critical clinical competencies in healthcare. Although the prescription for aseptic technique is universal, agreement on the aim, definition, description and application of aseptic technique is not (Preston 2005; NICE 2012; Gorski et al. 2016).

Historical and contemporary literature presents a confused hierarchy of terms and practices including sterile technique, aseptic technique, clean technique and non-touch technique, further compounded by interchangeable use and meaning (Aziz 2009; Rowley et al. 2010; Unsworth and Collins 2011). Internationally, it seems to have become 'fashionable' for guideline makers to address the historical confusion surrounding aseptic technique by simply prescribing the generic term 'aseptic technique', with virtually no meaningful explanation of what aseptic technique is or how it is to be applied to ensure patient safety (NICE 2012; Gorski et al. 2016; RCN 2016).

Such 'prescription without explanation' by major stakeholders appears to have undermined this critical clinical competency and potentially fuels the complacency associated with aseptic technique. In education, students and qualified staff are taught various educational concepts and practical methods of performing essentially the same activity using different methods and descriptors (Hartley 2005; Flores 2008; Aziz 2009; Rowley et al. 2010). But most concerning of all is the effect of a confused literature on clinical practice with poor standards of aseptic technique commonly and consistently reported (Hartley 2005; Flores 2008; Aziz 2009; Rowley et al. 2010; Unsworth and Collins 2011). As a result, concern for standards of aseptic technique has been reflected in a wide range of international initiatives concerned with improving infection prevention such as the Keystone project (Pronovost et al. 2006; Pronovost 2008), 5 Moments for Hand Hygiene (Sax et al. 2007), Saving Lives [UK] (DH 2007) and the 100,000 Lives Campaign [USA] (Berwick et al. 2006).

Given the significantly invasive nature of inserting indwelling medical devices and their ongoing care and maintenance, aseptic technique has always been of much concern in the field of intravenous therapy. However, despite this, historically and contemporaneously, the field of IV therapy fairs no better in aseptic technique than any other field of clinical practice. Moreover, given the incidence of particularly high-profile organisms such as MRSA, IV therapy has consistently been identified as a particularly problematic area for aseptic technique.

Perhaps of most concern is that despite more than a century of infection prevention that has paralleled many advances in IV therapy, there is a dearth of evidence supporting which specific aseptic technique provides the most effective prevention against the risk of infection. For example, in a partial update to Clinical Guideline 2 (replaced by CG139), the National Institute for Health and Care Excellence (NICE) was unable to identify any clinical or cost-effectiveness evidence to recommend the best technique when handling vascular access devices to reduce infection-related bacteremia, phlebitis, compliance, MRSA or C. diff reduction and mortality (NICE 2012). Subsequently, NICE and other stakeholders have recognized ANTT® as providing the prerequisite platform required for guideline development and research enquiry in aseptic technique (NICE 2012 [updated 2017]).

Right Aseptic Technique: ANTT®

To avoid any ambiguity regarding aseptic technique as discussed above, all references to aseptic technique throughout this book are articulated using the practice terms and principles explicitly defined in the ANTT® Clinical Practice Framework.

ANTT® is the most commonly used aseptic technique framework in healthcare today and is rapidly evolving as a global standard. As a result, it is increasingly becoming the recognized standardized practice (NICE 2012), providing meaningful, accurate practice language. The development of ANTT® has been closely associated with IV practice as the insertion and use of IVs is the most commonly performed invasive procedure in healthcare. There are two types of ANTT®: Surgical-ANTT and Standard-ANTT (for context, Surgical-ANTT reflects the so-called sterile technique, and Standard-ANTT is a rationalized approach to better describing a multitude of ambiguous practice terms).

11.2 Aseptic Non Touch Technique (ANTT®)

Originated by Rowley in the late 1990s (2001), the Aseptic Non Touch Technique (ANTT®) Clinical Practice Framework was designed to help address variable and poor standards of practice and ambiguous theory by providing a rationalized, contemporary, evidence-based framework to standardize this critical competency and help improve standards of practice. Notably, ANTT® is a clinical practice standard for the complete spectrum of invasive clinical procedures, from major surgery to intravenous access, from intravenous maintenance to simple first aid activities. The National Institute for Health and Clinical Excellence (NICE) describes ANTT® as 'a specific type of aseptic technique with a unique theory and practice framework' (NICE 2012). The unique theory refers to the original educational and practice concept of 'Key-Part and Key-Site Protection'. Used internationally in over 25 countries, ANTT® is now used frequently in the literature to describe aseptic technique practice and study and is commonly referenced or endorsed by international guidance including the *Australian Guidelines for the Prevention and Control of Infection in Healthcare* (NHMRC 2010), Public Health/NHS Wales (Welsh Government 2015), the National Institute for Health and Clinical Excellence (NICE 2012), the Health Protection Surveillance Centre Ireland (HPSC 2011) and the Infusion Nurses Society Infusion Therapy Standards of Practice (Gorski et al. 2016).

11.3 The ANTT® Clinical Practice Framework Explained

To address the historically confused and interchangeable use of terminology for aseptic technique, the ANTT® Clinical Practice Framework utilizes only achievable practice terms and accurately defines them as follows:

Aseptic—Free from pathogenic organisms (in sufficient numbers to cause infection)
Sterile—Free from (all) microorganisms
Clean—Free from visible marks and stains
Non-touch—The action of not touching critical or important parts of equipment and/or vulnerable or compromised parts of a patient

Often used interchangeably with the term 'aseptic' is the term 'sterile', a well-defined word that specifically means 'an absence of *all* microorganisms'. Unfortunately, sterile is simply not achievable in typical healthcare settings due to the multitude of microorganisms in the air environment. The term 'aseptic' refers to an absence of pathogenic microorganisms in sufficient quantity to cause infection and *is* achievable in the typical healthcare setting. These terms should not be used interchangeably as they are *not synonymous*. The term 'clean' is defined as the absence of visible marks and stains and, for the obvious reason that microorganisms are not visible to the naked eye, offers no measurable or safe practice definition for invasive procedures. Non-touch technique (NTT) is not a free-standing aseptic technique as such but rather represents a critical component of any safe aseptic practice.

The practice terms in the ANTT® Practice Framework provide an interrelated set of definitions that are technically accurate, achievable and applicable to any invasive clinical procedure. Using these definitions has aided in the development of standardized competency-based education and training for both novices and experienced clinicians. These accurate descriptors of practice allow risk assessment to be simplified and focus on rational practice-based factors rather than arbitrary and subjective variables, so that clinical practice is more consistently applied.

11.4 ANTT®: Key-Part and Key-Site Protection

The ANTT® Practice Framework established that the aim of infection prevention during invasive procedures or the maintenance of indwelling medical devices by definition is and can be no more and no less than the procedure being 'aseptic'. In ANTT®, maintaining an aseptic procedure is achieved by the fundamental concept and practical application of Key-Part and Key-Site Protection. The 'Key-Parts' of procedural equipment and the patients' vulnerable points of access are portals of entry for bacteria. 'Key-Parts' and 'Key-Sites' are maintained in an aseptic state at all times during invasive procedures. Key-Part and Key-Site Protection is achieved by a practical process that involves prerequisite basic infective precautions such as hand cleaning and personal protective equipment (PPE), the use of sterilized equipment and medical supplies and an appropriate combination of aseptic fields and a non-touch handling technique.

Key-Sites—Areas of skin penetration that provide a direct route for the transmission of pathogens into the patient and present a significant infection risk. Key-Sites include surgical wounds, skin breakdowns or exit sites from CVAD/PVC placement.

Key-Parts—Critical parts of medical devices/items of procedure equipment that, if contaminated, provide a route for the transfer of harmful microorganisms directly onto or into a patient. In IV therapy, these include any part of the equipment that comes into direct or indirect contact with the liquid infusion.

11.5 Aseptic Fields

The type of aseptic fields utilized in an aseptic procedure is dependent upon the type of procedure and aseptic technique utilized. To this end, ANTT® defines the utilization of the three different types of aseptic fields in common practice:

Critical Aseptic Field—Usually a sterilized drape, used when a single main aseptic field is required to house and protect all procedure equipment that is typically removed from individual packaging onto the field. A main Critical Aseptic Field is used to help *ensure* equipment is maintained in an aseptic state during procedures by providing essential and primary protection from the procedure environment. Critical Aseptic Fields require what can be termed 'critical management' or the prohibition of anything non-sterilized entering the field at any time during the procedure. Subsequently, sterilized gloves are required to maintain asepsis while manipulating equipment into and out of the field. Essentially, all equipment is 'handled' as Key-Parts (Fig. 11.1).

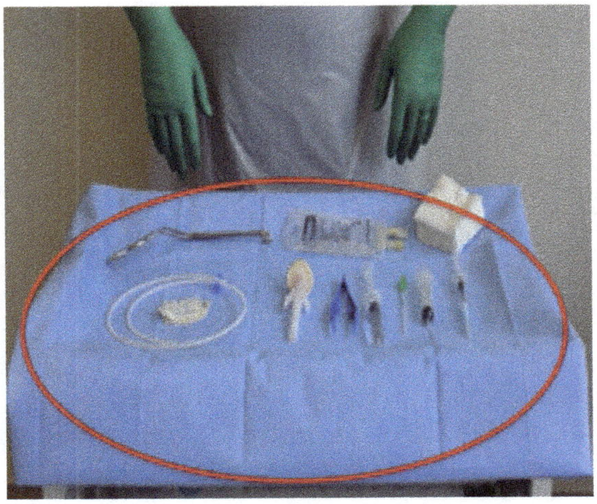

Fig. 11.1 Critical Aseptic Field (used with permission The Association for Safe Aseptic Practice – ASAP)

General Aseptic Field—Typically a decontaminated and disinfected surface (examples include plastic procedure trays or dressing trollies) or a single-use disposable product (examples include pulp paper or plastic trays). The main aseptic field that *promotes* asepsis during procedures by providing basic protection from the procedure environment. General Aseptic Fields are used when the procedure Key-Parts are easily and primarily protected using a type of Critical Field termed Micro Critical Aseptic Field (see below). General Aseptic Fields require 'general' rather than 'critical' management and are subsequently managed with non-sterilized gloves and non-touch technique (Fig. 11.2).

Micro Critical Aseptic Field (MCAF)—Examples include sterilized caps, covers and the inside of recently opened sterilized equipment packaging. Critical Aseptic Fields are used to protect Key-Parts individually, e.g. syringe cap or needle cover. They allow safe protection during less complex procedures while also affording a high level of cost-effective ANTT® (Fig. 11.2).

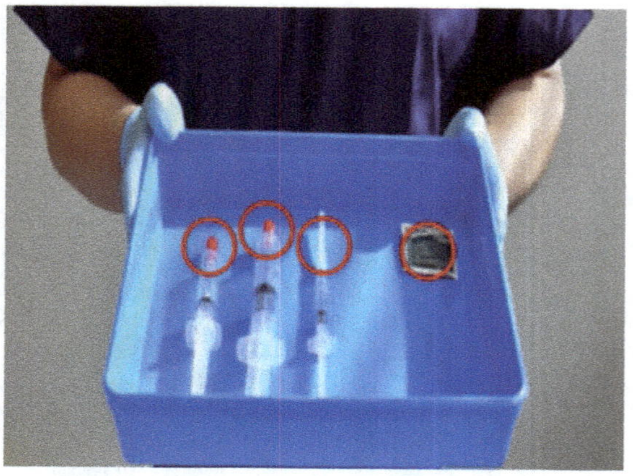

Fig. 11.2 General Aseptic Field with Micro Critical Aseptic Fields (used with permission The Association for Safe Aseptic Practice – ASAP)

11.6 Right Aseptic Technique: ANTT® Applied to IV Therapy

There are too many procedures and procedure variables to provide an exhaustive A–Z reference of ANTT® applied to IV therapy. Instead, the principles and practice terminology of the ANTT® Clinical Practice Framework have been outlined above, and broad examples of how the framework is applied to practice is outlined for four of the most common IV procedures below.

11.6.1 Right Aseptic Technique: ANTT® Applied to the Insertion of Central Venous Access Devices (CVAD)

11.6.1.1 Overview

The insertion of CVADs is a complex procedure with expert level of knowledge and competency-based skills required for safe and effective practice. Evidence-based consensus internationally supports insertion with a 'central venous line care bundle' and what has been termed 'maximal [sterile] barrier precautions' (O'Grady et al. 2011; Loveday et al. 2014; Gorski et al. 2016). Application of the ANTT® Risk Assessment supports this recommendation with central venous access always requiring Surgical-ANTT as explained below.

11.6.1.2 ANTT® Risk Assessment for CVAD Insertion

The process of ensuring asepsis (the absence of pathogenic organisms) during CVAD insertion is technically complex and involves having to protect numerous Key-Parts and one particularly large Key-Part, the CVAD itself. The procedure is highly invasive and may last an hour or more. These risk factors alone make it technically challenging to ensure asepsis throughout the procedure, and subsequently a Surgical-ANTT approach is required.

11.6.1.3 Basic Precautions *for CVAD Insertion*

Surgical-ANTT requires the practitioner to adopt a high level of precaution, such as a surgical hand scrub rather than a standard hand clean, and personal protective equipment (PPE) that includes the use of sterilized gloves, gowns, head wear and masks (Loveday et al. 2014).

Risk of airborne contamination at the bedside is reduced by ensuring the air environment has time to settle after any dust producing activities such as bed making or room cleaning prior to CVAD insertion.

11.6.1.4 Decontamination and Disinfection *for CVAD Insertion*

Most notably, Surgical-ANTT for CVAD insertion is typically performed using presterilized equipment and supplies and effective skin disinfection.

Skin disinfection starts with visibly clean skin prior to applying the antiseptic solution. Unless contraindicated,[1] the current evidence base supports the use of ≥0.5% chlorhexidine in 70% IPA (Loveday et al. 2014; Gorski et al. 2016) applied with a suitable single-use applicator and a systematic technique that follows manufacturer's recommendations. The disinfecting solution should be allowed to dry before insertion of a CVAD.

[1] For chlorhexidine sensitivity, consider povidone-iodine in alcohol, and use chlorhexidine with caution in infants. Consider the lowest effective concentration of chlorhexidine for premature infants and infants under 2 months of age (O'Grady et al. 2011; Gorski et al. 2016). Observe for hypersensitivity reactions or possible allergic responses to chlorhexidine gluconate.

11.6.1.5 Aseptic Fields *in CVAD Insertion*

Using Surgical-ANTT for CVAD insertions requires a large enough working area covered by a sterilized drape(s) to safely contain and protect all procedure equipment as aseptic. Large equipment used inter-procedure, such as ultrasound, is also covered in sterilized covers that enable aseptic handling by the operator.

11.6.1.6 Non-touch Technique *for CVAD Insertion*

Critical Aseptic Fields used in Surgical-ANTT CVAD insertion are managed critically, with sterilized gloves used to maintain aseptic continuity when handling all equipment and supplies. Due to the complexity of the procedure, a completely non-touch technique is not and cannot be mandated. However, the effective practitioner will be mindful that sterilized gloves and drapes are not infallible and can be inadvertently contaminated. With this in mind, the principle remains that the safest way to not inadvertently contaminate a Key-Part is to not touch it directly where practically possible. To this end, many CVAD inserters pay particular reverence to the major Key-Part, the CVAD that will be inserted deep into the patient and lay indwelling, and only handle this part indirectly via forceps or sterilized packaging.

11.6.2 Right Aseptic Technique: ANTT® Applied to the Insertion of Peripheral Venous Catheter

11.6.2.1 Overview

The risks of peripheral venous catheter (PVC) insertion and maintenance have arguably been understated compared to CVAD placement (Zingg and Pittet 2009; Webster et al. 2013). The most recent point prevalence survey in the English National Health Service (NHS) noted the use of PVCs (outside of ICU) was 38.6% compared with CVAD use of 5.9% of patients surveyed (Hopkins et al. 2012). A 6-year epidemiological study by DeVries and Valentine (2016) highlighted the difference in approach to peripheral and central venous management. Although PVCs naturally present less risk than CVADs, their considerably higher use resulted in similar numbers of bacteremia. Frequent manipulations of PVCs by different healthcare workers demand effective aseptic technique and regularly documented surveillance of the device site, such as the Visual Infusion Phlebitis (VIP) scale (Gorski et al. 2011), for early detection of any complications.

11.6.2.2 ANTT® Risk Assessment *for PVC Insertion*

It should be noted that type of ANTT® for PVC insertion is particularly dependent upon the vessel health and vein accessibility of individual patients. As a result, the competency and experience of the practitioner are particularly relevant in the ANTT® Risk Assessment and may often direct the practitioner to the Surgical-ANTT technique.

However, due to the technical ease of achieving asepsis for a relatively few number of Key-Parts, ANTT® Risk assessment typically determines that PVC insertion can be performed safely by a competent practitioner using Standard-ANTT. To this end, non-sterile gloves are indicated if the access site is not touched following skin antisepsis (O'Grady et al. 2011).

11.6.2.3 Basic Precautions *for PVC Insertion*

PVC insertion demands effective hand hygiene and the use of appropriate PPE to help protect the healthcare worker from exposure to blood-borne pathogens. Recommended PPE varies internationally. The most common PPE guidelines involve non-sterile or sterile glove usage depending upon the type of ANTT® utilized. In addition, disposable aprons are recommended in Epic3, but not universally. Loveday et al., through systematic review, identify a developing evidence base identifying a steady build-up of microorganisms on staff uniforms with some association to healthcare-associated infections (HAI) (Loveday et al. 2014).

All invasive procedures require appraisal of the aseptic technique integrity throughout the procedure. This principle is particularly relevant in PVC insertion as it can often be necessary to re-palpate the injection site. If performing Standard-ANTT, vein re-palpation requires recleaning of the puncture site; if vein detection continues to be problematic and it is not practical to reclean the skin after re-palpation, sterilized gloves should be introduced. If performing Surgical-ANTT and there is a need to insert the PVC immediately after re-palpation without recleaning the skin, the practitioner must consider the integrity of their sterilized gloves prior to proceeding and replace them if compromised.

11.6.2.4 Decontamination and Protection *for PVC Insertion*

If using a reusable procedure tray, the tray should be decontaminated and disinfected according to local policy pre- and post-procedure.

Prior to insertion, the skin, or Key-Site, should be cleaned and disinfected using a non-touch technique with a single-use applicator licensed for purpose. Solution should be applied with a frictional cross-hatch method using pressure to reach deep into the skin layers. The skin must be allowed to dry prior to insertion. If re-palpation is necessary, the site should be recleaned and managed as described above.

11.6.2.5 Aseptic Fields *in PVC Insertion*

PVC insertion using Standard-ANTT involves Key-Parts being primarily protected individually with Micro Critical Aseptic Fields such as sterilized caps and covers and the inside of sterilized equipment packaging. Secondary aseptic field protection is provided by containing all procedure equipment within a procedure tray serving as a General Aseptic Field.

Disposable trays used as General Aseptic Fields for PVC insertion should be large enough to provide a reasonable working area with high sides to contain spillage of liquids or sharps.

A sterilized drape may be considered for placement underneath the patient's arm to promote asepsis around the immediate procedure environment as well as to help contain any leakage of blood.

If Surgical-ANTT is selected for PIV insertion, full barrier precautions are not recommended by evidence-based guidance; however, there is consensus-based guidance suggesting an increased attention to skin disinfection and the use of sterilized gloves might be beneficial in the context of longer indwelling times for PVCs (Gorski et al. 2016). A modest-sized sterilized drape, large enough to cover a small treatment trolley or procedure tray, can adequately serve as a Critical Aseptic Field with sterilized gloves worn for all equipment handling.

11.6.2.6 Non-touch Technique *for PVC Insertion*

When using Standard-ANTT, non-touch technique for PVC equipment preparation and insertion is mandatory and technically straightforward. As already noted, asepsis of the Key-Site is compromised when the Key-Site requires re-palpation after skin disinfection. See above for the appropriate counter measures.

11.6.3 Right Aseptic Technique: ANTT® Applied to Intravenous Maintenance

11.6.3.1 Overview

The term intravenous maintenance is used below to describe the preparation and administration of intravenous drugs via infusion or injection. Any type of intravenous device, whether central or peripheral access, provides a portal of entry for microorganisms with a significant risk of infection. This risk is compounded by the frequency in which IV devices are handled and manipulated by many different and busy healthcare workers over long periods of time. Effective aseptic technique on every manipulation is of paramount importance. Although the risk of infection is significant, establishing and maintaining asepsis when connecting intravenous infusions or administering intravenous injections is not technically challenging and can warrant a relatively simple and efficient approach to aseptic technique.

11.6.3.2 ANTT® Risk Assessment *for IV Maintenance*

Standard-ANTT is most likely selected for IV maintenance on the basis that procedures are typically of short duration and will involve minimal numbers of small Key-Parts that are technically easy to protect with non-touch technique and individual Micro Critical Aseptic Fields. The risks of the invasive nature of an IV device can be reduced by the utilization of closed intravenous line systems (Graves et al. 2011).

11.6.3.3 Basic Precautions *for IV Maintenance*

In preparation for Standard-ANTT, the practitioner begins by performing important precautions such as hand cleaning and applying personal protective equipment (PPE) according to local policy. Given the volume and frequency of IV maintenance, the challenge for healthcare organizations is ensuring compliance with basic precautions, especially effective hand cleaning every time staff connect or access intravenous systems.

11.6.3.4 Decontamination and Protection *for IV Maintenance*

The most common aspects of decontamination for Standard-ANTT for IV maintenance are decontamination and disinfection of procedure trays / trolleys / surfaces and, particularly, disinfection of IV hubs.

11.6.4 Procedure Tray Disinfection

Due to a highly variable evidence base for this area of practice (Leas et al. 2015), there is a wide choice of disinfection wipes available. It is important that local policies be explicit regarding the expectancy for decontamination, disinfection, storage and usage of procedure trays.

Given that procedure trays are utilized to promote asepsis and not ensure it, pulp or paper trays can be acceptable; however, such trays should be large enough to serve as a General Aseptic Field and large enough to promote Key-Part protection, enable safe transport and handling of equipment as well as have sides high enough to contain any spillage of liquids or sharps. A clear, single system for safe storage of disposable trays is important as they cannot be decontaminated or disinfected prior to use.

Post-procedure decontamination and disinfection are important in preventing the potential for cross infection. Reusable medical equipment must not be stored without cleaning or while still wet to inhibit microorganism clustering and biofilm development while providing maximal effectiveness of the disinfection solution (NPSA 2009; HIRL 2006).

11.6.5 IV Hub Disinfection

When not in use, IV hubs are likely to come into contact with microorganisms from the patient or immediate environment. There is a strong and developing evidence base describing effective technique for disinfection of the IV hubs (Hibbard 2005; Kaler and Chinn 2007; Moureau and Flynn 2015; Gorski et al. 2016). It is widely accepted that best technique requires alcohol and chlorhexidine disinfection and adequate time spent 'scrubbing' the hub, creating friction (Kaler and Chinn 2007; Smith et al. 2012). Guidance still varies slightly concerning the type of disinfectant and the duration of scrubbing (Table 11.1). To this end, the user should be guided by local policy.

11.6.6 Passive IV Hub Disinfection

There is a growing body of evidence indicating that effective and routine IV hub disinfection is not universally achieved and that failure in hub disinfection is common (Moureau and Flynn 2015). To help address such 'human factors', so-called passive disinfection has been recommended as an alternative for effective and reliable IV hub disinfection (Gorski et al. 2016).

11.6.6.1 Aseptic Fields *in IV Maintenance*

Aseptic fields have a pivotal role in Key-Part protection, and typically, using Standard-ANTT for IV maintenance, Key-Parts are afforded primary

Table 11.1 Recommended hub disinfectant time and techniques per guidance documents

	Disinfectant	Time	Technique
Epic3 (Loveday et al. 2014)	• 2% CHG/70% IPA	≥15 s	Clean + allow to dry (follow manufacturer's recommendations)
CDC (O'Grady et al. 2011)	• >0.5% CHG/70% IPA • 70% IPA • Povidone-iodine	No recommendation	'Scrubbing'
INS (Gorski et al. 2016)	• >0.5% CHG/70% IPA • 70% IPA • Povidone-iodine	Various reported (i.e. between 5 and 60 s)	Vigorous mechanical scrubbing and allow to dry (follow manufacturer's recommendations)

protection by Micro Critical Aseptic Fields such as sterilized caps. For non-toxic medications, the sterilized inside of a syringe packet is also widely used for protecting syringe tip Key-Parts as they provide excellent Key-Part Protection and have the added advantage of positioning operator hands well away from the Key-Part. Secondary protection is typically provided by a plastic or disposable tray promoting asepsis, thus serving as a General Aseptic Field.

11.6.6.2 Non-touch Technique *for IV Maintenance*

IV maintenance typically involves technically simple non-touch technique of a few Key-Parts such as the connecting of a syringe to a needle-free connector. However technically simple, meticulous non-touch technique is paramount and mandatory. If compromised, equipment must be discarded or re-disinfected. Key-Parts should be assembled one at a time and immediately protected when not in use with individual Micro Critical Aseptic Fields such as sterilized caps and covers.

11.6.7 Right Aseptic Technique: ANTT® Applied to Central Line Dressing Change

11.6.7.1 Overview

Dressing changes are not necessarily invasive but do involve significant risk of infecting a patient through the transmission of harmful microorganisms (Ullman et al. 2015). Protecting a CVAD entry site requires ongoing Key-Site Protection involving CVAD dressings and site cleaning.

11.6.7.2 CVAD Dressings

Based on evidence, there is consensus across international guidance for the use of semipermeable clear dressings with integral or separate chlorhexidine and fixation (Loveday et al. 2014; Gorski et al. 2016). It should be noted that ANTT® considers the skin area beneath an intact aseptic dressing to be the Key-Site, not just the much smaller exit site.

Skin antisepsis is carried out during a dressing change using best practice guidance:

Use a single-use application of a solution of >0.5% chlorhexidine gluconate in 70% isopropyl alcohol (or povidone-iodine in alcohol for patients with sensitivity to chlorhexidine) to clean the CVAD insertion site during dressing changes, and allow to air dry (Loveday et al. 2014; Gorski et al. 2016).

11.6.7.3 ANTT® Risk Assessment *for CVAD Dressing Change*

The technical difficulty of maintaining asepsis during CVAD dressing change and the subsequent type of ANTT® utilized is largely dependent on the type and combination of medical supplies used. Complete and subsequently more complex CVAD dressing changes typically require Surgical-ANTT as there are a number of Key-Parts and a large Key-Site to manage aseptically: an old and new dressing, fixation devices that vary in handling complexity and a chlorhexidine disk if not integral to the dressing.

11.6.7.4 Basic Precautions *for CVAD Dressing Change*

Effective hand hygiene is followed by application of appropriate PPE such as aprons/protective gowns and gloves depending on the type of ANTT® used. Where Surgical-ANTT is utilized, non-sterile gloves can be used for dressing removal, and sterilized gloves are utilized thereafter.

11.6.7.5 Aseptic Fields *in CVAD Dressing Change*

Because CVAD dressing changes in many countries include sterile changes with CHG protective sponge and/or fixation devices, they require Surgical-ANTT, and thus application of the main Critical Aseptic Field with all the Key-Parts protected upon it would apply (Gorski et al. 2016).

11.6.7.6 Non-touch Technique *for CVAD Dressing Change*

When using Standard-ANTT and Micro Critical Aseptic Fields, the practitioner must be conscious throughout that maintaining asepsis depends on effective non-touch handling of Key-Parts and the Key-Site at all times.

Non-touch handling is promoted when skin cleaning is performed by using a purpose built and licensed applicator designed to keep the healthcare worker's fingers well away from the Key-Site.

Perhaps often forgotten, dressings should be removed with as much handling care as when applied. Carefully rolling the dressing up from the edges of the dressing is one such method of effective, controlled removal. As well as helping to prevent Key-Site contamination through non-touch technique, such care helps minimize the risks of adhesive-related skin injury. Application of a skin barrier solution may help reduce the risk of skin damage (Gorski et al. 2016).

11.6.7.7 Decontamination *for CVAD Dressing Change*

Skin antisepsis following existing dressing removal should be performed using evidence-based recommendations. Preferred disinfection, if not contraindicated*[1], is an alcoholic solution with >0.5% CHG (Gorski et al. 2016) in a single-use applicator (Loveday et al. 2014). The skin should be cleaned as per manufacturer's recommendations such as a firm cross-hatch technique (Moureau 2003) with a minimum cleaning time of 30 s (Gorski et al. 2016). For the cleaning solution to provide its most effective bacterial kill effect, it must be allowed to dry fully before a dressing is applied.

Efficacy has not been sufficiently demonstrated for the use of topical antimicrobial ointments (Loveday et al. 2014); however, the use of chlorhexidine-impregnated dressings or impregnated sponges is recommended (NICE 2012, 2015; Gorski et al. 2016).

11.7 ANTT® Clinical Governance: Competency, Compliance and Surveillance

Achieving and maintaining the effective delivery of ANTT® for every patient during every invasive interaction across large healthcare organizations naturally require a robust effective clinical governance framework that reflects the critical importance of effective ANTT® to patient outcome. Effective governance should include:

- Clear responsibilities and accountabilities
- A robust implementation program
- Clear expectations communicated to staff through policy and guidelines
- Standardized education and training
- Competency assessment
- Infection surveillance of relevant indicators
- Compliance audit

11.7.1 Competency

The Infusion Nurses Society describes competency for infusion therapy as something that '… goes beyond psychomotor skills and includes application of knowledge, critical thinking, and decision-making abilities' (Gorski et al. 2016). Similarly, ANTT® competency assessment includes assessment of theory and practice. The standard competency assessment tool for Surgical-ANTT and Standard-ANTT requires demonstration of effective Key-Part and Key-Site Protection but also the articulation of ANTT®

terms and principles. The inclusion of theory in a practical assessment helps organizations embed a common practice language for this important competency that has the additional benefit of being used internationally—helping generate more meaningful discussion about this critical competency (ANTT® Competency Assessment Tools are freely available from www.antt.org/competency assessment).

11.7.2 Implementation

ANTT® is typically implemented across healthcare organizations as a quality assurance-based audit cycle (Fig. 11.3) involving a suite of targeted resources and implementation tools. The standardization of clinical practice is further aided by a series of visual, risk-assessed and sequenced clinical practice guidelines (Fig. 11.4). These simple and adaptable guidelines communicate a wealth of practical information in a bite-sized user-friendly package. Translated into multiple languages, the ANTT® Clinical Practice Guidelines are the visual embodiment of the Clinical Practice Framework.

Effective implementation of any important clinical competency is dependent upon various organizational factors (Melle et al. 2017). Evaluation of ANTT® implementation across seven large hospitals identified executive board-level organizational support as a key indicator for effective implementation (Rowley et al. 2010). A recently published study looked at the essential elements of the ANTT-Approach 36 months after implementation and demonstrated significantly improved practice with best practice elements of aseptic technique (Clare and Rowley 2017).

11.7.3 Compliance

Just like any other critical clinical competency, once ANTT® has been established across an organization, it is necessary to maintain practice standards. Again, like any clinical competency, this is not an easy task and is best not underestimated. For perspective, despite huge investments of time and money in hand hygiene practice, compliance internationally is commonly reported at approximately ≤50% (Fuller et al. 2011; Kingston et al. 2015; Brühwasser et al. 2016). Soberingly, effective aseptic technique requires staff compliance with an additional of four or five essential key practice components.

ANTT® addresses this compliance challenge with a multifactorial approach including:

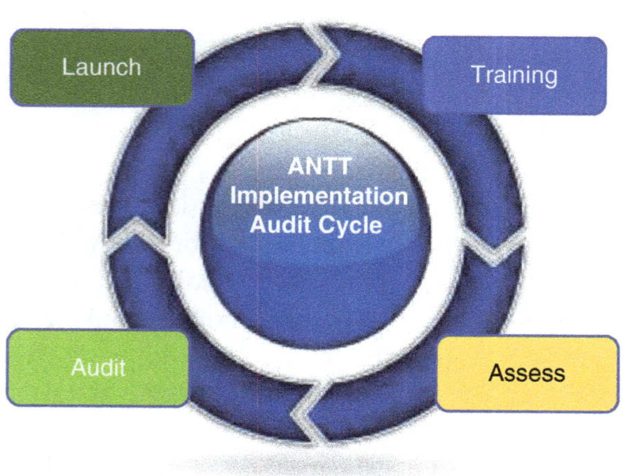

Phase	Suggested Resources (Freely available from www.antt.org)
Pre/Post Audit	The ANTT® Audit of Invasive Clinical Procedures The ANTT® Clinical Audit Tool(s)
Launch	Board level communication to all relevant staff
Training	ANTT Clinical Practice Framework ANTT Guidelines
Assess	The ANTT® Competency Assessment Tool (CAT)

Fig. 11.3 ANTT® audit cycle (used with permission The Association for Safe Aseptic Practice – ASAP)

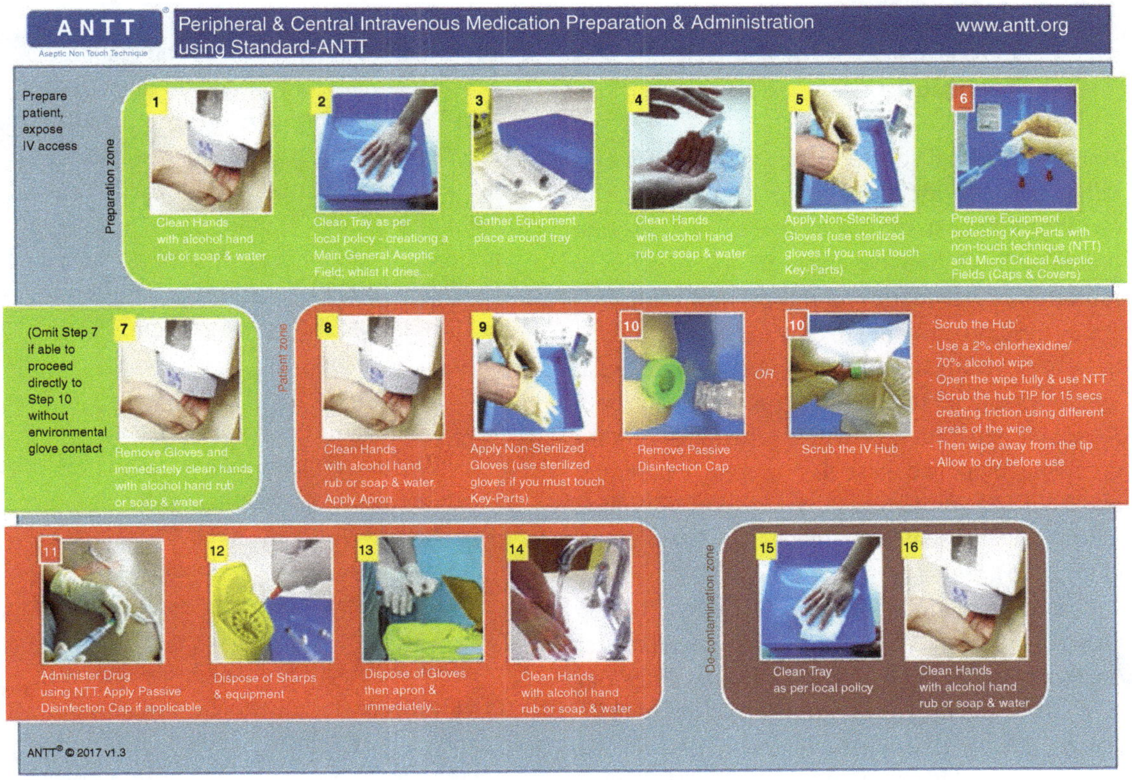

Fig. 11.4 ANTT® procedure guidelines (used with permission The Association for Safe Aseptic Practice – ASAP)

- Periodic assessment of ANTT® competency
- Simple but explicit picture-based ANTT® Guidelines visible in relevant practice areas to help make expectations explicit and measurable
- Surveillance—see below

11.7.3.1 Surveillance of Practice

Periodic 'snapshot' audit of various locations within a hospital can be an effective way of monitoring practice standards and informing the regularity of ANTT® competency reassessment.

11.7.3.2 Surveillance of Outcomes

It is important that healthcare organizations monitor for signs of poor standards of ANTT® by surveillance of relevant infective organisms. Point prevalence surveys (PPS) clearly demonstrate successes in reducing targeted organisms (Hopkins et al. 2012); however, they also illustrate the risks of only focusing on several high-profile harmful microorganisms and losing sight of the larger issue of the mechanisms and processes of infection prevention that help drive reductions in HAI across the board. In the most recently reported English NHS PPS from 2012, it was clear that the high-profile national targeting of MRSA bacteremia had reduced incidence considerably; however, it was also clear that other resistant organisms increased in prevalence (Hopkins et al. 2012).

Effective surveillance has highlighted the risks of not considering PVCs and CVADs as equally important in the context of healthcare-associated infections (DeVries and Valentine 2016), and the successful monitoring of the application of targeted resources is yielding improved outcomes (DeVries et al. 2016) along with a better understanding of adherence to best practice guidelines (Yagnik et al. 2017).

11.7.4 Developing a Meaningful Evidence Base for Aseptic Technique

As previously discussed, the pre-ANTT® evidence base for aseptic technique was weak and lacking in robust studies to define and describe practice. Since the development of ANTT®, a more robust, standardized and generalizable evidence base is beginning to develop as more countries and healthcare organizations implement a single practice standard for aseptic practice. Research generation provides a better and more complete evidence base for aseptic technique, and ANTT® is providing the framework for much of this development (Beaumont et al. 2016; Flynn et al. 2015).

The Association for Safe Aseptic Practice (ASAP) is a not-for-profit, non-governmental organization (NGO) based in the United Kingdom (UK) that promotes and administrates the ANTT® project. Using an epidemiological approach, the association produces standardized surveillance tools to assist in data collection, analysis and dissemination of ANTT® implementation and maintenance. A standard research protocol template aids in the design and implementation of local research studies helping to further develop a global evidence base for aseptic technique. It should be noted that ANTT® is trademarked to prevent variable alteration of the framework and standard approach. Utilization of ANTT® is very much encouraged and supported (see www.antt.org)!

Case Study

Nurse Smith was responsible for infection prevention at the hospital. As part of her objectives for the year, she identified aseptic practices with intravenous devices as a focus.

The first step in her initiative was to observe and document practices within the hospital (a pre-audit phase). After pinpointing gaps, confusion and compliance issues with aseptic technique, Nurse Smith contacted The-ASAP for advice and resources. Working collaboratively with The-ASAP/ANTT® Team she developed simple one-page educational sheets that emphasized the key points of the Aseptic Non Touch Technique (ANTT®). Nurse Smith, using a mixture of standardized ASAP and locally developed ANTT® resources, created a local multimodal form of education to roll out the key points.

- The education summary pages were used in department/unit huddles with a 5-min session of training with one page of the education per week.
- Posters were set up in locations around each unit, and observers were recruited to watch for opportunities to stimulate question and answer quick sessions with the nurses.
- ANTT® (visual) Clinical Practice Guidelines were deployed in clinical areas as education and training aids.
- Throughout the 3-month period, educational lectures from visiting clinicians were given to all the medical and nursing staff emphasizing the use of ANTT®.
- The ANTT-Approach was written into local policy and procedure documents, explicitly creating the expectation of standard aseptic practice.
- Nurse Smith used standardized assessment forms to competency assess clinical staff in ANTT®.

Follow-up observations and documentation revealed an 80% improvement in specific key points and practices of ANTT® and aseptic management of intravenous devices.

A long-term plan was developed to conduct periodic observation, using a checklist of key points and practices consistent with hospital policy, and to integrate annual aseptic education into the computer-based training already used for staff education.

Summary of Key Points

1. Aseptic technique involves a collection of infection prevention actions designed to protect patients from infection when undergoing invasive clinical procedures, including maintenance of indwelling medical devices.
2. The Aseptic Non Touch Technique (ANTT®) Clinical Practice Framework is quickly becoming the international standard when referring to aseptic technique.
3. The ANTT® Clinical Practice Framework utilizes only achievable practice terms and defines them as follows:
   (a) **Aseptic**—Free from pathogenic organisms (in sufficient numbers to cause infection)
   (b) **Sterile**—Free from (all) microorganisms (not possible in aseptic technique)
   (c) **Clean**—Free from visible marks and stains (useful for cleaning, but not an aim for aseptic technique)
   (d) **Non-touch**—The action of not touching critical or important parts of equipment and/or vulnerable or compromised parts of a patient
4. ANTT® focuses on a fundamental concept of Key-Part and Key-Site Protection to maintain an aseptic procedure.
5. The effectiveness of the ANTT® model has been demonstrated, but like any critical competency, its effectiveness depends on adherence to its principles and process by clinicians involved in inserting or manipulating/maintaining intravenous devices.
6. Compliance of ANTT® is enhanced through:
   (a) Periodic assessment of ANTT® competency
   (b) Picture-based ANTT® Guidelines visible in relevant practice areas to provide explicit and measurable expectations
   (c) Education, training and surveillance

Endorsement The Association for Safe Aseptic Practice (The-ASAP) oversees the development and dissemination of Aseptic Non Touch Technique (ANTT) intended for all invasive procedures and maintenance of invasive devices. Now used in over 30 countries and expanding, ANTT is the de facto international standard for aseptic technique. As editor, Nancy Moureau had the foresight to ensure that this contemporary book didn't articulate important matters of aseptic technique in historically variable terminology. Instead, the ANTT Practice Framework is defined comprehensively and used throughout. The-ASAP supports all healthcare organizations on matters of ANTT practice and implementation (www.antt.org).

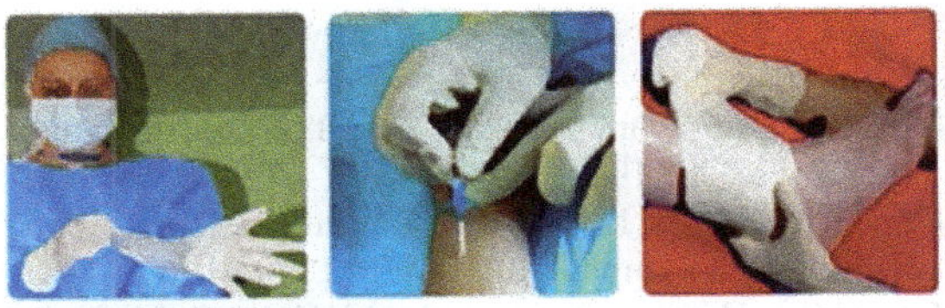

ASAP The Association for Safe Aseptic Practice

References

Aziz AM. Variations in aseptic technique and implications for infection control. Br J Nurs. 2009;18(1):26–31.

Beaumont K, Wyland M, Lee D. A multi-disciplinary approach to ANTT implementation: what can be achieved in 6 months. Infect Dis Health. 2016;21:67–71.

Berwick DM, Calkins DR, McCannon CJ, Hackbarth AD. The 100,000 lives campaign: setting a goal and a deadline for improving health care quality. JAMA. 2006;295(3):324–7.

Brühwasser C, Hinterberger G, Mutschlechner W, Kaltseis J, Lass-Flörl C, Mayr A. A point prevalence survey on hand hygiene, with a special focus on Candida species. Am J Infect Control. 2016;44:71–3.

Clare S, Rowley S. Implementing the Aseptic Non Touch Technique (ANTT®) clinical practice framework for aseptic technique: a pragmatic evaluation using a mixed methods approach in two London hospitals. J Infect Prev. 2017;19(1):6–15. Available: http://journals.sagepub.com/doi/abs/10.1177/1757177417720996 (accessed: September 2017).

DeVries M, Valentine M Bloodstream infections from peripheral lines: an underrated risk. American Nurse Today. (2016);11(1) https://www.americannursetoday.com/piv/. Accessed Sept 2017.

DeVries M, Valentine M, Mancos P. Protected clinical indication of peripheral intravenous lines: successful implementation. J Assoc Vasc Access. 2016;21:89–92.

DH. Department of Health, saving lives: reducing infection, delivering clean and safe care. 2007. http://webarchive.nationalarchives.gov.uk/+/http://www.dh.gov.uk/en/Publicationsandstatistics/Publications/PublicationsPolicyAndGuidance/DH_078134. Accessed Sept 2017.

Flores A. Sterile versus non-sterile glove use and aseptic technique. Nurs Stand. 2008;23:35–9.

Flynn JM, Keogh SJ, Gavin NC. Sterile vs aseptic non-touch technique for needle-less connector care on central venous access devices in a bone marrow transplant population: a comparative study. Eur J Oncol Nurs. 2015;19:694–700.

Fuller C, Savage J, Besser S, Hayward A, Cookson B, Cooper B, Stone S. "The dirty hand in the latex glove": a study of hand hygiene compliance when gloves are worn. Infect Control Hosp Epidemiol. 2011;32(12):1194–9.

Gorski L, Eddins J, INS. Infusion nursing standards of practice. JIN Suppl. 2011;34(1S):S1–110.

Gorski LA, Hadaway L, Hagle M, McGoldrick M, Orr M, Doellman D. Infusion therapy standards of practice. J Infus Nurs. 2016;39(Suppl 1):S1–S159.

Graves N, Barnett AG, Rosenthal VD. Open versus closed IV infusion systems: a state based model to predict risk of catheter associated blood stream infections. BMJ Open. 2011;1(2):e000188.

Hartley J. Aseptic technique to be part of essence of care guidance. Nurs Times. 2005;101:6.

Hibbard JS. Analyses comparing the antimicrobial activity and safety of current antiseptic agents: a review. J Infus Nurs. 2005;28:194–207.

HIRL. Bactericidal efficacy tests (EN1276) phase 2, step 1—Sani-Cloth® 7. Disposable disinfectant wipes for medical devices (PDI®). Hospital Infection Research Laboratory; 2006.

Hopkins S, Shaw K, Simpson L. English National Point Prevalence Survey on healthcare-associated infections and antimicrobial use. Health Protection Agency. 2012. http://webarchive.nationalarchives.gov.uk/20140714095446/http://www.hpa.org.uk/webc/HPAwebFile/HPAweb_C/1317134304594. Accessed Sept 2017

HPSC. Health Protection Surveillance Centre: guidelines for the prevention of catheter-associated urinary tract infection. 2011. https://www.hpsc.ie/a-z/microbiologyantimicrobialresistance/infectioncontrolandhai/guidelines/File,12913,en.pdf. Accessed Sept 2017.

Kaler W, Chinn R. A matter of time and friction. J Assoc Vasc Access. 2007;12(3):140–2.

Kingston L, O'Connell NH, Dunne CP. Hand hygiene-related clinical trials reported since 2010: a systematic review. J Hosp Infect. 2015;92(4):309–20.

Leas BF, Sullivan N, Han JH, et al. Environmental cleaning for the prevention of healthcare-associated infections [Internet]. Rockville: Agency for Healthcare Research and Quality (US); 2015. Technical briefs no 22. https://www.ncbi.nlm.nih.gov/books/NBK316174/. Accessed Sept 2017

Loveday HP, Wilson JA, Pratt RJ, Golsorkhi M, Tingle A, Bak A, Browne Prieto J, Wilcox M. epic3: national evidence-based guidelines for preventing healthcare-associated infections in NHS Hospitals in England. J Hosp Infect. 2014;86(S1):S1–S70.

Melle EV, Gruppen L, Holmboe ES, Flynn L, Oandasan I, Frank JR, for the International Competency-Based Medical Education Collaborators Academic Medicine. Using contribution analysis to evaluate competency-based medical education programs: it's all about rigor in thinking. Acad Med. 2017;92(6):752–8.

Moureau NL. Is your skin-prep technique up-to-date? Nursing. 2003;33(11):17.

Moureau NL, Flynn J. Disinfection of needleless connector hubs: clinical evidence systematic review. Nurs Res Pract. 2015;2015:1–20.

National Health and Medical Research Council. Australian Commission on Safety and Quality in Healthcare: Australian Guidelines for the Prevention and Control of Infection in Healthcare Commonwealth of Australia. 2010. https://www.nhmrc.gov.au/_files_nhmrc/publications/attachments/cd33_infection_control_healthcare_140616.pdf. Accessed Nov 2015.

NICE. Clinical guideline 139—healthcare-associated infections: prevention and control in primary and community care. 2012. https://www.nice.org.uk/guidance/cg139/evidence/control-full-guideline-pdf-185186701. Accessed Sept 2017.

NICE. The 3M Tegaderm CHG IV securement dressing for central venous and arterial catheter insertion sites. 2015. https://www.nice.org.uk/guidance/mtg25. Accessed Sept 2017.

NPSA. National Patient Safety Agency: the revised healthcare cleaning manual. 2009. http://www.nrls.npsa.nhs.uk/EasySiteWeb/getresource.axd?AssetID=61814. Accessed Sept 2017.

O'Grady NP, Alexander M, Burns LA, Dellinger EP, Garland J, O'Heard S, Lipsett PA, Mansur H, Mermel LA, Pearson ML, Raad II, Randolph A, Rupp ME, Saint S, The Healthcare Infection Control Practices Advisory Committee (HICPAC). Guidelines for the prevention of intravascular catheter-related infections. 2011. https://www.cdc.gov/hai/pdfs/bsi-guidelines-2011.pdf. Accessed Sept 2017.

Preston R. Aseptic technique: evidence-based approach for patient safety. Br J Nurs. 2005;14(10):540–6.

Pronovost P. Interventions to decrease catheter-related bloodstream infections in the ICU: the Keystone

Intensive Care Unit Project. Am J Infect Control. 2008;36(10):S171.e1–5.

Pronovost P, Needham D, Berenholtz S, Sinopoli D, Chu H, Cosgrove S, Sexton B, Hyzy R, Welsh R, Roth G, Bander J, Kepros J, Goeschel C. An intervention to decrease catheter-related bloodstream infections in the ICU. N Engl J Med. 2006;355:2725–32.

RCN. Royal College of Nursing: standards for infusion therapy. 4th ed. 2016. https://www.rcn.org.uk/professional-development/publications/pub-005704. Accessed Sept 2017.

Rowley S. Theory to practice: aseptic non-touch technique. Nurs Times. 2001;97:VI–VIII.

Rowley S, Clare S, Macqueen S, Molyneux R. ANTT v2: an updated practice framework for aseptic technique. Br J Nurs. 2010;19(5):S5–S11.

Sax H, Allegranzi B, Uckay I, Larson E, Boyce J, Pittet D. 'My five moments for hand hygiene': a user-centred design approach to understand, train, monitor and report hand hygiene. J Hosp Infect. 2007;67:9–21.

Smith J, Irwin G, Viney M, Watkins L, Morris S, Kirksey K, Brown A. Optimal disinfection times for needleless intravenous connectors. J Assoc Vasc Access. 2012;17:137–43.

Ullman AJ, Cooke ML, Mitchell M, Lin F, New K, Long DA, Mihala G, Rickard CM. Dressings and securement devices for central venous catheters (CVC). Cochrane Database Syst Rev. 2015;(9). Art. No.: CD010367. https://doi.org/10.1002/14651858.CD010367.pub2.

Unsworth J, Collins J. Performing an aseptic technique in a community setting: fact or fiction? Prim Health Care Res Dev. 2011;12:42–51.

Webster J, Osborne S, Rickard CM, New K. Clinically-indicated replacement versus routine replacement of peripheral venous catheters. Cochrane Database Syst Rev. 2013;(4). Art. No.: CD007798. https://doi.org/10.1002/14651858.CD007798.pub3.

Welsh Government. Welsh health circular. WHC/2015/026. 2015. http://www.primarycareservices.wales.nhs.uk/sitesplus/documents/1150/WHC%202015.026.pdf.

Yagnik L, Graves A, Thong K. Plastic in patient study: prospective audit of adherence to peripheral intravenous cannula monitoring and documentation guidelines, with the aim of reducing future rates of intravenous cannula-related complications. Am J Infect Control. 2017;54:34–8.

Zingg W, Pittet D. Peripheral venous catheters: an under-evaluated problem. Int J Antimicrob Agents. 2009;34(4):S38–42.

12

CLABSI Surveillance and Definition

Michelle DeVries

Abstract

Surveillance is an active process which requires proactively reviewing data sources indicative of an infection with the most common starting point through review of positive blood cultures. Based on the model of surveillance in the United States, if it is determined the bloodstream infection is associated with the central venous access device, mandatory data is collected. Other parts of the world do not have mandatory reporting. The surveillance data is used in a variety of ways including rating of hospitals for patient satisfaction, reimbursement/value-based purchasing percentages, comparison to other hospitals of similar bed size, central line device utilization ratio to determine if a hospital is using an inordinate ratio of central catheters, and determination of a standardized infection ratio. This chapter aims to define how surveillance is performed and the various uses of the gathered/reported information.

M. DeVries (✉)
Methodist Hospitals, Gary, IN, USA

Menzies Health Research Institute—Alliance for Vascular Access Teaching and Research (AVATAR) Group, Griffith University, Brisbane, QLD, Australia
e-mail: infectionprevention@comcast.net

Keywords

CLABSI surveillance · CLABSI reporting · CLABSI definition · CLABSI rate · Central line utilization ratio · Standardized Infection Rate

12.1 Surveillance Definition

12.1.1 CDC CLABSI Protocol

The National Healthcare Safety Network (NHSN) of the Centers for Disease Control and Prevention (CDC) publishes surveillance definitions for a broad range of healthcare-associated infections (HAI) (Horan et al. 2008). These definitions are reviewed and may be slightly revised annually and serve as the standard surveillance criteria for infections included in public reporting mandates through state regulations and federal Centers for Medicare and Medicaid Services (CMS) requirements for value-based purchasing (CDC 2017). They are also used for reporting into Press Ganey/National Database of Nursing Quality Indicators (NDNQI), which serves as the data repository for hospitals seeking Magnet™ designation. With minor variations, the Australian Commission on Safety and Quality in Health Care has implemented the same definitions throughout their country (Healthcare 2015).

Surveillance for CLABSIs is recommended in all areas of healthcare facilities that care for patients with CVADs and is required by Joint Commission to be conducted facility-wide rather than in a targeted manner (T. J. Commission 2012). Surveillance is an active process which requires proactively reviewing data sources indicative of an infection rather than relying on coded data or provider self-reporting of infections. The most common starting point is through review of positive blood cultures. Based on whether the organism is classified as a pathogen or a commensal (defined by CDC), the appropriate next steps are followed. Pathogens do not require symptoms in addition to the positive culture, but the patient record must be reviewed to rule out other potential sources of infection, which may cause the bacteremia to be defined as secondary to another site of infection. There are specific criteria to be followed when determining whether a suspected infection can be labeled as a secondary infection rather than a CLABSI. A pathogen requires only one positive culture to be considered an infection; organisms identified as commensals (i.e., coagulase-negative staphylococcus or diphtheroids) require two positive cultures collected at different times, in addition to clinical symptoms of infection such as fever or hypotension.

Equally important to the above infection surveillance is the collection of accurate denominators to allow for risk-adjusted CLABSI rates and ratios. Central line days are used as the standardized denominator for reporting CLABSI across units, expressed as the number of CLABSI/1000 central line days historically. Each unit has a mean rate of infection to which comparisons are made. More recently, public reporting has created a need for a standardized infection ratio (SIR) which allows for a single number to be used to reflect overall hospital CLABSI performance while allowing appropriate risk adjustment to take place to account for differing patient populations and other facility considerations. To collect these denominator days (regardless of whether using rates or SIRs), each unit provides a count at the same time every day of how many patients on the unit have one or more central lines at that specific point in time. Each patient only counts once, even if they have more than one central line. (Of note, neonatal ICU and nursery locations require stratification by birth weight, and specialty areas such as dialysis and oncology require stratification by temporary and permanent central lines). Those counts are totaled and reported once a month. Of interest to some organizations, there is now an option to collect this data by doing a once-a-week sample to extrapolate monthly line days. Electronic data capture is permitted for denominator calculations as well, but only after successful pre-validation for 3 months. Each unit must complete its own validation, confirming that electronic counts are within ±5% of the manually collected numbers. Ensuring the accuracy of denominator collection cannot be overemphasized (CDC 2017).

The protocol details may change annually. The most recent protocol is always available at https://www.cdc.gov/nhsn/pdfs/pscmanual/4psc_clabscurrent.pdf with compliance with the new version becoming required starting January first of each year for state and federal reporting. Each spring, the CDC offers a free, detailed training on the surveillance protocol to ensure that the definitions are strictly adhered to by all participating organizations. There is a lottery to attend the event live, but it is available for all to participate via webstream. Those training materials are archived and readily accessible for anyone interested at https://www.cdc.gov/nhsn/training/patient-safety-component/index.html. Infection preventionists and any others involved in collection of the data must remain up-to-date with the protocols and related reporting requirements as they evolve.

12.2 Understanding the Goals and Limitations of Surveillance Definitions

CLABSI is a surveillance definition only. It is not synonymous with the catheter-related bloodstream infection (CRBSI) definition and is not intended to offer guidance regarding patient care decisions for the patient who has been classified as meeting the definition. Use of standardized surveillance protocols allows for data to be compared (with appropriate risk adjustment) across facilities and within organizations for performance improvement. Because of limitations of surveillance definitions in their ability to identify the central line as the true source of infection, it may overestimate the true burden of disease. CLABSI does not have any elements which assess which device (if any) is the true source of the infection, nor do paired cultures or time to positivity studies play a role in ruling in or ruling out an infection which has otherwise met the definition. This can create discomfort with treatment teams and vascular access experts, but the importance of adherence to the protocol is crucial, particularly with regulatory and accreditation requirements for accurate data collection.

12.3 Using CDC Protocol Beyond Central Lines

Although hospitals commonly use the laboratory-confirmed bloodstream infection (LCBI) definitions only for CLABSI reporting, the actual definition is not specific to only central lines. A LCBI is reported as a CLABSI when the patient has a central line in for greater than 2 days and is in place the day of or the day before the first sign or symptom used to meet the definition. That same LCBI definition is appropriate for bloodstream infections that do not have a central line present. Some organizations identify those infections as CLABSI vs. non-CLABSI; others apply the line designation with other devices in the same manner as central lines are evaluated to make the determination of CLABSI. That same rationale can be applied to short peripheral catheters and midlines. It should be noted that the requirement for greater than 2 days of dwell time does not require a single catheter to account for that; in the case of peripherals, it may be seen that a patient has a series of devices during that time interval. If there is not a full calendar day without a device in place, the dwell time can be met using sequential devices. At the time of this writing, CDC has a proposal open for comment which considers expanding surveillance to include all hospital onset bacteremia, of which CLABSI would be a subset.

12.4 Brief Primer on How to Interpret Surveillance Data

With NHSN data as the standard method of collecting and reporting hospital-acquired infections throughout the United States and mirrored in many other countries, there is robust data available through the required database. Partnering with infection prevention teams at the organization to provide reports on a routine basis helps guide the vascular access team to areas for focused education or monitoring.

12.4.1 CLABSI Rate

Historically, CLABSI incidence was analyzed by reviewing an individual unit's incidence of CLABSI expressed as a rate per 1000 central line days. Using historic data (within an institution, system-wide aggregate performance, state-based goals, or national benchmarks), the performance can be easily evaluated and compared to other similar units. The CDC publishes descriptions of the different unit types which require carefully "mapping" each unit in the hospital to identify the appropriate comparison group. Each type of unit and specialty within many types of units (i.e., critical care has many different risk types based on the primary patient population served) will have published information on the average rate of infection in that population. Reports run from within NHSN historically also specify where a hospital's performance is on the bell curve of all other similar units in the reporting period, based on percentile distribution.

12.4.2 Central Line Device Utilization Ratio

Central line utilization is a required element for existence of a CLABSI, with many recent publications assessing the appropriateness of specific line choices. As part of the CLABSI rate reports available within NHSN, information is also shared on central line utilization for each individual unit. This is expressed as a ratio of central line days over patient days for the unit. Similar to what is produced for CLABSI comparisons, there is data that allows facilities to compare their central line utilization ratios to other similar units to see if there is potential for decreasing excess central line utilization. Most recently, there are now reports on standardized utilization ratios (SUR) which represent a hospital's device utilization compared to what is predicted based on the types of patients seen. This new measure allows for aggregate review of device utilization opportunities as well as a more detailed review at the unit level. There is more discussion on how to interpret the ratios in the section below regarding infection ratios.

12.4.3 Standardized Infection Ratio

Standardized infection ratios (SIR) allow for aggregate data to be used to produce a single number reflecting the performance of an entire hospital or a group of units. This is the figure that is used for public reporting on Hospital Compare and for evaluation of hospital performance as part of the Centers for Medicare and Medicaid Services (CMS) value-based purchasing (VBP). This ratio allows for complicated risk adjustment to take place "behind the scenes" and allows for a simple comparison against expected performance. A SIR of "1" indicates that performance is consistent with what is predicted based on the patient population included in the report. Numbers of less than one indicate that patients in the assessed population experienced fewer infections than predicted, and similarly a SIR of greater than one indicates that the assessed population observed more infections than were predicted. This is qualified with tests of statistical significance. It is possible to run SIR reports for individual units, for specified groupings of units, and for an entire organization to provide whichever overview is most useful.

12.5 Understanding Variations and Limitations in Technique for Diagnosing CRBSI

The need to determine the role of the central venous catheter as the underlying source of infection may have clinical relevance to inform treatment decisions by the medical team. Depending on available laboratory resources, options may include culturing of the catheter tip, reviewing differential time to positivity between blood cultures collected from the implicated device and from a peripheral stick, and quantitative assessment of culture results. There is no recommendation for routinely culturing catheter tips on removal in the absence of a suspected infection.

The Infectious Diseases Society of America publishes recommendations for diagnosis and treatment of vascular catheter-related bloodstream infections. They describe preferential culturing of catheter tips and avoidance of broth culturing techniques and define interpretation of roll plate (>15 CFU from a 5 cm segment) and sonication techniques (>10^2 CFU) when assessing for colonization. CRBSI diagnosis can be made when culture results identify the same organism in at least the culture obtained as a peripheral stick and from a culture of the catheter tip. If the catheter is left in place, the diagnosis can be made if there are two blood samples being drawn (one from the catheter and one from a peripheral stick) that meet specific criteria for quantitative blood cultures or differential time to positivity. For multi-lumen catheters, quantitative cultures may be obtained through multiple lumens; results at least 3 times higher through one of the lumens are suggestive of CRBSI (Mermel et al. 2009).

Recommendations regarding treatment and possible removal or replacement of CVCs suspected of infection are based on several factors including pathogen, underlying health conditions, and consultation with infectious disease specialists (Center for Disease Control 2017; Chopra et al. 2015).

12.6 Summary

The surveillance for CLABSI and the required reporting of those results provide useful information to determine if a facility is operating within common averages. The information is used to compare one hospital CLABSI rate to another, compare central line device utilization ratios to see if a particular unit is using a higher percentage of central lines compared to similar units in other hospitals, and to determine a standardized infection ratio for each hospital to be used when comparing facilities.

While surveillance for CLABSIs does not provide information regarding how to treat the infections, it does provide information allowing facilities to determine what may be causing higher than normal CRBSIs at their facility (e.g., higher central line usage rates).

Case Study

As part of the hospital's annual infection control risk assessment, CLABSI is listed as a priority based on performance of the organization not meeting value-based purchasing thresholds. The infection prevention team provides a detailed breakdown of the standardized infection ratio as well as central line standardized utilization ratio to target specific units which are high outliers for either or both infections or excess device utilization. Working collaboratively with vascular access and professional development, the team can use this information to create meaningful action plans and a standard method of assessment for improvement against institutional as well as accreditation and regulatory goals.

Summary of Key Points

1. Surveillance for CLABSI is an active process which requires proactively reviewing data sources indicative of an infection.
2. CLABSI is a surveillance definition only. It is not synonymous with CRBSI and is not intended to offer guidance regarding patient care decisions. It is for the collection of data.
3. Blood is tested when there is a clinical suspicion of bloodstream infection. When a positive blood culture is present, the organism is classified as a pathogen or a commensal, and the appropriate next steps are followed.
4. There are specific criteria to be followed when determining whether a suspected infection is labeled as a CLABSI or a secondary infection. The need to determine the role of the central venous catheter as the underlying source of infection may have clinical relevance to inform treatment decisions by the medical team.
5. Surveillance data can be used to help guide the vascular access team to areas for focused education or monitoring. The data is useful to:
   (a) Compare one population's CLABSI incidence to another in a risk-adjusted manner.
   (b) Compare central line device utilization ratios to see if a particular unit or population is using a higher percentage of central lines compared to similar units in other hospitals.

References

CDC. Bloodstream infection event (Central line-associated bloodstream infection and non-central line-associated bloodstream infection) [Online]. 2017. https://www.cdc.gov/nhsn/pdfs/pscmanual/4psc_clabscurrent.pdf. Accessed 9 July 2017.

Center for Disease Control, C. Updating the guideline methodology of the healthcare infection control practices advisory committee (HICPAC) [Online]. 2017. https://www.cdc.gov/hicpac/pdf/guidelines/2009-10-29HICPAC_GuidelineMethodsFINAL.pdf: CDC. Accessed 17 Feb 2017.

Chopra V, Flanders SA, Saint S, Woller SC, O'grady NP, Safdar N, Trerotola SO, Saran R, Moureau N, Wiseman S, Pittiruti M, Akl EA, Lee AY, Courey A, Swaminathan L, Ledonne J, Becker C, Krein SL, Bernstein SJ, Michigan Appropriateness Guide for Intravenouse Catheters, P. The michigan appropriateness guide for intravenous catheters (MAGIC): results from a multispecialty panel using the RAND/UCLA appropriateness method. Ann Intern Med. 2015;163:S1–40.

Commission, T. J Preventing central line–associated bloodstream infections: a global challenge, a global perspective [Online]. 2012.

Healthcare, A. C. O. S. a. Q. I. Implementation-guide-for-surveillance-of-central-line-associated-bloodstream-infection-2016-edition.pdf [Online].

2015. https://www.safetyandquality.gov.au/wp-content/uploads/2016/04/Implementation-Guide-for-Surveillance-of-Central-Line-Associated-Bloodstream-Infection-2016-Edition.pdf. Accessed 10 July 2017.

Horan TC, Andrus M, Dudeck MA. CDC/NHSN surveillance definition of health care-associated infection and criteria for specific types of infections in the acute care setting. Am J Infect Control. 2008;36:309–32.

Mermel LA, Allon M, Bouza E, Craven DE, Flynn P, O'grady NP, Raad I, Rijnders BJ, Sherertz RJ, Warren DK. Clinical practice guidelines for the diagnosis and management of intravascular catheter-related infection: 2009 update by the Infectious Diseases Society of America. Clin Infect Dis. 2009;49:1–45.

Part V

Health and Preservation: Pediatric Vessels

13

Pediatrics and the Importance of Vascular Access

Amanda Ullman and Tricia Kleidon

Abstract

A high-quality vascular access practice is of utmost importance in the area of pediatrics to ensure the preservation of vessel health. Pediatric clinicians must ensure that a focus on vessel health and preservation is evident from the child's earliest exposure to healthcare. The ability to ensure long-term vessel health and preservation from infancy into adulthood and the prevention of complications associated with VAD in pediatrics are key components to ensure successful, efficient, lifelong healthcare.

Keywords

Pediatric developmental stages · VHP for adolescents

A. Ullman (✉)
Alliance for Vascular Access Teaching and Research (AVATAR) Group, Menzies Health Institute Queensland, School of Nursing and Midwifery, Griffith University, Brisbane, QLD, Australia
e-mail: a.ullman@griffith.edu.au

T. Kleidon
Alliance for Vascular Access Teaching and Research (AVATAR), Queensland Children's Hospital, Brisbane, QLD, Australia
e-mail: tricia.kleidon@health.qld.gov.au

13.1 Introduction

The vessels that children are born with are the only vessels they will have throughout their entire lifetime. Once injured, vessels rarely fully recover. Internationally, a growing number of children are reliant upon vascular access devices (VADs) for extended periods of time. Severe, life-threatening chronic health conditions, such as intestinal failure and cystic fibrosis, require children to be dependent on VADs for their entire lifespan. In addition, children undergoing treatment for complex conditions such as cancer often require additional intravenous access to treat the unintended complications of anticancer therapies. These children continue to progress through healthcare systems as adolescents and then adults, undergoing treatment for further health conditions later in life.

13.2 Vascular Access-Related Anatomical, Physiological, and Developmental Variations by Age Group

Children undergo rapid changes throughout the first 18 years of their life. The anatomical, physiological, and developmental differences between children, adolescents, and adults impact the way illnesses and diseases present. These differences determine what type of healthcare is provided at

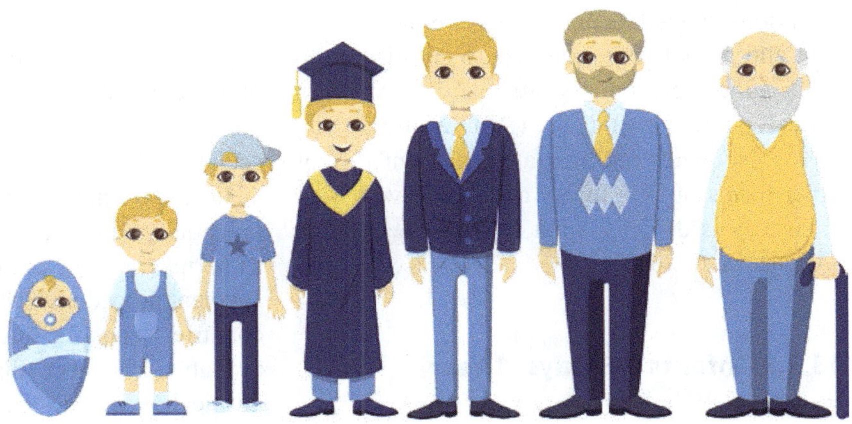

Fig. 13.1 Aging life cycle

various stages for the growing child (see Fig. 13.1). These differences also have an impact on how vessel health and preservation is supported. Throughout all stages, parents and other primary caregivers should be recognized as partners with clinicians when planning, inserting, and managing VADs.

13.2.1 Neonatal (<28 Days)

For approximately the first week of life, the umbilical vascular network is a viable means of central venous and arterial therapy. A range of VADs are utilized for neonates in the special care or neonatal intensive care setting to facilitate therapies associated with preterm delivery, low birthweight, congenital disease, or abnormality and/or to treat infection. A definition of the common terms used in the neonatal period can be found in Table 13.1.

The neonatal vascular network continues to mature throughout the first year of life after term delivery (Mccullen and Pieper 2006). The developing vein structure includes decreased muscle diameter, meaning clinicians need to use smaller, size-appropriate catheters for both peripheral and central devices (Franck et al. 2001). This is explored further in Chap. 14.

Table 13.1 Definitions (Rudolf et al. 2011)

Preterm delivery	Infant born before 37 completed weeks of gestation
Very low birthweight (VLBW)	A baby born with a birthweight of 1500 g or less
Extremely low birthweight (ELBW)	A baby born with a birthweight of 1000 g or less

An important consideration for vascular access and infusion therapy is the neonates' low circulating blood volume. The total blood volume is relative to body weight and neonatal development. In the immediate post-birth neonatal period, blood volume varies from 85 mL/kg at birth rising to a peak of 105 mL/kg by the end of the first month and then drops over the ensuing months (Sorge et al. 2016). This means the average, full-term neonate has a circulating blood volume of between 250 and 400 mL. Careful monitoring of fluid balance in the neonatal period is critical as the infusion of multiple continuous and intermittent medications such as antibiotics, blood products, and fluid can unintentionally and dramatically increase the neonates' fluid intake, which may result in fluid overload. Conversely, excessive blood sampling can also be associated with harm, including iatrogenic anemia (Ullman et al. 2016).

Many other physiological attributes of neonates significantly increase their risk for vascular access-associated harm. An immature immune system places the neonate at significant increased risk of developing infection. Functional skin maturation continues until the second year of life; therefore, neonatal skin is thin and structurally immature (Visscher et al. 2017). A thin stratum corneum increases the risk of absorption of procedural solutions (e.g., chlorhexidine or alcohol) leading to burns and irritations as well as potential systemic absorption and associated harm. These solutions and other adhesive products are likely to result in adhesive-related injuries (Ponnusamy et al. 2014). Neonates are also at significant risk of other forms of skin injury associated with vascular access devices, such as pressure injuries (August et al. 2017).

13.2.2 Infants (28 Days–1 Year)

Infancy involves a more rapid rate of growth than at any other age (Rudolf et al. 2011). As discussed within the previous section, the infant's immature vascular network, immune system, skin structure, and circulating blood volume continue to develop over the ensuing year, providing challenges when providing vascular access and infusion therapy.

The infant's rapid growth and development also necessitates changes in pediatric vascular access practice. Rapid growth, including increased adiposity during infancy and toddler years, can make it difficult to visualize and palpate veins, making the insertion of VADs challenging. Vein visualization technology, such as ultrasound and infrared, can be useful in this age group. In particular, the insertion and management of jugular CVADs can be challenging due to increased adiposity and the limited amount of space in an infant's neck. In emergent situations when intravenous access is not possible, intraosseous (IO) infusions are sometimes necessary in this age group (Tobias and Ross 2010). The regular assessment of all VADs for signs of dysfunction and complication is especially relevant for this age group due to their inability to communicate discomfort and alert the clinician to a potential complication.

13.2.3 Toddler (1–3 Years)

The toddler years involve an expansion in mobility and social interaction. Within vascular access, this provides new challenges regarding procedural compliance. Various resources are available to reduce anxiety and promote compliance during VAD insertion, management, and removal procedures. Within North America, child life specialists (CLS) provide expertise in child psychosocial and cognitive development to reduce anxiety and improve experiences associated with potentially painful and stressful procedures, such as peripheral vein cannulation and CVAD management procedures (Murag et al. 2017). In other countries and facilities where CLS are not available, cognitive, distractive, behavioral, and physical strategies are used to assist pediatric patients within these situations. Localized and/or generalized pain relief during the insertion and management procedures should always be incorporated, as with other populations. The insertion of CVADs (including PICCs) into toddlers without appropriate sedation is difficult and may result in suboptimal outcomes.

Additional strategies should also be incorporated to ensure the safety of the clinician, VAD, and thereby the toddler, during mobilization and episodes of non-compliance. This includes the use of additional security devices and circumspect placement. For example, a PIVC or PICC into the leg of a newly mobile toddler is likely to be quickly dislodged.

13.2.4 Preschool to School-Age Children (3–12 Years)

Motor, language, and social skills continue to develop during the preschool and school years (Rudolf et al. 2011). Procedural compliance varies between children and ages. As communication improves, so does the need to ensure children are properly consulted throughout vascular access decision-making. CLS (if available) or their professional equivalent should be engaged early during the assessment and intervention phase of VAD insertion to ensure involvement. Distraction therapies are useful in this age group to assist in reducing anxiety and promoting procedural success (Murag et al. 2017). Device placement should be planned to ensure minimal disruption to the preschool and school-age child's ability to continue with usual play activities. This will ensure better compliance with the inserted device and reduce the risk of complications such as inadvertent dislodgement.

13.2.5 Adolescents (13–18 Years)

Starting from as early as 9 years of age, adolescence is characterized by a physical, psychological, and social maturity which occurs under the influence of rising hormone levels (Rudolf et al. 2011). Puberty culminates when an individual becomes physiologically capable of sexual reproduction. While many of the anatomical and physiological differences between pediatric and adult patients which impact vascular access and infusion therapy have plateaued by adolescence, there are developmental attributes which necessitate specialized care. Additionally, children with chronic illness may have exhausted many of the traditional vascular access routes by this age. This situation necessitates complex management of their vasculature, including the insertion of nontraditional vascular access routes.

As emerging adults, adolescents are generally more able to participate in decision-making about their own care and have opinions and views which can challenge those of their family and healthcare providers. It is necessary to find the most appropriate way to work with each adolescent on an individual basis, ensuring the adolescent is sufficiently involved in his/her vascular access decision-making, including choices surrounding device type, location, insertion procedure, management, and many other aspects. For adolescents with chronic health conditions, they are likely to be the expert of their own health condition, and consideration of their opinion is likely to make an important contribution to the success of the device.

13.3 Common Pediatric Conditions Which Are Vascular Access Dependent

The pediatric health conditions described in this section are not an exhaustive list. The list provides a short summary of common, complex, and chronic pediatric conditions that are heavily reliant on vascular access for management over prolonged time periods.

13.3.1 Short Bowel (Gut) Syndrome

Short bowel, or gut, syndrome commonly occurs in pediatric patients as a sequela of necrotizing enterocolitis, which can occur within the first few weeks of any newborn but is most commonly found in premature infants. Chronic intestinal failure results from a bowel resection that leaves a short residual length of small bowel (Nightingale and Woodward 2006). Many children with short gut syndrome are highly dependent upon vascular access for prolonged periods of time due to their reliance on parenteral nutrition. This occurs due to severe intestinal failure and/or reduced intestinal absorption so that macronutrient and/or water and electrolyte supplements are needed to maintain health/growth (Nightingale and Woodward 2006). If untreated, undernutrition and dehydration ensue, resulting in impaired growth and development.

The safe administration of parenteral nutrition commonly requires the insertion of a CVAD (M. Pittiruti et al., Pittiruti et al. 2009). International clinical practice guidelines recommend the use of parenteral nutrition if a patient absorbs less than one third of the oral energy intake, if there are high energy requirements and absorption is 30–60%, or if increasing oral/enteral nutrient intake causes a socially unacceptable amount of diarrhea or a large volume of stomal output (Nightingale and Woodward 2006).

There are many other acute and chronic causes of intestinal failure which may result in a short- or long-term dependency on parenteral nutrition (see Fig. 13.2).

There are emerging treatment strategies for end-stage intestinal failure and incurable gastrointestinal disorders, such as short bowel syndrome, including the use of intestinal transplantation (Abu–Elmagd 2006). However, consequences associated with the historically heavy immunosuppression schedules have meant that widespread use has been limited. An alternative to organ transplant in patients with short bowel syndrome is the serial transverse entero-

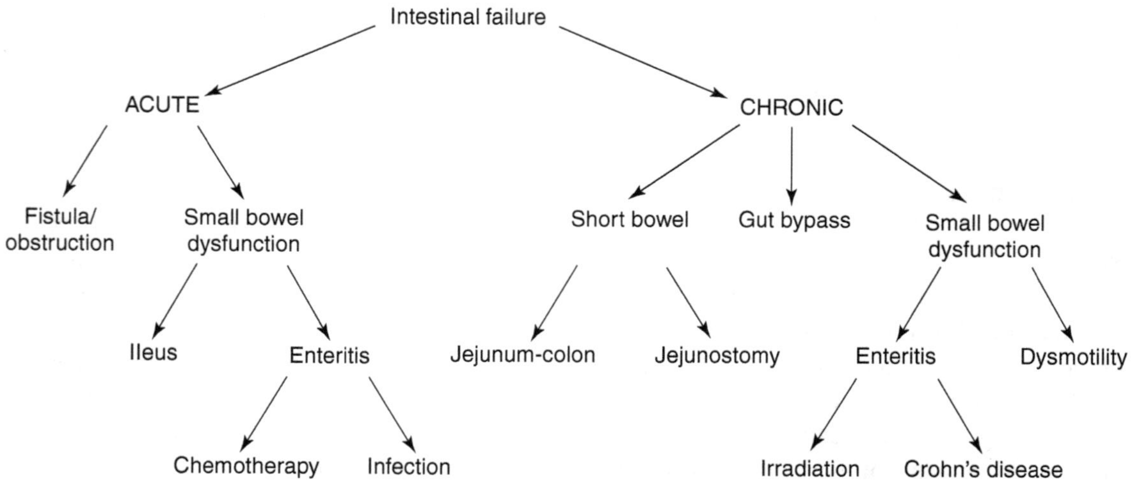

Fig. 13.2 Reasons for intestinal failure (Nightingale and Woodward 2006) (used with permission of BMJ)

plasty (STEP) procedure (Chang et al. 2006) which aims to increase intestinal absorption by optimizing intestinal function and motility, so that patients can better tolerate nutrition through the gastrointestinal tract and eventually wean from parenteral nutrition.

13.3.2 Cystic Fibrosis

Cystic fibrosis (CF) is a life-limiting, complex, multi-organ, congenital disorder affecting 1 in 3500 births in Australia, Europe, and the United States (Flume et al. 2010; Pedersen et al. 2015; World Health Organization 2012). CF is characterized by dehydration of the airway surface liquid and impaired mucociliary clearance (Flume et al. 2010). As a result, individuals with the disease have difficulty clearing pathogens from the lung and experience chronic pulmonary infections and inflammation.

Specialized CF care has led to a dramatic improvement in survival and quality of life (Smyth et al. 2014). An important element of early and ongoing supportive therapy is the administration of intravenous antibiotics to treat pulmonary exacerbations caused by infections. Reliable vascular access enables protocolized administration of antibiotics; a range of devices are used depending upon the patients' vessel availability, duration of treatment, severity of illness, and personal preference.

13.3.3 Hematological Disorders

Hematological conditions are disorders of any aspect of the blood, bone marrow, or lymph nodes. These include malignant and nonmalignant conditions which may be either acute or chronic. Chronic or life-threatening conditions frequently require repetitive vascular access due to frequent testing and the administration of treatments and supportive therapies (e.g., blood transfusions).

13.3.4 Nonmalignant Hematological Disorders

Common nonmalignant (benign) conditions requiring vascular access in pediatrics include:

- **Sickle cell anemia:** Sickle cell anemia is the most severe form of sickle cell disease, a genetic disorder of the red blood cell. Sickle cell disease is caused by abnormal hemoglobin, called hemoglobin S (or sickle hemoglobin, HbS). Several sickle cell disease genotypes exist. The most prevalent genotype, HbSS, and the much less common HbSβ0-thalassemia are both commonly referred to as sickle cell anemia (SCA) because they are phenotypically very similar and are associated with the most severe clinical manifestations (Yawn et al. 2014). A wide variety of acute complications occur in sickle cell disease reflecting the complex pathophysiology of vaso-occlusion, infection, anemia, and infarction (Ware et al. 2017). The main treatments for the disease are red blood cell transfusions and hydroxycarbamide, with cure possible with stem cell transplantation (Ware et al. 2017).

- **Aplastic anemia:** Aplastic anemia (AA) is a rare and heterogenous disorder of the bone marrow in which hematopoietic stem cells get destroyed by either drugs, idiopathic or inherited autoimmune process (Barone et al. 2015). It is defined as a pancytopenia with a hypocellular bone marrow in the absence of an abnormal infiltrate, major dysplasia, or marrow fibrosis (Bhatnagar and Samarasinghe 2015). The management of AA includes platelet and red blood cell transfusions and the prevention and treatment of infections (including antibiotic prophylaxis, with severe neutropenia). Treatment choices include stem cell transplantation and immunosuppressive therapy (Bhatnagar and Samarasinghe 2015).
- **Hemophilia:** Hemophilia is a congenital bleeding disorder caused by a deficiency of coagulation factor VIII (in hemophilia A) or factor IX (in hemophilia B) (Srivastava et al. 2013). The deficiency is the result of mutations of the respective clotting factor gene. The severity of bleeding in hemophilia is generally correlated with the clotting factor level (Srivastava et al. 2013). The treatment of hemophilia is complex, and overall indwelling VADs are to be avoided whenever possible. However, some children with severe disease are heavily reliant on their VAD for the administration of blood components and clotting factor concentrates.

13.3.5 Malignant Hematological Disorders

Blood cancers, or hematological malignancies, include leukemias, lymphomas, and myeloma. The mortality rates associated with hematological malignancies have decreased over the last 30 years (Inaba et al. 2013); however, intensive, complex, vascular-access-dependent treatments are necessary. Hematological malignancies common to pediatrics include:

- **Acute lymphoblastic leukemia (ALL):** ALL is characterized by an overproduction of lymphocytes (immature white blood cells). These cells crowd the bone marrow, which prevent it from producing normal blood cells. Approximately 60% of patients with ALL are less than 20 years of age (Inaba et al. 2013). Treatments for ALL are highly protocolized, typically span 2–2.5 years, and are comprised of three phases: induction of remission, intensification (or consolidation), and continuation (or maintenance). Reliable vascular access is key during all phases of treatment. Risk factors related to device complication vary dependent on the treatment phase and should be considered with device choice. In addition to treatment, supportive care is also intensive, including infection prevention and frequent blood product administration. Stem cell transplantation is an option for children with very high risk or persistent disease. Central nervous system (CNS) disease control, through a combination of systemic chemotherapy and risk-based early intensive intrathecal chemotherapy, plays a substantial role in prevention of relapse (Inaba et al. 2013).
- **Acute myeloid leukemia (AML):** AML involves the expansion of undifferentiated, immature, myeloid cells (Tarlock and Meshinchi 2015). Like in ALL, these cells reduce/prevent the production of normal blood cells. AML is more common in adult populations; however, pediatric AML has a genomic and epigenetic profile distinct from adult AML (Tarlock and Meshinchi 2015). Protocolized treatments and supportive care are somewhat similar in structure to ALL and are also highly vascular access dependent.
- **Hodgkin's lymphoma (HL):** HL is cancer of the lymphatic system, where developing lymphocytes become lymphoma cells, which include a Reed-Sternberg cell, and multiply aggressively. It is the most common of the pediatric lymphatic neoplasias, however is

considered one of the most curable cancers, with long-term survival rates now exceeding 90% after treatment (Mauz-Körholz et al. 2015). The staging classification of HL (I–IV) delineates severity of spread between lymph node regions and extralymphatic organs or sites (Lister et al. 1989). The treatment of pediatric HL is primarily through tailored radiation and chemotherapy (Mauz-Körholz et al. 2015).
- **Non-Hodgkin lymphomas (NHL):** NHL also affect the lymphatic system and originate in lymphocytes. The cancer starts in the lymphoid tissue but can originate outside the lymph nodes. Pediatric NHL are a diverse group of diseases in morphological and clinical characteristics (Sorge et al. 2016). The two main types of NHL are B-cell (in the lymph nodes in the neck, head, throat, and abdomen) and T -cell (in the lymph nodes in the chest). Treatment of NHL varies between NHL types and is principally through traditional chemotherapy, radiotherapy, and biological therapies (e.g., monoclonal antibodies) (Sorge et al. 2016).

13.3.6 Oncological Conditions

While hematological malignancies such as leukemia and lymphoma are the most common individual types of cancer, over 50% of cancers originate outside of the hematological system. These include:

- **Brain and CNS tumors**: including astrocytoma, brain stem glioma, craniopharyngioma, ependymoma, medulloblastoma, glioma, and others
- **Neuroblastoma:** cancer forming in certain types of nerve tissues, frequently in the adrenal glands, neck, chest, abdomen, or spine and common in children less than 5 years of age
- **Wilms tumor:** cancer of the kidney(s) that is also known as the nephroblastoma, mostly occurring before 10 years of age
- **Childhood rhabdomyosarcoma:** cancer developing from rhabdomyoblasts which form skeletal muscles; develop in either children or young adults
- **Retinoblastoma:** a genetic and congenital cancer developing from immature cells of the retina, common in young children (<2 years)
- **Osteosarcoma**: a cancerous tumor in a bone, common to teenagers and young adults

13.4 Conclusion

Vascular access has a fundamental role to the successful treatment and management of these complex health conditions. While the reliance on vascular access varies, a focus on vessel health and preservation is necessary throughout the entire treatment period to ensure children with these conditions can receive treatment and support for as long as necessary, including into adulthood if necessary.

Case Study

Cassie, a 13-year-old girl, is undergoing the insertion of a tunneled, cuffed CVAD to facilitate treatment and supportive therapies associated with her relapsed acute lymphoblastic leukemia (ALL). She is in the early stages of puberty, including the development of breasts.

What considerations should be made when planning this device?

Summary of Key Points

1. A high-quality vascular access practice is of utmost importance in the area of pediatrics to ensure the preservation of vessel health.
2. The anatomical, physiological, and developmental differences between children, adolescents, and adults impact the way illnesses and diseases present.
3. Developmental differences determine what type of healthcare is provided at various stages for the growing child.

These differences also impact how vessel health and preservation is supported.

4. Throughout all stages, parents and other primary caregivers should be recognized as partners with clinicians when planning, inserting, and managing VADs.
5. Vascular access has a fundamental role to the successful treatment and management of these complex health conditions.

References

Abu-Elmagd KM. Intestinal transplantation for short bowel syndrome and gastrointestinal failure: current consensus, rewarding outcomes, and practical guidelines. Gastroenterology. 2006;130:S132–7. https://doi.org/10.1053/j.gastro.2005.09.069.

August DL, New K, Ray RA, Kandasamy Y. Frequency, location and risk factors of neonatal skin injuries from mechanical forces of pressure, friction, shear and stripping: a systematic literature review. J Neonatal Nurs. 2017;24(4):173–80. https://doi.org/10.1016/j.jnn.2017.08.003.

Barone A, Lucarelli A, Onofrillo D, Verzegnassi F, Bonanomi S, Cesaro S, Fioredda F, Iori AP, Ladogana S, Locasciulli A, Longoni D, Lanciotti M, Macaluso A, Mandaglio R, Marra N, Martire B, Maruzzi M, Menna G, Notarangelo LD, Palazzi G, Pillon M, Ramenghi U, Russo G, Svahn J, Timeus F, Tucci F, Cugno C, Zecca M, Farruggia P, Dufour C, Saracco P. Diagnosis and management of acquired aplastic anemia in childhood. Guidelines from the Marrow Failure Study Group of the Pediatric Haemato-Oncology Italian Association (AIEOP). Blood Cell Mol Dis. 2015;55:40–7. https://doi.org/10.1016/j.bcmd.2015.03.007.

Bhatnagar N, Samarasinghe S. Diagnosis and management of childhood aplastic anaemia. Paediatr Child Health. 2015;25:343–9. https://doi.org/10.1016/j.paed.2015.04.001.

Chang RW, Javid PJ, Oh J-T, Andreoli S, Kim HB, Fauza D, Jaksic T. Serial transverse enteroplasty enhances intestinal function in a model of short bowel syndrome. Ann Surg. 2006;243:223. https://doi.org/10.1097/01.sla.0000197704.76166.07.

Flume PA, Mogayzel PJ Jr, Robinson KA, Rosenblatt RL, Quittell L, Marshall BC. Cystic fibrosis pulmonary guidelines: pulmonary complications: hemoptysis and pneumothorax. Am J Respir Crit Care Med. 2010;182:298–306. https://doi.org/10.1164/rccm.201002-0157CI.

Franck L, Hummel D, Connell K, Quinn D, Montgomery J. The safety and efficacy of peripheral intravenous catheters in ill neonates. Neonatal Netw. 2001;20:33–8. https://doi.org/10.1891/0730-0832.20.5.33.

Inaba H, Greaves M, Mullighan CG. Acute lymphoblastic leukaemia. Lancet. 2013;381:1943–55. https://doi.org/10.1016/S0140-6736(12)62187-4.

Lister T, Crowther D, Sutcliffe S, Glatstein E, Canellos G, Young R, Rosenberg S, Coltman C, Tubiana M. Report of a committee convened to discuss the evaluation and staging of patients with Hodgkin's disease: cotswolds meeting. J Clin Oncol. 1989;7:1630–6. https://doi.org/10.1200/JCO.1989.7.11.1630.

Mauz-Körholz C, Metzger ML, Kelly KM, Schwartz CL, Castellanos ME, Dieckmann K, Kluge R, Körholz D. Pediatric hodgkin lymphoma. J Clin Oncol. 2015;33:2975–85. https://doi.org/10.1200/JCO.2014.59.4853.

Mccullen KL, Pieper B. A retrospective chart review of risk factors for extravasation among neonates receiving peripheral intravascular fluids. J Wound Ostomy Cont Nurs. 2006;33:133–9. https://doi.org/10.1097/00152192-200603000-00006.

Murag S, Suzukawa C, Chang TP. The effects of child life specialists on success rates of intravenous cannulation. J Pediatr Nurs. 2017;36:236–40. https://doi.org/10.1016/j.pedn.2017.03.013.

Nightingale J, Woodward JM. Guidelines for management of patients with a short bowel. Gut. 2006;55:iv1–iv12. https://doi.org/10.1136/gut.2006.091108.

Pedersen MG, Jensen-Fangel S, Olesen HV, Tambe SDP, Petersen E. Outpatient parenteral antimicrobial therapy (OPAT) in patients with cystic fibrosis. BMC Infect Dis. 2015;15:290. https://doi.org/10.1186/s12879-015-1019-4.

Pittiruti M, Hamilton H, Biffi R, Macfie J, Pertkiewicz M. ESPEN Guidelines on parenteral nutrition: central venous catheters (Access, Care, Diagnosis and Therapy of Complications). Clin Nutr. 2009;28:365–77. https://doi.org/10.1016/j.clnu.2009.03.015.

Ponnusamy V, Venkatesh V, Clarke P. Skin antisepsis in the neonate: what should we use? Curr Opin Infect Dis. 2014;27:244–50. https://doi.org/10.1097/QCO.0000000000000064.

Rudolf M, Lee T, Levene M, editors. Paediatrics and child health. Chichester: Wiley; 2011.

Smyth AR, Bell SC, Bojcin S, Bryon M, Duff A, Flume P, Kashirskaya N, Munck A, Ratjen F, Schwarzenberg SJ, Sermet-Gaudelus I, Southern KW, Taccetti G, Ullrich G, Wolfe S. European cystic fibrosis society standards of care: best practice guidelines. J Cyst Fibros. 2014;13(Suppl 1):S23–42. https://doi.org/10.1016/j.jcf.2014.03.010.

Sorge C, Mcdaniel J, Xavier A. Targeted therapies for the treatment of pediatric non-hodgkin lymphomas: present and future. Pharmaceuticals. 2016;9:28. https://doi.org/10.3390/ph9020028.

Srivastava A, Brewer AK, Mauser-Bunschoten EP, Key NS, Kitchen S, Llinas A, Ludlam CA, Mahlangu JN, Mulder K, Poon MC, Street A, Treatment Guidelines Working Group the World Federation of Hemophilia. Guidelines for the management of hemophilia. Haemophilia. 2013;19:e1–e47. https://doi.org/10.1111/j.1365-2516.2012.02909.x.

Tarlock K, Meshinchi S. Pediatric acute myeloid leukemia. Pediatr Clinics North Am. 2015;62:75–93. https://doi.org/10.1016/j.pcl.2014.09.007.

Tobias JD, Ross AK. Intraosseous infusions: a review for the anesthesiologist with a focus on pediatric use. Anesth Analg. 2010;110:391–401. https://doi.org/10.1213/ANE.0b013e3181c03c7f.

Ullman AJ, Keogh S, Coyer F, Long DA, New K, Rickard CM. 'True Blood' The Critical Care Story: an audit of blood sampling practice across three adult, paediatric and neonatal intensive care settings. Aust Crit Care. 2016;29(2):90–5. https://doi.org/10.1016/j.aucc.2015.06.002.

Visscher MO, Burkes SA, Adams DM, Hammill AM, Wickett RR. Infant skin maturation: preliminary outcomes for color and biomechanical properties. Skin Res Technol. 2017;23(4):545–51. https://doi.org/10.1111/srt.12369.

Ware RE, De Montalembert M, Tshilolo L, Abboud MR. Sickle cell disease. Lancet. 2017;390:311–23. https://doi.org/10.1016/S0140-6736(17)30193-9.

World Health Organisation. Genes and human disease [Online]. 2012. Accessed 31 Aug 2017.

Yawn BP, Buchanan GR, Afenyi-Annan AN, et al. Management of sickle cell disease: summary of the 2014 evidence-based report by expert panel members. JAMA. 2014;312:1033–48. https://doi.org/10.1001/jama.2014.10517.

14

Assessment and Selection of VADs in Pediatrics

Tricia Kleidon and Amanda Ullman

Abstract

Achieving vascular access in infants and pediatrics can be physically and emotionally challenging; therefore, every attempt to mitigate unnecessary venous access should be considered. The *Infusion Nursing Standards of Practice* recommends that, after assessment of all pertinent factors, the least invasive device to facilitate the prescribed treatment for the required time be inserted.

Keywords

Pediatric device selection · Device assessment · Intravenous · Catheter

T. Kleidon (✉)
Queensland Children's Hospital and Alliance for Vascular Access Teaching and Research (AVATAR), Brisbane, QLD, Australia
e-mail: tricia.kleidon@health.qld.gov.au

A. Ullman
Alliance for Vascular Access Teaching and Research (AVATAR) Group, Menzies Health Institute Queensland, School of Nursing and Midwifery, Griffith University, Brisbane, QLD, Australia
e-mail: a.ullman@griffith.edu.au

14.1 Introduction

Interdisciplinary discussion should precede any vascular access decision to ensure the right device is inserted for the pediatric patient at the right time to enable the necessary treatment. Vascular access devices (VADs) should only be used when necessary, and other treatment options such as oral antibiotics, intranasal analgesia, and enteral fluid therapy should be considered when appropriate. If a VAD is necessary, choice is based on the indication, duration, and frequency of treatment, the properties of the infusate, and, when possible, the preference of the patient or caregiver. Chopra et al. (2015) recently published the Michigan Appropriateness Guide for Intravenous Catheters (MAGIC) to develop appropriateness criteria for VAD selection, care, and management (Chopra et al. 2015). While the algorithms contained within this study were based on the needs of adult patients, the study emphasizes the usefulness and necessity of a device selection algorithm to guide VAD choice. While selection of the right vascular access device is not always obvious, and many device decisions will fall outside the bounds of the most comprehensive algorithm, an algorithm should be used as a guide to generate interdisciplinary discussion regarding the right device choice for the patient. Figure 14.1 illustrates a pediatric VAD decision-making algorithm which has been used successfully in tertiary pediatric facilities to guide this complex decision-making.

Please see Vascular Access Device (VAD) Decision Tree below. The VAD Decision Tree is a guide to the most appropriate device for your patient and should guide device selection when VAMS NP is not available.

Central Venous Access Devices (CVAD) in Children
The following VAD Decision Tree should be used as a guide only and all other CVAD enquiries directed to VAMS NP

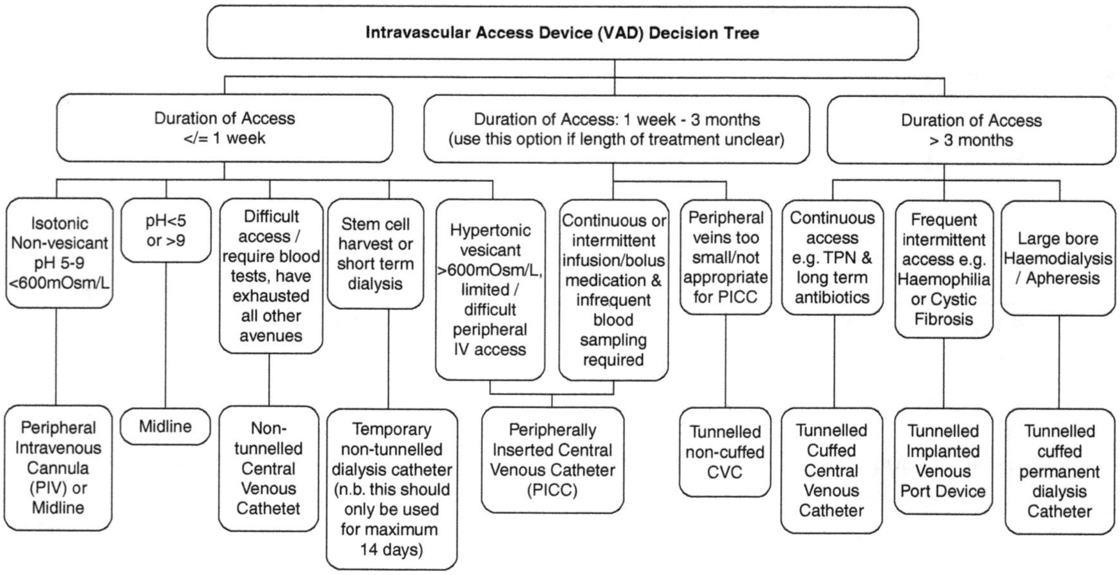

Decision for venous access device should be made using the Decision Tree as a **guide only**. For complex cases, especially neonatal lines, device selection should be made in conjuction with all clinical teams involved in care, including VAMS NP when available.
When choosing the most appropriate device the following principles must be adhered to:
1. Right device inserted first time
2. Smallest possible device for completion of treatment
3. Minimum number of lumens required for completion of treatment

Fig. 14.1 VAD decision-making algorithm (used with permission from Children's Health Services (2016))

14.2 Device Options

14.2.1 Peripheral Intravenous Cannula (PIVC)

A peripheral intravenous cannula (PIVC) is the most commonly used VAD in hospitalized patients and is primarily used for the infusion of fluid and fluid resuscitation, administration of antibiotics, some chemotherapy, and the administration of other parenteral medications (Alexandrou et al. 2015; Marsh et al. 2015; Kleidon et al. 2019). It is estimated that approximately 47% of hospitalized pediatric patients have a PIVC (Ullman et al. 2016). Placement of a PIVC in infants and young children is time-consuming and difficult due to smaller, less visible, or palpable veins, reduced procedural cooperation, increased adipose tissue, vasoconstriction, and parental anxiety (Malyon et al. 2014; Kleidon et al. 2019). Pediatric inpatients report PIVC insertions as the leading source of procedure-related pain while in hospital (Zempsky 2008). For these reasons, it is important to ensure that the PIVC is the most appropriate device to facilitate the necessary treatment.

Criteria for Appropriate PIVC Use

- Short term.
- Inserted into small peripheral vessels of the upper and lower limbs.
- Scalp veins have been used previously in infants and neonates; however, with the availability and use of technology to assist peripheral vein identification and PIVC insertions,

fewer scalp vein insertions are necessary (Benkhadra et al. 2012; Juric and Zalik 2014) (see Chap. 15).

- Suitable for a variety of nonirritant infusion therapies.
- Minimally invasive.
- Almost all doctors and nurses are skilled in this procedure.

PIVCs range from 24 gauge (which is the smallest and most commonly used in neonates and infants) to 14 gauge, which is infrequently used in pediatric patients but may be required in various situations including trauma, fluid resuscitation, or blood transfusion in adolescents as they accommodate greater flow and limit hemolysis (Gorski et al. 2016; L'Acqua and Hod 2015). Table 14.1 further describes the characteristics and indications of PIVC gauges in pediatrics.

PIVCs are short devices, ranging from 2 to 6 cm in length. New, longer PIVCs are available in 20 gauge or greater, with some countries (e.g., the United States) also having a longer 22-gauge PIVC available. The benefit of these longer devices is the ability to access veins that are deep to the skin surface while still ensuring enough cannula is anchored in the vessel to reduce the risk of dislodgement. This is commonly referred to as "vessel purchase." Ideally half of the PIVC will be situated within the actual vessel itself, while the remainder is within the subcutaneous layer (Pandurangadu et al. 2018). See Fig. 14.2—looking down the right-hand side of the ultrasound image, you will note numeric markings indicating depth in centimeters. The red arrow indicates the vessel to be punctured is 1 cm deep. Due to the size of this vessel, direct puncture is required to ensure half of the PIVC is within the vessel, reducing the risk of dislodgement.

Table 14.1 PIVC size and use

Gauge and length	Usual age	Purpose
24G	Neonates Infants	Most infusions Day infusion Small superficial vessel
22 g (short)	Toddlers and school age	Most infusions Minimal adiposity
22 g (long)	Toddlers and school age	Ultrasound-guided insertion Excessive adipose tissue
20 g (short)	School age Older school age and adolescence	Intraoperative Trauma, fluid resuscitation Blood sampling on insertion Most infusions Minimal adiposity
20 g (long)	Older school age and adolescence	Ultrasound-guided insertion Excessive adipose tissue
>20 g and up to 14 g	Older school age and adolescence	Intraoperative Trauma, fluid resuscitation Blood sampling on insertion Most infusions

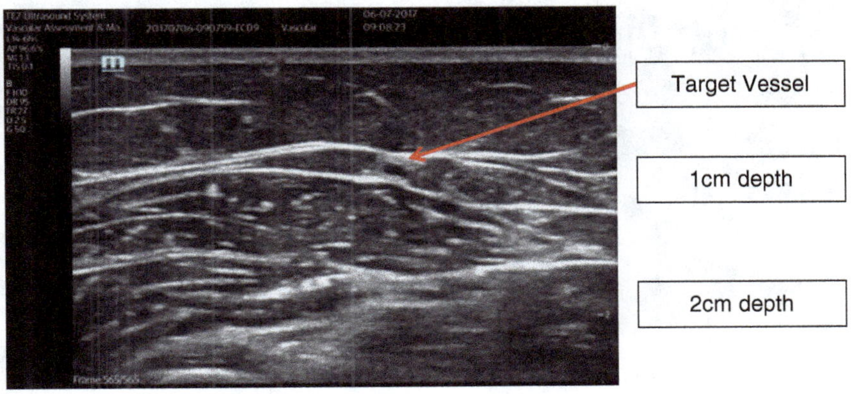

Fig. 14.2 Ultrasound imaging showing vessel depth (used with permission T. Kleidon)

Inappropriate use of PIVC includes:

- Infsuion of vesicants or other irritants, which should be infused through a central venous access device will be discussed later in this chapter. Inadvertent administration of irritants or vesicants into a peripheral vein can result in tissue-damaging necrosis requiring surgical intervention to treat (see Figs. 14.3 and 14.4).
- Routine blood sampling, other than initial insertion bloods.
- Just in case—the continued need for PIVC should be reviewed daily. If the PIVC is no longer necessary, it should be removed (Kleidon et al. 2019).

PIVCs should be reviewed daily to assess:

- Function: Does the PIVC still infuse; is there any leakage evident at the site?
- Complication: Any signs of local complication such as infiltration, extravasation, phlebitis, or dislodgement (see Figs. 14.5 and 14.6).
- Necessity: Is the PIVC still clinically indicated?

If any of these criteria are met, the PIVC must be removed and replaced, if necessary. Most pediatric hospitals have never routinely replaced PIVCs at regular 72–96-h intervals. High-quality research has confirmed this as best practice. Clinicians should replace pediatric PIVCs when clinically indicated rather than at routine intervals; this practice does not lead to an increased risk of complications (Rickard et al. 2012; Webster et al. 2015). Pediatric nurses are now tasked with exploring insertion-related factors that may prolong the functional duration of PIVCs including the use of ultrasound for insertion and placement of PIVCs in the forearm rather than those of the hand, wrist, or feet.

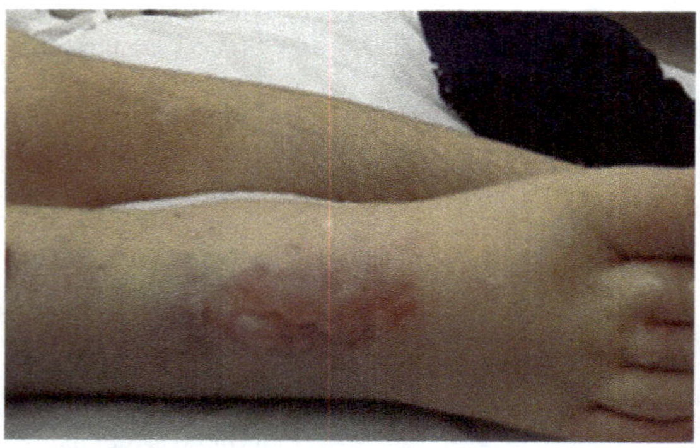

Fig. 14.3 Extravasation (used with permission T. Kleidon)

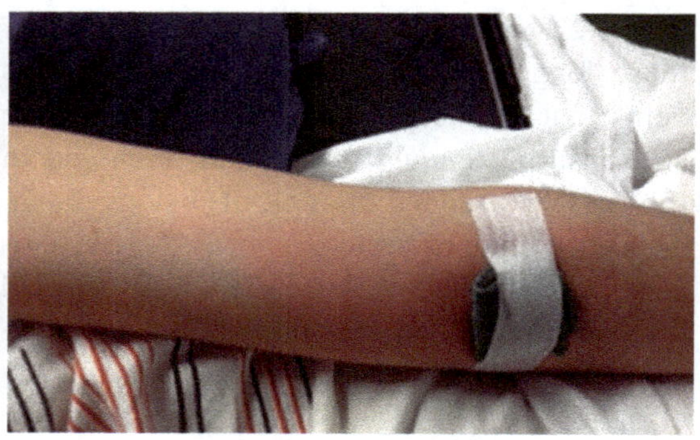

Fig. 14.5 Phlebitis (used with permission T. Kleidon)

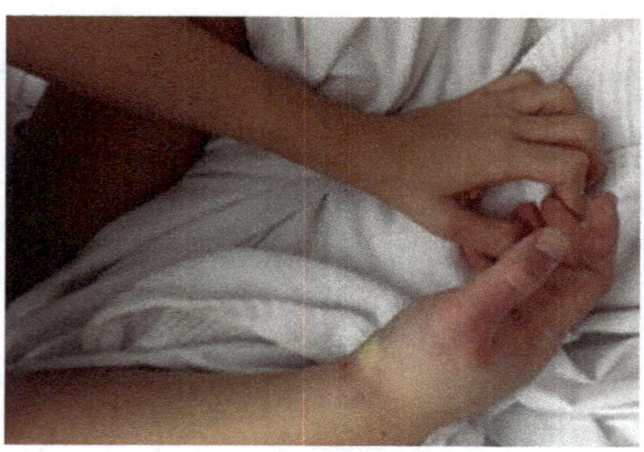

Fig. 14.4 Infiltration (used with permission T. Kleidon)

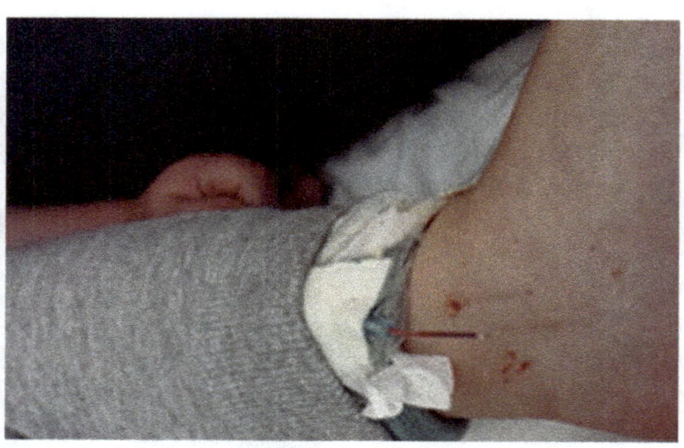

Fig. 14.6 Dislodgement. Dressing no longer clean, dry, or intact (used with permission T. Kleidon)

14.2.2 Midlines

A midline (see Fig. 14.7) is an alternative to a PIVC and should be considered when intravenous medications such as antibiotics are prescribed for a period of time greater than the average dwell time of a PIVC in your institution. The tip of a midline typically sits in the basilic, brachial, or cephalic veins at or below the axillary fold, distal to the shoulder (Gorski et al. 2016). The comparative properties of PIVC, midlines, and PICCs are displayed in Table 14.2.

Midlines come in a variety of sizes and are not yet uniform. Some midlines are sized by gauge (G), while others have been converted to French (Fr).

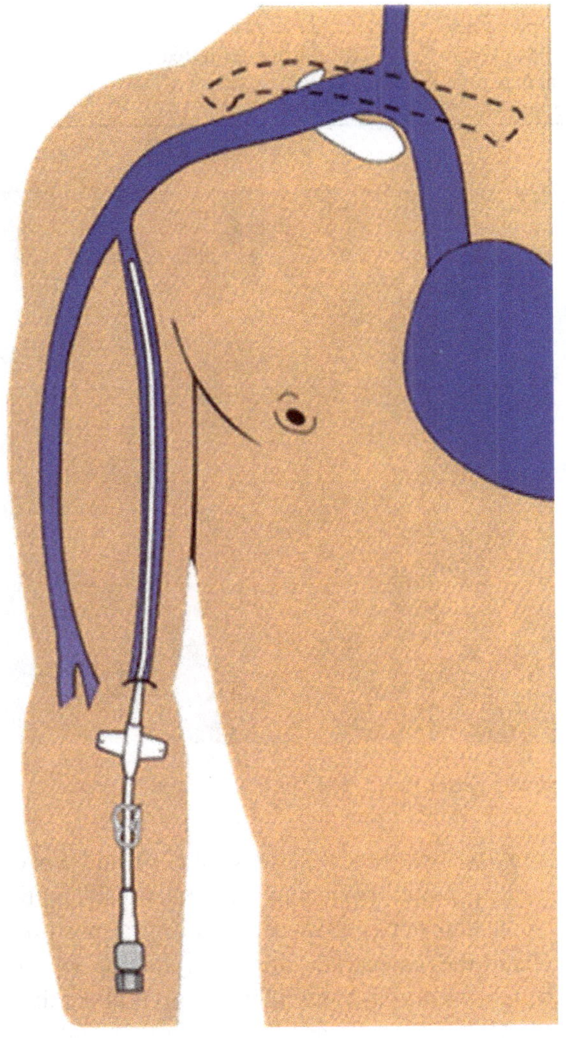

Fig. 14.7 Placement of a midline catheter (used with permission N. Moureau, PICC Excellence)

There is limited choice in some countries, and availability depends on the relevant regulatory approvals in your country such as US Food and Drug Approval (FDA), European "Conformité Européenne" (CE marking), or the Australian Therapeutic Goods Administration (TGA). To minimize the risk of thrombosis, most pediatric patients will be best suited to a 22–20G or 3–4Fr catheter. Catheter to vein ratio will be discussed in the PICC section of this chapter but should also be considered when selecting an appropriately sized midline.

Criteria for Appropriate Midline Use

Overall, limited evidence regarding the efficacy of midlines is available. However, general indications include:

- Extended dwell peripheral intravenous therapy—longer dwell times than standard PIVCs (see Table 14.2) (Gorski et al. 2016).
- Intravenous infusions of 1–4 weeks duration.
  - The increased length of a midline compared to a PIVC might reduce the risk of dislodgement. Additionally, the larger diameter of the vein where the midline terminates reduces the risk of phlebitis and occlusion compared to the smaller vein locations of PIVCs (Caparas and Hu 2014; Tagalakis et al. 2002).
- Avoid infusions with irritating properties. Consider pH and characteristics of medication (Caparas and Hu 2014; Gorski et al. 2015).
  - Short durations (<6 days) of diluted medications such as vancomycin, which typically has a pH of 4, may be infused through a midline that has its tip terminating in a larger, proximal upper arm vessel (Caparas and Hu 2014).
- Midlines *are not* indicated for continuous vesicant therapy, parenteral nutrition where dextrose is >10% and protein >5%, or infusates with an osmolarity greater than 900 mOsm/L (Gorski et al. 2016; Royal College of Nursing 2016).
- Administration of intermittent vesicant medication through a midline should be performed with extreme caution due to the risk of undetected extravasation.

Table 14.2 Properties of PIVC, midline, and PICC

Property	PIVC	Midline	PICC
Size	24G–14G	3Fr or 4Fr 22G or 20G	1Fr, 2Fr, 3Fr, 4Fr, 5Fr (single lumen) 2Fr (neonates), 4Fr, 5Fr 6Fr (triple lumen)
Length	Variable, usually 2–6 cm	4–12 cm (may be longer in adults)	55–60 cm Can be trimmed to appropriate length
Insertion position	Peripheral vessel of upper or lower limb	Upper arm Basilic, brachial, cephalic	Upper arm Basilic, brachial, cephalic
Tip position	Peripheral	Distal to axillar	SVC/RA junction (upper arm insertion) IVC (lower limb insertion)
Tip confirmation	Not necessary	No imaging necessary use measurement to ensure correct tip positioning	Tip confirmation with X-ray or ECG
Flow rates around tip	20–40 mL/min	100–150 mL/min	2 L/min
Clinical indication	Day infusion Short-term therapy, usually 2–5 days	Infusion greater than 5 days Medication/infusions up to 2 weeks (may be indicated up to 4 weeks) Dilute infusions when pH<5/>9 Modified parenteral nutrition, i.e., </= 10% Dextrose, protein 5%	Vesicants Continuous chemotherapy Parenteral nutrition Long-term treatment >2 weeks

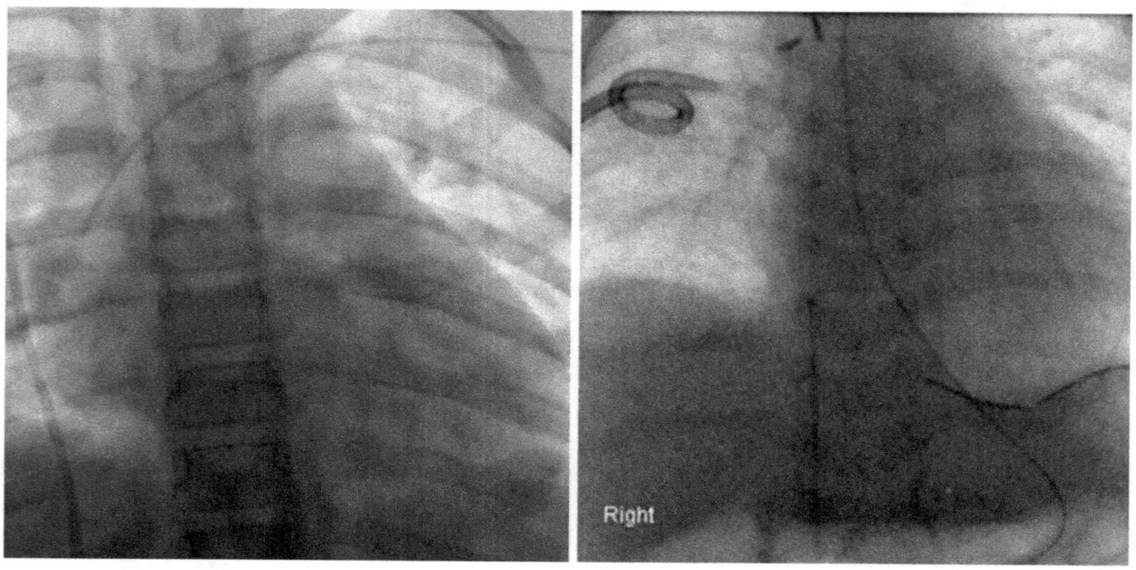

Fig. 14.8 PICC terminal tip placement (SVC and IVC) (used with permission T. Kleidon)

14.2.3 Peripherally Inserted Central Catheters (PICCs)

A peripherally inserted central catheter (PICC) is a long catheter that is approximately 55–60 cm untrimmed, with most trimmable to a more appropriate length for pediatric patients. PICCs are inserted into peripheral veins of the upper arm (basilic, brachial, or cephalic) and lower limbs (greater saphenous) in pediatrics. The tip of the catheter is advanced to a central position, either the cavoatrial junction (junction of the superior vena cava and right atrium) if upper limb PICC insertion (image on the left) or inferior vena cava if inserted from the lower limbs (Fig. 14.8). Because the tip of a PICC terminates in a central vessel, the blood flow around the catheter is high, usually 2 L or more per minute. This provides immediate dilution of the infusate and helps protect the vessel walls from chemical irritation from the prescribed intravenous medication.

Criteria for Appropriate PICC Use

- Central venous access for patients in acute care and home care or outpatient facilities.
- Extended venous access dwell is necessary and may remain in situ for weeks, months, and sometimes years (Hatakeyama et al. 2011).
- Reliable alternative to short-term central venous catheters with presumably fewer complications.
  - If multiple infusions including those only suitable for central infusion are required, insertion of a PICC has less complication compared to a catheter that has its origin in a neck vessel. For example, complications such as pneumothorax, hemothorax, and uncontrolled bleeding are comparatively less likely to occur during PICC insertions (Hatakeyama et al. 2011; Westergaard et al. 2013).
  - While PICCs have a lower complication profile, they're not innocuous, and experienced clinicians suggest vascular access professionals should adopt a more considered approach to the situations that are suitable for PICC insertion (Chopra et al. 2015).

PICCs range in size from 3Fr to 6Fr and are single- or multi-lumen devices. Just as the decision to insert the right device should be made collaboratively, so should the decision regarding the number of lumens that are required to provide the necessary treatment. A good question to ask yourself and your colleagues requesting PICC insertion is "How many lumens do you *need*" rather than how many lumens do you *want*. This is especially relevant in pediatrics where vessel size is so small. A multi-lumen PICC will surely make medication administration easier in complex patients requiring multiple therapies. However, it is these complex patients that are at a higher risk of developing complications such as infection, occlusion, and thrombosis (Raffini et al. 2009). Collaboration with healthcare professionals such as pharmacists will assist in planning medication administration to better utilize single lumen devices and avoid the unnecessary risk of complications related to multiple lumen PICCs. Additionally, the strong association between catheter/vein ratio and PICC-related thrombosis should be considered when choosing an appropriately sized PICC to insert (Sharp et al. 2015). The PICC should occupy no more than 45% of the selected vessel at its smallest point to ensure there is adequate blood flow through the vessel where the PICC is situated (Gorski et al. 2016). An easy rule of thumb is a 3Fr PICC requires a 3 mm vessel, 4Fr PICC requires a 4 mm vessel, and so forth. Prevention, recognition, and early management of thrombosis are increasingly important to ensure vessel health and preservation in these complex pediatric patients who will require lengthy and sometimes lifelong vascular access.

14.3 Catheter Materials and Design

Performance and reliability of a PICC is reliant on catheter material that is suitably flexible to reduce vessel irritation and patient discomfort and has adequate flow rates and structural integrity to achieve successful infusion therapy. This combination can be difficult to achieve in catheters that are small enough for pediatric vessels. Traditional silicone catheter material is soft, requiring more plastic in the outer wall to ensure stability of the catheter. As the size of the PICC is determined by the outer diameter of the catheter, a thicker outer wall limits the size of the inner lumen which in turn affects flow rates. This is clinically significant in pediatric catheters 3Fr and smaller as viscous infusions or high-volume infusions might be more difficult.

An alternative to silicone is polyurethane, a hardier material that does not require the same degree of thickness in its outer walls to provide catheter integrity. Polyurethane is now the material of choice for PICCs, providing a stronger catheter with a larger internal lumen that can provide better flow rates, especially in small pediatric catheters (Poli et al. 2016). Much variability exists in polyurethane, and Carbothane™ is a third-generation polyurethane that increases conformability within the vein (May et al. 2015).

Thrombosis and intraluminal occlusions are the most common cause of PICC failure in pediatric patients (Menendez et al. 2016; Morgenthaler and Rodriguez 2016). A recent development in PICC material involves the incorporation of antithrombogenic material (Endexo™) throughout the catheter—the inside, the outside, and the cut surface. Therefore, when PICCs are trimmed to a more suitable length for pediatric patients (Interface Biologics 2017), the risk of thrombotic complications including occlusion is greatly reduced. A recent randomized control trial in pediatric inpatients demonstrated a 50% reduction in PICC failure when antithrombogenic catheters were used compared to a power injectable polyurethane PICC (Kleidon et al. 2018). Additionally, significantly fewer complications such as occlusion occurred in patients with antithrombogenic PICCs.

PICCs with an antimicrobial coating have been associated with fewer central line-associated bloodstream infections (CLABSI) and should be considered in high-risk patients or when prolonged therapy is anticipated (Kramer et al. 2017). Children requiring insertion of PICCs are often immunocompromised or have comorbidities or an existing infection that increases their risk for developing CLABSI.

Traditionally, PICCs have had a clamp to reduce blood reflux. An alternative to a clamp is a valve positioned either at the distal or proximal PICC end. An inbuilt valve in pediatric PICCs might be preferential to an external clamp that children can play with and potentially undo, allowing blood to reflux into the unclamped catheter and increase the risk of occlusion within the PICC lumen.

14.4 Tunneling

Novel insertion techniques are often required in pediatric patients because their infusion needs require a catheter that is greater than their peripheral vessels can accommodate. Additionally, when multiple infusions are required, a multiple lumen catheter may be required, necessitating a larger vessel to accommodate this. Non-tunneled central venous catheters are often used in these situations; however, pediatric patients have small necks making care and maintenance of multi-lumen, non-tunneled central venous catheters difficult. Situations that might require novel insertion techniques include:

- Peripheral vessels too small to insert an appropriately sized catheter to complete treatment.
- Axillar or femoral most appropriate peripheral vein.
- Stenosis between axillar and subclavian.
- Renal disease that requires preservation of peripheral veins for future fistula.

In the above situations where a PICC is not able to be inserted in the traditional manner, the actual catheter can be used to instead insert a tunneled PICC. The advantage of this is that the femoral or axillary vein is punctured, but the exit site or point of skin puncture is more distal, mid-upper arm or mid-thigh (see Fig. 14.9). The advantages to this technique include lower microbial load and increase in comfort and postoperative care and maintenance. A long subcutaneous tunnel is created from the point of skin entry to the point of vein entry in either the femoral or axillary vein (Fig. 14.9) (Ostroff and Moureau 2017). A variation to this is a tunneled non-cuffed

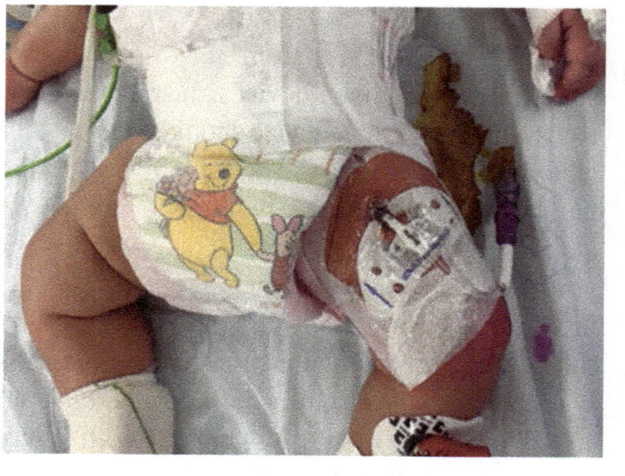

Fig. 14.9 Post-insertion tunneled PICC placement. PICC exists mid-thigh; long subcutaneous tunnel to femoral vein at its largest point to accommodate 3Fr catheter in 3.2 kg baby (used with permission T. Kleidon)

Table 14.3 Centrally inserted central catheters

Property	Non-tunneled central venous catheter (nt-CVC)	Tunneled cuffed central venous catheter (Tc-CVC)	Totally implanted venous port device (TIVPD)
Size	4Fr–8Fr Single and multiple lumen	2.7Fr–12.5Fr Single and multiple lumen	5Fr–9.6Fr Single and double lumen
Length	Variable, 4–12 cm	Variable, cut to length	Variable, cut to length
Insertion position	Neck or groin	Neck	Neck
Tip position	Central	SVC/RA junction	SVC/RA junction
Tip confirmation	Confirmation of venous placement	CXR	CXR
Advantages	• Short term • Quick procedure • Rapid infusion • Blood sampling • Hemodynamic monitoring • Multiple infusions possible	• Long-term device • (usually ≥3 months) • External device • No needles required to access • Multiple lumens • Tunnel reduces infection risk • Tunnel placement to patient preference • Cuff to stabilize catheter • Long-term, frequent use (e.g., anticancer treatment)	• Long-term device • (usually ≥3 months) • Totally implanted • Reduced risk profile when not accessed • Less interference with patient lifestyle when not accessed • Tunnel placement to patient preference • Long-term, infrequent use (e.g., cystic fibrosis, hemophilia)
Disadvantages	• Usually placed high on neck, difficult to manage • Insertion directly into vessel increases infection risk	• Complications of long-term external device – Fracture – Dislodgement – Infection • Weekly care and maintenance	• Needle phobia • Port body erosion • Weekly needle change when in use

central venous catheter, whereby a central vessel such as the internal jugular is punctured, and the PICC is tunneled and exists in the anterior chest wall. It is important to differentiate between the two and avoid simply calling the procedure a tunneled PICC. In a true tunneled PICC, a central vessel, which has an extended complication profile including the risk of pneumothorax, uncontrolled bleeding, etc., is punctured rather than a peripheral vessel.

14.4.1 Short CVADs

Despite the difficulties in managing short or non-tunneled central venous catheters (CVCs), they have a place in pediatric infusion therapy. They are traditionally placed immediately prior to anesthetic in the pediatric intensive care unit and, in some circumstances, in the emergency department. The subclavian, jugular, brachiocephalic, or femoral vein is the origin of access, and the catheter tip is ideally placed in a large central vein, enabling safe administration of various drugs including vesicants as well as hemodynamic monitoring and blood sampling. The advantage of these catheters in the pediatric setting is the large caliber, multi-lumen catheter, and the short length, enabling multiple, rapid infusions if necessary (see Table 14.3). Short CVCs or non-tunneled central venous catheters (nt-CVCs) are typically used for 1–2 weeks but may remain in situ for longer if necessary and show no signs of complication such as infection.

14.4.2 Catheter Material

As with PICCs, various materials have been used to coat and impregnate CVCs to reduce the risk of infection and occlusion. As previously mentioned, children need smaller central venous catheters which tend to occlude more readily than larger catheters. Additionally, the most common route of infection is migration of skin organisms at the insertion site into the catheter tract. Newborn infants and low birth weight infants are especially susceptible to infection due to their immature immune system and thin immature skin. Additionally, infants and pediatric patients in the intensive care unit receive multiple medications and require frequent monitoring, necessitating more frequent catheter manipulation, further increasing their risk of infection. To prevent these complications and reduce healthcare costs, various impregnated central venous catheters have been trialed in the pediatric setting. These include heparin-bonded catheters, chlorhexidine and silver sulfadiazine, and minocycline-rifampin. These treatments have shown a reduction in catheter-related bloodstream infection (CR-BSI); however, risks associated with the use of these treatments including resistance to chlorhexidine, previously induced in vitro, chlorhexidine anaphylaxis, and antimicrobial resistance have not been discounted. Therefore, use of coated and impregnated catheters should be reserved for instances where risk of infection is high (Balain et al. 2015; Gilbert et al. 2016; Shah and Shah 2014; Timsit et al. 2011).

14.4.3 Tunneled and Totally Implanted Devices

Long-term tunneled central venous catheters are characterized by whether they are an external device such as a tunneled cuffed central venous catheter (tc-CVC) or a totally implanted venous port device (TIVPD). Tunneled catheters that are external have a Dacron cuff to prevent migration of microorganisms along the subcutaneous tract as well as provide an anchor to reduce the risk of dislodgement once the cuff adheres to the subcutaneous tract. TIVPDs have a port body and septum that is implanted on the anterior upper chest wall. A catheter is attached to the port body hub and tunneled through the subcutaneous tract and enters the venous system in the supraclavicular region, usually via the jugular route. The catheter tips of tc-CVC and TIVPD terminate in a central position making them ideal for the long-term administration of all infusions.

Tc-CVCs are single and multi-lumen devices predominantly used in pediatric patients requiring long-term, frequent central venous access, i.e., those patients requiring central venous access for 3 months or longer and receiving anticancer treatment and bone marrow transplant or requiring long-term parenteral nutrition (see Table 14.3). Traditionally these catheters are large bore, capable of providing high-volume infusion and reliable blood sampling, and reduce the need for venipuncture in pediatric patients, which is often a difficult, anxiety-provoking, and time-consuming process. Tc-CVCs have a reduced incidence of infection compared to nt-CVCs due to the separation of insertion and exit points of the catheter.

A TIVPD is an ideal device for children and adults who require long-term intermittent central venous access capable of delivering reliable infusions and blood sample, because when it is not in use, it has no external accessories, reducing the risk of complications such as infection, dislodgement, and fracture (Kulkarni et al. 2014). However, this reduced risk is negated when the device is in use. Traditionally, TIVPDs are suitable for patients with cystic fibrosis and hematological conditions requiring infrequent infusion and blood sampling. TIVPD requires access via a special slant cut Huber needle inserted through the skin into the port body septum; therefore, TIVPDs may not be suitable for patients with needle phobia.

14.5 When to Consider Alternatives

Children who have had multiple previous vascular access procedures may now have venous occlusion, limiting the use of traditional vascular access sites. Occlusion of large central veins can occur when neonates have extended intensive care admissions requiring large vascular access devices to provide the necessary emergent therapy during their intensive care admission. Additionally, children who have required multiple vascular access procedures due to previously failed central venous access may also have limited venous access.

14.5.1 Nontraditional Routes

Large collateral veins will eventually develop in the neck when one or both of the internal jugular veins become occluded. Potential collateral veins include the anterior jugular and inferior thyroid veins and the jugular arch, which can often be used for vascular access if an established connection with the brachiocephalic vein and superior vena cava is formed (Lorenz et al. 2001; Shankar et al. 2002; Willetts et al. 2000; Wragg et al. 2014).

The right and left brachiocephalic veins may remain patent in the presence of an ipsilateral jugular and subclavian occlusion. When the ultrasound is placed in the supraclavicular position with caudal tilt, it is easy to identify the brachiocephalic vein in infants and pediatric patients. In situations where the jugular and subclavian veins are small due to prematurity or vessel anomaly, or if a large catheter is required to provide the necessary medical treatment, use of the larger brachiocephalic vein is a better alternative to the smaller jugular and subclavian veins (Badran et al. 2002).

Transhepatic and translumbar catheters have been used in the past to provide a route for vascular access when all veins of the neck and groin have been exhausted. Today, with the use of ultrasound, fewer venous occlusions resulting in venous insufficiency occur, and this route is almost never required. If venous insufficiency occurs, discussion with the interdisciplinary team should include interventional radiology to discuss these extended options (Barnacle 2014).

14.5.2 Recanalization

Large veins that have been occluded for some time can often be recanalized with the use of a dilator and guidewire following puncture of a vein peripheral to the occlusion. Recanalization is time-consuming and costly and should only be attempted by experienced personnel such as interventional radiologists (Barnacle et al. 2008; Barnacle 2014).

14.6 Summary

Numerous vascular access options exist for pediatric patients, and selecting the right device can be difficult, complicated by the often uncertain prognostic and treatment trajectories. It is important to clarify the clinical needs of the patient and involve all relevant clinicians in the decision-making process to ensure the right device is inserted to ensure safe practice and vessel health and preservation.

Case Study

Tessa is a 10-month-old toddler; her mom has brought her to the emergency department. Tessa presents with fever, a swollen left forearm, and miserable with coryzal symptoms. Although she has been crawling for the past 3 months, she now refuses to weight bear. The provisional diagnosis is osteomyelitis, and you are tasked with inserting a PIVC. Tessa weighs 12 kg, has limited venous access sites to the naked eye, and sucks her right thumb.

1. What are the venous access options that might be suitable for Tessa?
2. What site would you consider for placement?
3. Are you confident in successful PIVC insertion?
   (a) What are your options if you are not?

Case Study

Max is 6-year-old boy with a compound fractured tibia. Postoperative recovery has been complicated with infected pin sites from his external fixation device. Max is prescribed 250 mg vancomycin three times per day. Max had a PIVC inserted intraoperatively that has now stopped working after receiving his second dose of vancomycin.

1. What are the venous access options that might be suitable for max?
2. As his vascular access specialist, what factors do you need to consider prior to choosing a suitable device?
3. Which interdisciplinary healthcare workers might it be appropriate to discuss Max's options with to help you choose the right vascular access device for max?

Case Study

Lily is born at 38 weeks gestation, a presumably normal birth and uncomplicated delivery. At 1 day of age, Lily is noted to be pale and lethargic. A blood test reveals anemia and thrombocytopenia. Lily does not have a genetic reason for this abnormality. Initial treatment with packed red blood cells and platelets did not improve Lily's platelet count. Due to uncontrolled thrombocytopenia, her medical team chose a PICC to treat Lily rather than insertion of a centrally inserted central venous catheter. The measurements of Lily's basilic and axillary veins are 1.4 mm and 2.1 mm, respectively.

1. What are the venous access options that might be suitable for lily?
   (a) Is it appropriate to insert a 3Fr PICC in an upper arm vessel?
2. What other options might be available if a 3Fr PICC is not suitable in Lily's upper arm vessels?
3. Lilly's femoral vein is measured 3.0 mm.
   (a) Given Lily's thrombocytopenia, is it safe to puncture a femoral vessel?
   (b) What are the risks of inserting a catheter in the femoral vein in an infant?

In collaboration with Lily's hematologist, oncologist, intensivist, and vascular access specialist, the decision to insert a PICC via the femoral vein was made. If bleeding occurs, it is easy to apply pressure to the femoral vein. The risk of infection is high in catheters inserted in the nappy area in infants. Lily's vascular access specialist inserted the PICC by beginning the puncture mid-thigh, then creating a long subcutaneous tunnel before puncturing the femoral vein.

Case Study

Jeffrey is a 5-year-old boy who is about to start school. He was born with short gut secondary to necrotizing enterocolitis and subsequently is reliant on nutrition through his central venous access device. Jeffrey was fed through his tc-CVC. Jeffrey has had several complications related to his tc-CVC including infection, dislodgement, and fracture. Jeffrey presents to the emergency department with a fractured catheter. Jeffrey finds his current tc-CVC limiting on his lifestyle as he would like to play football and swim.

1. What vascular access options are available to Jeffrey?
2. What are the various risk factors to consider with each device?
3. How important is it to consider Jeffrey's lifestyle for his device choice?
4. Consider which interdisciplinary healthcare professionals you could consult regarding the most appropriate device for Jeffrey.

Case Study

Grace is a 6-month-old baby recently diagnosed with infant ALL. Grace will require intensive anticancer therapy and possibly a bone marrow transplant. Grace was born at 32 weeks gestation and spent 12 weeks in the neonatal intensive care unit, requiring multiple vascular access devices to support nutritional feeding initially. However, several line occlusions and fractures resulted in sepsis and extended inpatient stay. Grace ultimately required insertion of a femoral vein catheter due to multiple neck vein occlusions of the subclavian and jugular veins.

1. Are there any potential complicating factors to Grace's vasculature?
2. What vascular access options are available to grace?
3. What size line and how many lumens is grace likely to need to complete her anticancer therapy?
4. Consider which interdisciplinary healthcare professionals you could consult to determine the most appropriate type of device and placement of device.

Summary of Key Points

1. Pediatric patients have small veins, and this must be considered when determining the most appropriate vascular access plan to successfully complete treatment.
2. Some pediatric treatments will necessitate a larger device; novel insertion techniques should be considered to facilitate treatment with the least risk of complication.
3. There are a variety of devices available to the vascular access clinicians, and choice is not always obvious; however, interdisciplinary consultation will ensure all treatments and vascular access requirements are considered.
4. Tip positioning is important to reduce the risk of device complication and failure.
5. Multi-lumen devices are associated with increased complications and should only be inserted when absolutely necessary.
6. Patient lifestyle and device preference should be considered when possible.
7. Some patients require lifelong vascular access; therefore, every attempt to insert the right device and reduce potential complications to ensure vessel health and preservation should be considered.

References

Alexandrou E, Ray-Barruel G, Carr PJ, Frost S, Inwood S, Higgins N, et al. International prevalence of the use of peripheral intravenous catheters. J Hosp Med. 2015;10(8):530–3. https://doi.org/10.1002/jhm.2389.

Badran DH, Abder-Rahman H, Abu Ghaida J. Brachiocephalic veins: an overlooked approach for central venous catheterization. Clin Anat. 2002;15(5):345–50. https://doi.org/10.1002/ca.10046.

Balain M, Oddie SJ, McGuire W. Antimicrobial-impregnated central venous catheters for prevention of catheter-related bloodstream infection in newborn infants. Cochrane Database Syst Rev. 2015;(9):Cd011078. https://doi.org/10.1002/14651858.CD011078.pub2.

Barnacle AM. Interventional radiology in infancy. Early Hum Dev. 2014;90(11):787–90. https://doi.org/10.1016/j.earlhumdev.2014.08.017.

Barnacle A, Arthurs OJ, Roebuck D, Hiorns MP. Malfunctioning central venous catheters in children: a diagnostic approach. Pediatr Radiol. 2008;38(4):363–78 . quiz 486-367. https://doi.org/10.1007/s00247-007-0610-2.

Benkhadra M, Collignon M, Fournel I, Oeuvrard C, Rollin P, Perrin M, et al. Ultrasound guidance allows faster peripheral IV cannulation in children under 3 years of age with difficult venous access: a prospective randomized study. Paediatr Anaesth. 2012;22(5):449–54. https://doi.org/10.1111/j.1460-9592.2012.03830.x.

Caparas JV, Hu JP. Safe administration of vancomycin through a novel midline catheter: a randomized, prospective clinical trial. J Vasc Access. 2014;15(4):251–6. https://doi.org/10.5301/jva.5000220.

Children's Health Services. IVAD procedure—intravascular access device, management of (peripheral and central venous access devices). Brisbane: Queensland Government; 2016.

Chopra V, Flanders S, Saint S, Woller S, O'Grady N, Safdar N, et al. The Michigan appropriateness guide for intravenous catheters (MAGIC): results from a multispecialty panel using the RAND/UCLA appropriateness method. Ann Intern Med. 2015;163(6 Suppl):S1–40. https://doi.org/10.7326/M15-0744.

Gilbert RE, Mok Q, Dwan K, Harron K, Moitt T, Millar M, et al. Impregnated central venous catheters for prevention of bloodstream infection in children (the CATCH trial): a randomised controlled trial. Lancet. 2016;387(10029):1732–42. https://doi.org/10.1016/s0140-6736(16)00340-8.

Gorski LA, Hagle ME, Bierman S. Intermittently delivered IV medication and pH: reevaluating the evidence. J Infus Nurs. 2015;38(1):27–46. https://doi.org/10.1097/nan.0000000000000081.

Gorski L, Hadaway L, Hagle M, McGoldrick M, Orr M, Doellman D. Infusion therapy: standards of practice (supplement 1). J Infus Nurs. 2016;39(1S):S1–S159.

Hatakeyama N, Hori T, Yamamoto M, Mizue N, Inazawa N, Igarashi K, et al. An evaluation of peripherally inserted central venous catheters for children with cancer requiring long-term venous access. Int J Hematol. 2011;94(4):372–7. https://doi.org/10.1007/s12185-011-0928-2.

Interface Biologics. Surface modification technology platform; 2017. http://www.interfacebiologics.com/endexo.htm.

Juric S, Zalik B. An innovative approach to near-infrared spectroscopy using a standard mobile device and its clinical application in the real-time visualization of peripheral veins. BMC Med Inform Decis Mak. 2014;14:100. https://doi.org/10.1186/s12911-014-0100-z.

Kleidon TM, Ullman AJ, Zhang L, et al. How does your PICCOMPARE? A pilot randomized controlled trial comparing Various PICC materials in pediatrics. J Hosp Med. 2018. E1-e9

Kleidon TM, Cattanach P, Mihala G, Ullman AJ. Implementation of a paediatric peripheral intravenous catheter care bundle: a quality improvement initiative. J Paediatr Child Health. 2019.

Kramer RD, Rogers MA, Conte M, Mann J, Saint S, Chopra V. Are antimicrobial peripherally inserted central catheters associated with reduction in central line-associated bloodstream infection? A systematic review and meta-analysis. Am J Infect Control. 2017;45(2):108–14. https://doi.org/10.1016/j.ajic.2016.07.021.

Kulkarni S, Wu O, Kasthuri R, Moss JG. Centrally inserted external catheters and totally implantable ports for the delivery of chemotherapy: a systematic review and meta-analysis of device-related complications. Cardiovasc Intervent Radiol. 2014;37(4):990–1008. https://doi.org/10.1007/s00270-013-0771-3.

L'Acqua C, Hod E. New perspectives on the thrombotic complications of haemolysis. Br J Haematol. 2015;168(2):175–85. https://doi.org/10.1111/bjh.13183.

Lorenz JM, Funaki B, Van Ha T, Leef JA. Radiologic placement of implantable chest ports in pediatric patients. Am J Roentgenol. 2001;176(4):991–4. https://doi.org/10.2214/ajr.176.4.1760991.

Malyon L, Ullman AJ, Phillips N, Young J, Kleidon T, Murfield J, Rickard CM. Peripheral intravenous catheter duration and failure in paediatric acute care: a prospective cohort study. Emerg Med Australas. 2014;26(6):602–8. https://doi.org/10.1111/1742-6723.12305.

Marsh N, Webster J, Mihala G, Rickard C. Devices and dressings to secure peripheral venous catheters to prevent complications. Cochrane Database Syst Rev. 2015;(6):CD011070. https://doi.org/10.1002/14651858.CD011070.pub2.

May RM, Magin CM, Mann EE, Drinker MC, Fraser JC, Siedlecki CA, et al. An engineered micropattern to reduce bacterial colonization, platelet adhesion and fibrin sheath formation for improved biocompatibility of central venous catheters. Clin Transl Med. 2015;4:9. https://doi.org/10.1186/s40169-015-0050-9.

Menendez JJ, Verdu C, Calderon B, Gomez-Zamora A, Schuffelmann C, de la Cruz JJ, de la Oliva P. Incidence and risk factors of superficial and deep vein thrombosis associated with peripherally inserted central catheters in children. J Thromb Haemost. 2016;14(11):2158–68. https://doi.org/10.1111/jth.13478.

Morgenthaler TI, Rodriguez V. Preventing acute care-associated venous thromboembolism in adult and pediatric patients across a large healthcare system. J Hosp Med. 2016;11(Suppl 2):S15–s21. https://doi.org/10.1002/jhm.2662.

Ostroff M, Moureau N. Report of modification for peripherally inserted central catheter placement: subcutaneous needle tunnel for high upper arm placement. J Infus Nurs. 2017;40(4):232–7. https://doi.org/10.1097/nan.0000000000000228.

Pandurangadu AV, Tucker J, Brackney AR, Bahl A. Ultrasound-guided intravenous catheter survival impacted by amount of catheter residing in the vein. Emerg Med J. 2018;35(9):550–5.

Poli P, Scocca A, Di Puccio F, Gallone G, Angelini L, Calabro EM. A comparative study on the mechanical behavior of polyurethane PICCs. J Vasc Access. 2016;17(2):175–81. https://doi.org/10.5301/jva.5000452.

Raffini L, Huang YS, Witmer C, Feudtner C. Dramatic increase in venous thromboembolism in children's hospitals in the United States from 2001 to 2007. Pediatrics. 2009;124(4):1001–8. https://doi.org/10.1542/peds.2009-0768.

Rickard C, Webster J, Wallis M, Marsh N, McGrail M, French V, et al. Routine versus clinically indicated replacement of peripheral intravenous catheters: a randomised controlled equivalence trial. Lancet. 2012;380(9847):1066–74.

Royal College of Nursing. Standards for infusion therapy. London, United Kingdom; 2016.

Shah PS, Shah N. Heparin-bonded catheters for prolonging the patency of central venous catheters in children. Cochrane Database Syst Rev. 2014;(2):Cd005983. https://doi.org/10.1002/14651858.CD005983.pub3.

Shankar KR, Abernethy LJ, Das KS, Roche CJ, Pizer BL, Lloyd DA, Losty PD. Magnetic resonance venography in assessing venous patency after multiple venous catheters. J Pediatr Surg. 2002;37(2):175–9.

Sharp R, Cummings M, Fielder A, Mikocka-Walus A, Grech C, Esterman A. The catheter to vein ratio and rates of symptomatic venous thromboembolism in patients with a peripherally inserted central catheter (PICC): a prospective cohort study. Int J Nurs Stud. 2015;52(3):677–85. https://doi.org/10.1016/j.ijnurstu.2014.12.002.

Tagalakis V, Kahn SR, Libman M, Blostein M. The epidemiology of peripheral vein infusion thrombophlebitis: a critical review. Am J Med. 2002;113(2):146–51.

Timsit J-F, Dubois Y, Minet C, Bonadona A, Lugosi M, Ara-Somohano C, et al. New materials and devices for preventing catheter-related infections. Ann Intensive Care. 2011;1(1):34. https://doi.org/10.1186/2110-5820-1-34.

Ullman AJ, Cooke M, Kleidon T, Rickard CM. Road map for improvement: point prevalence audit and survey of central venous access devices in paediatric acute care. J Paediatr Child Health. 2016; https://doi.org/10.1111/jpc.13347.

Webster J, Osborne S, Rickard CM, New K. Clinically-indicated replacement versus routine replacement of peripheral venous catheters. Cochrane Database Syst Rev. 2015;8:CD007798. https://doi.org/10.1002/14651858.CD007798.pub4.

Westergaard B, Classen V, Walther-Larsen S. Peripherally inserted central catheters in infants and children—indications, techniques, complications and clinical recommendations. Acta Anaesthesiol Scand. 2013;57(3):278–87. https://doi.org/10.1111/aas.12024.

Willetts IE, Ayodeji M, Ramsden WH, Squire R. Venous patency after open central-venous cannulation. Pediatr Surg Int. 2000;16(5–6):411–3.

Wragg RC, Blundell S, Bader M, Sharif B, Bennett J, Jester I, et al. Patency of neck veins following ultrasound-guided percutaneous Hickman line insertion. Pediatr Surg Int. 2014;30(3):301–4. https://doi.org/10.1007/s00383-013-3416-3.

Zempsky WT. Optimizing the management of peripheral venous access pain in children: evidence, impact, and implementation. Pediatrics. 2008;122(Suppl 3):S121–4. https://doi.org/10.1542/peds.2008-1055c.

15

Vascular Access and Pediatric Site Selection

Tricia Kleidon and Amanda Ullman

Abstract

Venous access is one of the most basic yet critical components of patient care in both inpatient and ambulatory healthcare settings. Safe and reliable venous access is vital to patients and their families to ensure timely and complication-free treatment. Obtaining reliable access in the pediatric patient can be challenging due to various factors including physical (small, mobile veins, excessive subcutaneous tissue) and emotional (pediatric patients are often less cooperative, especially in the awake patient). The use of ultrasound to insert both peripheral and central venous access devices has improved success rates of insertions and reduced complications associated with insertions.

A variety of vascular access options exist, and selection of the most appropriate site helps to ensure vessel health and preservation and should be tailored to each individual patient need. Prior to selecting the insertion site, clinicians should consider the patient's condition, developmental age (discussed further in Chap. 13), skin condition, previous vascular access history, duration of infusion therapy, and patient preference where possible.

Keywords

Pediatric site selection · Pediatric technologies · Pediatric considerations for VAD placement

T. Kleidon (✉)
Alliance for Vascular Access Teaching and Research (AVATAR), Queensland Children's Hospital, Brisbane, QLD, Australia
e-mail: tricia.kleidon@health.qld.gov.au

A. Ullman
Alliance for Vascular Access Teaching and Research (AVATAR) Group, Menzies Health Institute Queensland, School of Nursing and Midwifery, Griffith University, Brisbane, QLD, Australia
e-mail: a.ullman@griffith.edu.au

15.1 Site Selection for Peripheral Devices

15.1.1 Peripheral Intravenous Cannula (PIVC)

15.1.1.1 Vein Options

A detailed understanding of the venous systems of the upper and lower extremities facilitates successful cannulation. The upper extremities have two primary venous systems: the cephalic and basilic veins (Fig. 15.1).

When choosing the best vein for each individual patient, consider the length of treatment (e.g., one-off infusion versus IV therapy for multiple

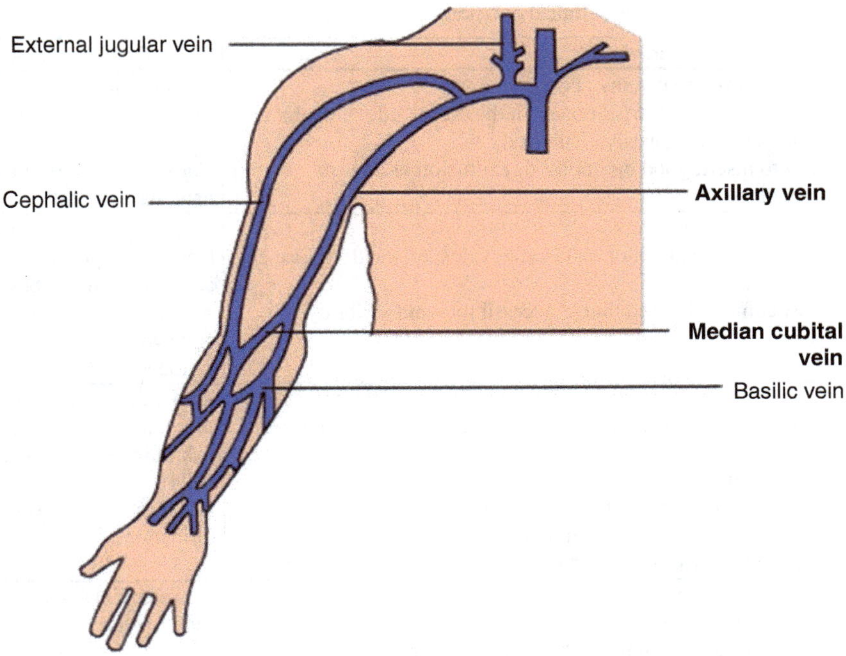

Fig. 15.1 Veins of the upper arm (used with permission N. Moureau PICC Excellence)

days), type of treatment to be infused (such as pH, viscosity, and osmolarity), as well as vein assessment (full, bouncy, straight).

15.1.1.2 Site Location

When choosing a site for PIVC insertion in the pediatric patient, consideration must be given to the site that is going to least interrupt the child's usual play and activity as they are less likely to be protective of their PIVC as an adult patient might—see Table 15.1. In particular, avoid placing a PIVC in the hand of the thumb that they might suck for comfort and in areas of flexion such as the wrist and antecubital fossa. The preferred cannulation sites are the veins of the non-dominant forearm. These veins are often easy to palpate in older children but might be more difficult in the chubby toddler. The use of technology such as ultrasound, which will be discussed later in this chapter, might be of assistance in this instance.

When upper extremity veins are inaccessible, the dorsal veins of the foot or the saphenous veins of the lower extremity may be used in toddlers that are not yet mobile. Other alternative intravenous cannulation sites that have been used in neonates and young infants include the scalp veins.

Contraindications to an insertion site in the body may include edema, infection, phlebitis, sclerosed veins, previous intravenous infiltration, burns, skin injury such as eczema, or traumatic injury proximal to the insertion site and surgical procedures affecting the extremity.

When traditional PIVC insertion techniques such as palpation fail and multiple attempts at vascular access are unsuccessful, the use of visual aids such as ultrasound and other ultraviolet light might be required. Practitioners have described increased success when PIVCs are inserted into deeper vessels with the aid of longer catheters in adults (Fabrizio Elia et al. 2012), and ultrasound guidance is similarly beneficial in both the adult and pediatric population (Benkhadra et al. 2012; Stolz et al. 2015). The use of technology to assist in PIVC insertion in children with difficult intravenous access (DIVA) will be discussed later in this chapter.

15.2 Midlines

15.2.1 Vein Options

Midlines can be inserted in both the upper and lower extremities. The ultimate goal of midline insertion is to extend the dwell of the infusion therapy device for medication that can be deliv-

Table 15.1 PIVC sites: clinical and practical considerations in pediatrics

Location/characteristics	Clinical considerations
Dorsal metacarpal veins Between the metacarpal bones on the dorsal side of the hand Superficial veins, easily visualized Easy to insert, good option for day infusion or one-off procedure	For short-term access only Tip of catheter should not extend over the wrist joint Consider the impact that restricting the use of the hand will present
Dorsal venous network Formed by the union of metacarpal veins, on the dorsal aspect of the forearm Most commonly used due to accessibility and visibility	Comfortable site for patient Not always prominent, difficult to visualize particularly in chubby infants and toddlers Avoid placement over the wrist/prominent ulna bone which can cause mechanical phlebitis or dislodgement
Cephalic vein Runs the length of the arm from the wrist to the lateral aspect of the upper arm to the shoulder Easy to palpate Does not restrict patient activity as hands are free Easy to secure and maintain on the forearm Preferred site for prolonged peripheral intravenous therapy	Radial nerve runs parallel Avoid insertion in the wrist area due to increased risk of inadvertent arterial puncture (Lirk et al. 2004) Avoid in patients who might require future fistula formation
Median cubital vein Crosses the antecubital fossa Preferred site during urgent/trauma management due to easy access and capacity to accommodate large-bore PIVC Commonly used to draw blood	Nerve endings in this area may result in painful venipuncture Brachial artery lies medial; therefore caution should be taken to avoid inadvertent arterial puncture Limits patient's mobility due to joint articulation Prone to failure due to movement, blockage, dislodgement, infiltration, and infection
Accessory cephalic vein Branches off the cephalic vein Joins the cephalic again at the antecubital fossa PIVC insertion at this site does not restrict movement Easily stabilized	Avoid catheter tip placement at joint articulation
Basilic vein Runs the entire length if the arm from the wrist to axilla Runs along the medial aspect of the upper forearm Runs deep above the elbow and combines with the brachia veins to form the axillary vein First choice for PICC insertion	Vein rotates around the arm and requires firm skin tension to stabilize vein Avoid use for short-term devices if longer-term device might be required
Great and small saphenous vein Generally visible, palpable, and easily accessible Best used in patients not yet walking Straight, easy to secure	Decreases mobility in active toddler Often deep within tissues and requires ultrasound insertion
Dorsal venous arch Superficial vessel on dorsum of foot Best used in patients not yet walking Avoid tip crossing ankle joint	Decreases mobility in active toddler

ered into the peripheral venous system. Ideally, a midline will be inserted into a vein in the upper arm or upper thigh region, so the tip, while still situated in a peripheral vein, is ideally situated in a large peripheral vein to increase natural hemodilution of intravenous medication. As veins move proximally toward the heart, they increase in size.

15.2.2 Site Location

The optimal insertion site is the non-dominant arm within the middle third of the upper arm. For the pediatric patient population, the fixed length of midlines currently available requires the insertion site to be tailored to the length of the catheter. For example, if an 8 cm midline is all that is available, the insertion site should start 8 cm below the axillary vein which is ideally where the tip will be positioned. Alternatively, a lower limb insertion should commence at a distance equal to the length of the midline, just distal to the femoral vein for ideal midline tip placement.

Catheters placed within the lower limb have an increased risk of complications such as infection due to close proximity to the nappy area in infants and toddlers and thrombosis (Greene et al. 2015). Placement of midlines in the lower limbs should only be considered as a last resort.

The use of ultrasound to support midline placement has clear benefits as the vein chosen can be assessed for patency along its entire length. Ultrasound also provides additional venous access options that would previously be too deep to palpate using blind punctures and enables site placement proximal to the antecubital fossa which has the advantage of siting the catheter outside the elbow joint.

15.2.3 Central Venous Access Devices (CVADs)

The remainder of this chapter will review the catheter, site, vein, and technology choice for insertion of various central venous access devices or central venous catheters to ensure vessel health and preservation throughout the child's lifespan and through to adulthood. A central venous access device (CVAD) is defined as a catheter placed with the tip positioned within the region of the cavoatrial junction (Silberzweig et al. 2003). When placing a CVAD with its insertion in the neck, the cavoatrial junction is defined as two vertebral body units below the carina. This is a reliable marker in the adult and adolescent patient; however, variability might be found in younger pediatric patients and should be used with caution as an absolute marker (Baskin et al. 2008; Song et al. 2015).

Patient assessment prior to choice of vein, site, and device should include information of previous indwelling CVADs and reason for use and removal that might limit available sites for future access. Likewise, it is also recommended that documentation at the conclusion of CVAD insertion should include relevant demographic and procedural CVAD information including patient consent, selection and exclusion criteria for device and site choice, reason for device insertion, and intended length of use (Silberzweig et al. 2003).

15.3 PICCs

15.3.1 Vein Options

PICCs are inserted into peripheral veins of the upper arm (basilic, brachial, or cephalic) with the tip of the catheter advanced to the cavoatrial junction. If placement of PICC in the upper limb is not possible, lower limb PICC insertion is necessary. The vein of choice is usually the greater saphenous found on the medial aspect of the lower limb, and the tip of the catheter is then advanced to the inferior vena cava, located above the level of the diaphragm (Gorski et al. 2016) (Chap. 14). Cannulation of the lower limb veins for PICC insertion is associated with a higher incidence of thrombosis; however, as with midlines, this risk is lower in children and infants than in adults. Therefore this is an acceptable alternative when cannulation of the upper extremities has failed in a child or infant (Spentzouris et al. 2012).

15.3.2 Site Location

The ideal site for insertion of PICC in the upper limb is in the middle third of the upper arm (Dawson 2011; Simcock 2008). In some pediatric patients, finding a suitable vein in this location can be challenging. This might be due to venous thrombosis or stenosis resulting from multiple previous PICC insertions; anatomical limitation including nerves and artery located anterior to the intended vein; or, in the very small neonate, vein size is simply not large enough to accommodate an appropriate sized PICC for the treatment required. In this situation, veins closer to the axilla may be more appropriate to access; however, placing a PICC insertion site at the axilla makes care and maintenance challenging. To avoid this suboptimal exit site, tunneling the PICC distal to the insertion site has proven successful (Ostroff and Moureau 2017). In this way, the PICC insertion/exit site is appropriately placed in the middle third of the upper arm, and the vessel accessed in the axillar region is sufficient for the intended treatment.

When PICC placement via an upper limb vessel is not possible in neonates and pediatric patients, it is acceptable to place a PICC via a lower limb vessel such as the greater saphenous, popliteal, or common femoral vein. The obvious limitation to placing a PICC/small-bore catheter in the lower limb is mobility and soiling in the diaper area which should be considered when choosing a site. If, after thorough venous assessment, the common femoral vein is the most appropriate vein for PICC insertion, tunneling the PICC away from the insertion site will remove the insertion/exit site from the threat of contamination from the nappy and may increase the ease of site visibility and care and maintenance—see Fig. 15.2.

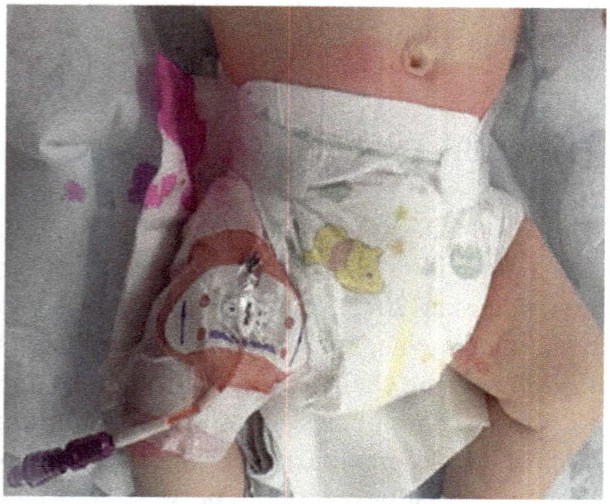

Fig. 15.2 Tunneled femoral CVAD (used with permission T. Kleidon)

15.4 Non-Tunneled CVCs

15.4.1 Vein Options

Short, non-tunneled CVCs are usually inserted into the neck (internal jugular, external jugular, subclavian, and brachiocephalic) or groin (great saphenous and common femoral).

15.4.2 Site Location

Securing a CVC in pediatric patients can prove challenging due to anatomical limitations of small neck size and the potential for contamination from the nappy if the CVC is placed in the groin. Cannulation of the internal jugular has predominantly been achieved by utilizing the short-axis view (i.e., ultrasound probe is placed in cross section to the internal jugular vein, and the needle puncture is in-line with jugular but out of plane with the probe). While the advantage to this approach is increased cannulation success, post-insertion can be problematic when trying to secure a dressing and maintain CVC function in the pediatric population (Gorski et al. 2016). An alternative approach is to place the ultrasound probe in the supraclavicular notch (out of plane to the vein) and utilizing an out-of-plane approach to the vein, approach the internal jugular from the lateral edge of the probe (in line with the ultrasound probe), and achieve access from a low jugular approach which improves the nurses' ability to secure the catheter to the anterior chest wall (Fig. 15.3).

A similar approach is used to puncture the subclavian vein. Using a long-axis view, the ultrasound probe is often placed in an infraclavicular position, and the needle is placed as close as possible to the lateral edge of the probe and enters the axillar vein or subclavian under direct visualization.

15.5 Approach to Insertion

Patient position can impact the likelihood of a successful central venous access procedure. Place the patient in the Trendelenburg position

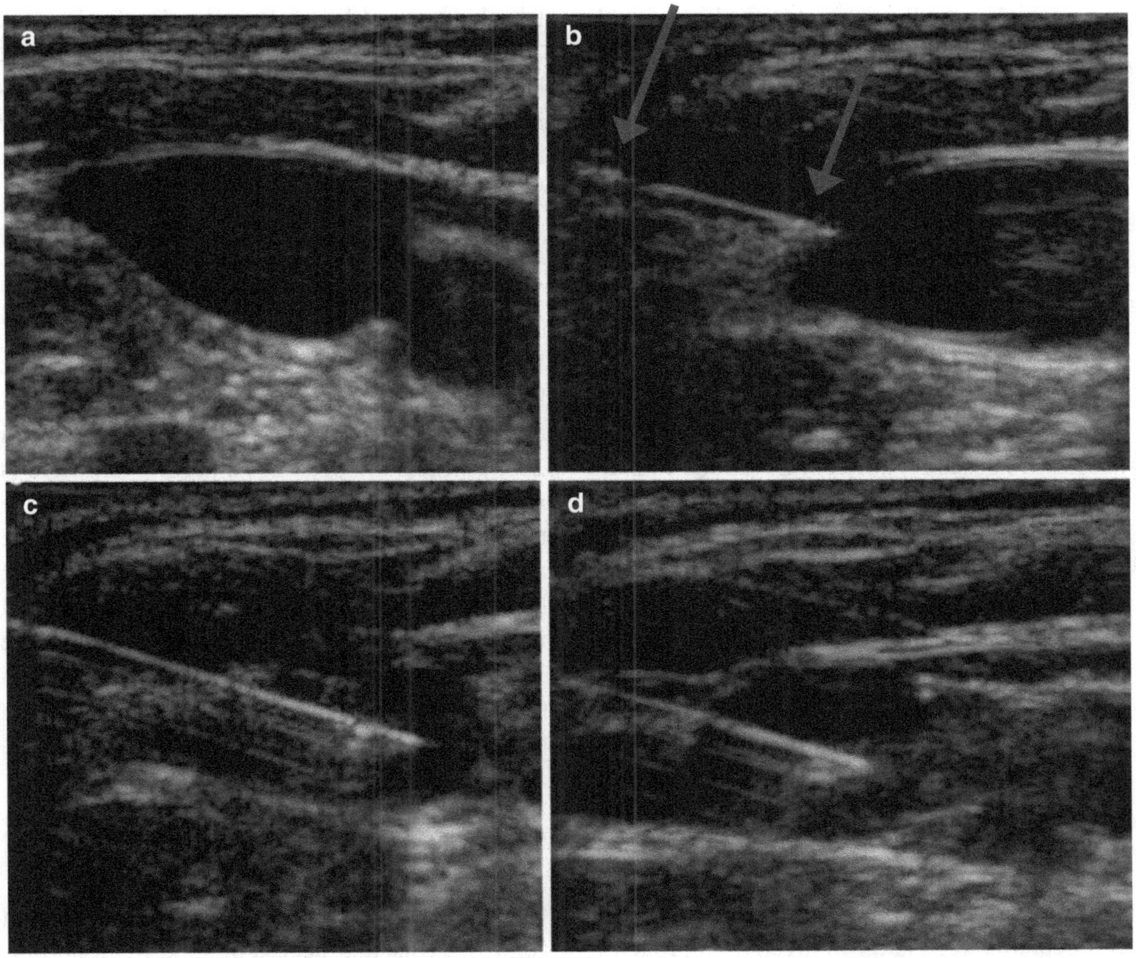

Fig. 15.3 (**a–d**) Ultrasound image showing RIJV lying lateral to common carotid artery; (**b**) needle indenting wall of the vein (**c**) successful cannulation of the IJV shown by needle moving freely within the vessel (**d**) aspiration of blood confirming successful cannulation (used with permission T. Kleidon)

or have a small roll placed under their shoulders (unless contraindicated due unstable c-spine that may occur due to injury or disease) for central vein cannulation of veins in the neck region. Trendelenburg position allows gravity to enhance central venous filling to create a larger target for venipuncture and minimize risk of air embolus (Bannon et al. 2011). A roll under the hip will elevate the common femoral vein and aid cannulation; however initiating the reverse Trendelenburg position will not substantially increase femoral vein size.

External landmarks, venography, and ultrasound are used to localize central vessels including internal and external jugular, subclavian, axillary, common femoral, and brachiocephalic (innominate) veins. The ultrasound-guided approach to cannulation of the internal jugular vein has been shown to have a lower complication rate, time to insertion, and increased first time success compared to landmark-guided puncture (Lau and Chamberlain 2016).

The Society of Interventional Radiology reporting standards for central venous access insertion (Silberzweig et al. 2003) recommends reporting the method and route of venous access, including patient position, technique for vein localization, and venous puncture site selection. Furthermore, also report the number of catheterization attempts, defined as the passing of a needle through the skin with the intent to obtain venous access, and any inadvertent arterial punctures. Venous anomalies such as stenosis and occlusion should also be reported.

15.6 Tunneled and Totally Implanted Devices

15.6.1 Vein Options

The right internal jugular vein is considered the access site of choice for central venous cannulation. Advantages include a superficial location, easy visualization with ultrasound, and a straight trajectory to the superior vena cava. Additionally, cannulation of the internal jugular rather than subclavian vein avoids “pinch-off syndrome” and avoids potential stenosis of the subclavian vein (Bannon et al. 2011). This is an important vessel health and preservation consideration in pediatric patients with chronic renal disease, as they may require formation of an arteriovenous fistula in the future, as a means of providing hemodialysis.

Cannulation of the innominate vein or brachiocephalic vein is an innovative approach to central venous access. Place the ultrasound probe in the supraclavicular notch, and angle the probe caudally to obtain a longitudinal view of the junction of the internal jugular vein, subclavian vein, and brachiocephalic vein. This is a useful puncture site when the internal jugular veins are small or absent bilaterally or if previous attempts to puncture the jugular vein have failed.

15.6.2 Site Location

The tunneled catheter exit site or implanted port pocket is usually placed over the upper anterior chest or the inner aspect of the upper extremity (Barnacle et al. 2008). Reports have described alternative access routes for tunneled central venous catheter including transfemoral, translumbar, and transhepatic (Roebuck et al. 2005b). Circumstances where this route might be required are in extreme cases of venous insufficiency whereby all traditional sites have been used and are no longer available (Barnacle et al. 2008).

15.7 Technology Emergence

Ultrasound technology has been found to be invaluable in vascular access procedures, particularly for deep veins (Lamperti and Pittiruti 2013; Simon and Saad 2012). However, there is now a range of near-infrared devices available that are useful for peripheral cannulation of the more superficial veins (Lamperti et al. 2014; Moureau et al. 2013). This technology is still fairly new, and although there have been some evaluations, to properly understand the potential benefits of this technology, further evaluations are necessary (Phipps et al. 2012).

15.7.1 Near-Infrared (nIR)

Near-infrared is light technology that aids in achieving vascular access of superficial peripheral veins in neonates, patients with complex medical conditions and the severely dehydrated patient (Gorski et al. 2016). nIR technology captures an image of the veins and reflects it back to the skin’s surface. nIR can be used as a real-time cannulation technique or as an aid to identify viability of peripheral venous sites as well as offering more information about vein selection (i.e., bifurcation, tortuous vessels, and viable palpable vein -v- thrombosed vein).

15.7.2 Ultrasound

Ultrasound evaluation of veins is an invaluable resource to assess venous course, identify underlying structures such as arteries and nerves and ensure venous patency before venous puncture (Fig. 15.4). Real-time ultrasound guidance has been shown to reduce complications, procedure time, and improve first time puncture and overall technical success of both peripheral and central venous catheter placement (Benkhadra et al. 2012; Lau and Chamberlain 2016).

Additionally, the use of ultrasound for PIVC insertion in pediatrics facilitates the operator to choose a catheter length that will ensure sufficient catheter is residing within the vein lumen. The ultrasound screen indicates vessel depth (Fig. 15.5); therefore a vessel that is 1 cm deep should have a catheter that is equal to or greater than 2 cm long to ensure half of the catheter is anchored within the vessel.

The use of technology to identify CVAD tip position intraoperatively has the advantage of increased accuracy, reduced delays to start of treatment, and reduced complications such as dislodgement and risk of contamination if catheter repositioning is required.

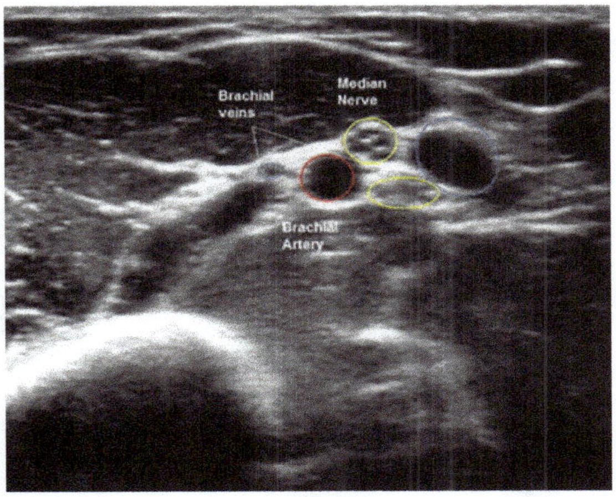

Fig. 15.4 Identification of vein in relation to underlying structures (used with permission T. Kleidon)

15.7.3 Fluoroscopy

Ideally the catheter tip of a CVAD that is placed in the upper body is advanced to the cavoatrial junction. For lower body insertions, the catheter tip should be positioned in the inferior vena cava, above the level of the diaphragm (Gorski et al. 2016). This ensures a tip position with high blood flow which prevents thrombosis and is also positioned external to the atrium to prevent arrhythmias and pericardial erosion and cardiac tamponade. The radiographic surface landmarks that correspond to this position are less clear in the pediatric patient than the adult patient. The carina and inferior border of the right main bron-

Fig. 15.5 Ultrasound image indicating vessel depth. This information should be used to choose appropriate length PIVC (used with permission T. Kleidon)

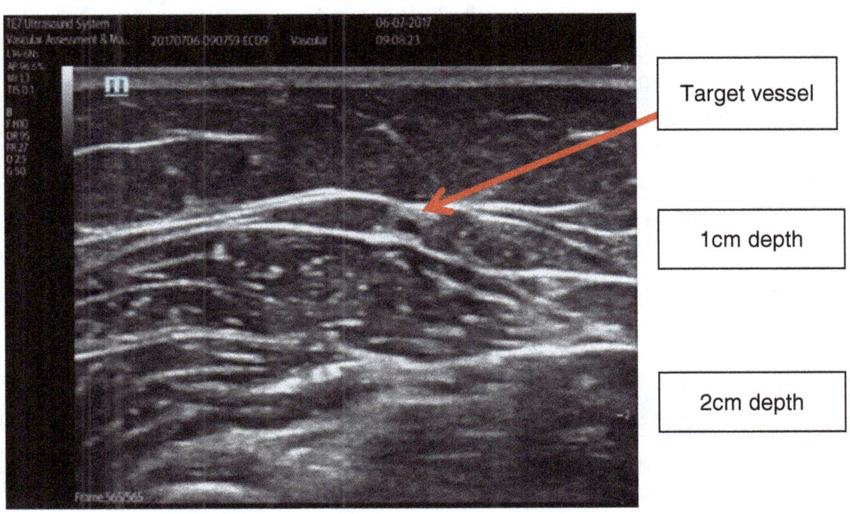

chus are appropriate landmarks in pediatrics to ensure safe positioning of the catheter tip (Gorski et al. 2016).

15.7.4 Electrocardiogram (ECG)

Electrocardiogram is a recent accurate and safe alternative to the use of fluoroscopic-guided tip position for insertion of CVAD. Although this technology has not been evaluated as widely in pediatrics as it has in the adult population, small, multicenter studies have demonstrated safety and accuracy in the pediatric population (Rossetti et al. 2015). This technology allows the inserter to identify accurate tip placement within the cavoatrial junction with corresponding changes in ECG trace. Caution should be employed when using this technology for patients with known history of cardiac dysrhythmias and an absence or alteration in the P-wave (Chap. 7).

15.8 Conclusion

The percutaneous technique to cannulate central veins reduced the need for open, surgical cut-down procedures and the associated morbidity that can result from the large incision wound and vein trauma (Roebuck et al. 2005a, b). Traditionally, the use of the percutaneous technique to successfully cannulate a central vessel was reliant on the relationship between surface anatomic landmarks and the anatomic structures beneath the skin. Contemporary approaches to percutaneous cannulation of central vessels have involved the use of real-time ultrasound visualization which enhances the safety of puncturing the internal jugular, brachiocephalic, and femoral veins. Ultrasound also offers the axillary vein as a "visible" alternative to blind subclavian approach which is difficult to visualize with ultrasound due to overlying bony structures (Sharma et al. 2004). In today's modern healthcare, pediatric patients are living longer and many into adulthood. This means they have increasingly complex comorbidities that will often require long term and possibly lifelong intravenous treatment. The ultimate goal of the vascular access healthcare professional should be to ensure long-term viability of vessels through careful assessment, planning, insertion, and management.

Case Study

Geoffrey is a 2-year-old boy who requires a 5-day course of intravenous antibiotics to treat cellulitis of the right thumb. Geoffrey still sucks his left thumb. Consider the potential sites available for PIVC insertion in this instance. What considerations should be made when planning for device insertion?

Abbie is a 12-year-old girl with rheumatoid arthritis. Abbie attends the outpatient department for monthly infusions of rituximab. What different considerations can you see in the two scenarios?

Case Study

Claire is a 3-year-old recently admitted with disseminated infected eczema. Most of Claire's face and upper and lower limbs are affected, especially over areas of flexion. In addition to administration of intravenous flucloxacillin, Claire has wet wraps to her limbs as part of her treatment plan.

As Claire's vascular access nurse, what are the clinical considerations when choosing a vascular access device for her treatment? How can you reduce the risk of vascular access device failure and ensure its longevity for the entire treatment?

Case Study

Billy is a 12-year-old with cystic fibrosis who requires insertion of PICC for 14–28 days of intravenous antibiotics. Billy has recently commenced high school and has become non-compliant with his medication and physiotherapy, and this is his third admission for chest optimization this year.

Ultrasound assessment of Billy's upper limbs reveals a large basilic vein in the region of the antecubital fossa that narrows significantly as it advances proximally and becomes large again at the axilla. It is difficult to visualize beyond the axilla due to normal anatomical placement of bony structures such as the clavicle; however, there is no evidence of superficial, collateral vessels on the chest wall.

What are your considerations when placing a PICC for Billy?

Case Study

Audrey is a 14-year-old who has recently been diagnosed with acute myeloid lymphoma. Prior to diagnosis, Audrey led an active teenage lifestyle and is a member of her college water polo team. Audrey will require intensive chemotherapy, infusion of blood and blood products, multiple blood tests, and eventual bone marrow transplant. As Audrey's infusion nurse specialist, you are discussing the various CVAD options with Audrey and her family.

1. What CVAD options do you consider appropriate for this treatment?
2. What are some of the advantages and disadvantages of the various devices you will discuss with Audrey and her family?
3. What are the practical considerations of inserting a CVAD in a prepubescent/pubescent female?

Case Study

Xavier is a 2-week-old baby transferred to your hospital with a history of thrombocytopenia, neutropenia, and uncorrected coagulopathy. Xavier currently has no peripheral or central venous access as multiple attempts by the intensivist to insert a PIVC have failed. You have been asked to insert a vascular access catheter that will provide reliable, medium to long-term access for blood, and blood product transfusion and sampling.

1. What are your immediate considerations and potential risk factors?
2. What are the potential vascular access options suitable for this patient?

Case Study

You are a nurse in a medical day unit. The majority of your patients attend the unit on a regular basis ranging from weekly, monthly, to quarterly appointments for infusion of medication for prevention and treatment of various disease processes. Some of these patients are becoming increasingly difficult to place a PIVC due to multiple PIVC insertions and side effects of their treatment increasing their adiposity.

You don't currently have a vascular access team in your hospital, and medical officers rotate through this unit on a 3–6 monthly basis.

1. What processes can you implement to reduce the pain and discomfort of multiple PIVC insertion attempts?
2. What technology factors might be useful in this setting?
3. What patient factors might improve PIVC insertion?

Summary of Key Points

1. Prior to selecting the insertion site, clinicians should consider the patient's condition, developmental age, skin condition, previous vascular access history, duration of infusion therapy, and patient preference where possible.
2. Determining site placement requires different considerations with pediatrics versus adults. Some considerations include:
   (a) Mobility
   (b) Skin integrity
   (c) Thumb sucking
   (d) Diaper use
   (e) Activities (older children)
3. The introduction of technologies such as nIR, ultrasound, fluoroscopy, and EKG has increased the success rates of VAD insertions with pediatric patients and should be used as a mean of vessel health and preservation, reducing the number of sticks required for successful access.
4. The ultimate goal of the vascular access healthcare professional working with pediatric patients should be to ensure long-term viability of vessels through careful assessment, planning, insertion, and management.

References

Bannon MP, Heller SF, Rivera M. Anatomic considerations for central venous cannulation. Risk Manage Healthcare Policy. 2011;4:27.

Barnacle A, Arthurs OJ, Roebuck D, Hiorns MP. Malfunctioning central venous catheters in children: a diagnostic approach. Pediatr Radiol. 2008;38(4):363–78. https://doi.org/10.1007/s00247-007-0610-2. quiz 486-367.

Baskin KM, Jimenez RM, Cahill AM, Jawad AF, Towbin RB. Cavoatrial junction and central venous anatomy: implications for central venous access tip position. J Vasc Interv Radiol. 2008;19(3):359–65. https://doi.org/10.1016/j.jvir.2007.09.005.

Benkhadra M, Collignon M, Fournel I, Oeuvrard C, Rollin P, Perrin M, et al. Ultrasound guidance allows faster peripheral IV cannulation in children under 3 years of age with difficult venous access: a prospective randomized study. Paediatr Anaesth. 2012;22(5):449–54. https://doi.org/10.1111/j.1460-9592.2012.03830.x.

Dawson RB. PICC zone insertion method™ (ZIM™): a systematic approach to determine the ideal insertion site for PICCs in the upper arm. J Assoc Vasc Access. 2011;16(3):162–5. https://doi.org/10.2309/java.16-3-5.

Elia F, Ferrari G, Molino P, Converso M, De Filippi G, Milan A, Aprà F. Standard-length catheters vs long catheters in ultrasound-guided peripheral vein cannulation. Am J Emerg Med. 2012;30(5):712–6. https://doi.org/10.1016/j.ajem.2011.04.019.

Gorski L, Hadaway L, Hagle M, McGoldrick M, Orr M, Doellman D. Infusion therapy: standards of practice. J Infus Nurs. 2016;39(1S):S1–S159.

Greene MT, Flanders SA, Woller SC, Bernstein SJ, Chopra V. The association between PICC use and venous thromboembolism in upper and lower extremities. Am J Med. 2015;128(9):986–93.e1. https://doi.org/10.1016/j.amjmed.2015.03.028.

Lamperti M, Pittiruti M. II. Difficult peripheral veins: turn on the lights. Br J Anaesth. 2013;110(6):888–91. https://doi.org/10.1093/bja/aet078.

Lamperti M, Moureau N, Kelly LJ, Dawson R, Elbarbary M, van Boxtel AJ, Pittiruti M. Competence in paediatric central venous lines placement. Br J Anaesth. 2014;112(2):383. https://doi.org/10.1093/bja/aet557.

Lau C, Chamberlain R. Ultrasound-guided central venous catheter placement increases success rates in pediatric patients: a meta-analysis. Pediatr Res. 2016;80(2):178–84. https://doi.org/10.1038/pr.2016.74.

Lirk P, Keller C, Colvin J, Colvin H, Rieder J, Maurer H, Moriggl B. Unintentional arterial puncture during cephalic vein cannulation: case report and anatomical study. Br J Anaesth. 2004;92(5):740–2. https://doi.org/10.1093/bja/aeh118.

Moureau N, Lamperti M, Kelly L, Dawson R, Elbarbary M, van Boxtel J, Pittiruti M. Evidence-based consensus on the insertion of central venous access devices: definition of minimal requirements for training. Br J Anaesth. 2013;110(3):333–46.

Ostroff M, Moureau N. Report of modification for peripherally inserted central catheter placement: subcutaneous needle tunnel for high upper arm placement. J Infus Nurs. 2017;40(4):232–7. https://doi.org/10.1097/nan.0000000000000228.

Phipps K, Modic A, O'Riordan MA, Walsh M. A randomized trial of the vein viewer versus standard technique for placement of peripherally inserted central catheters (PICCs) in neonates. J Perinatol. 2012;32(7):498–501. https://doi.org/10.1038/jp.2011.129.

Roebuck D, Kleidon T, McLaren CA, Barnacle A. Internal jugular vein (IJV) patency after central venous (CV) access [abstract]. Pediatr Radiol. 2005a;35(suppl 1):s76.

Roebuck D, Kleidon T, Mclaren C, Barnacle A. Central venous access by recanalization of occluded central veins [abstract]. Pediatr Radiol. 2005b;35(Suppl 1):S76.

Rossetti F, Pittiruti M, Lamperti M, Graziano U, Celentano D, Capozzoli G. The intracavitary ECG method for positioning the tip of central venous access devices in pediatric patients: results of an Italian multicenter study. J Vasc Access. 2015;16(2):137–43. https://doi.org/10.5301/jva.5000281.

Sharma A, Bodenham AR, Mallick A. Ultrasound-guided infraclavicular axillary vein cannulation for central venous access. Br J Anaesth. 2004;93(2):188–92. https://doi.org/10.1093/bja/aeh187.

Silberzweig JE, Sacks D, Khorsandi AS, Bakal CW. Reporting standards for central venous access. J Vasc Interv Radiol. 2003;14(9 Pt 2):S443–52.

Simcock L. No going back: advantages of ultrasound-guided upper arm PICC placement. J Assoc Vasc Access. 2008;13(4):191–7. https://doi.org/10.2309/java.13-4-6.

Simon PO Jr, Saad WE. Ultrasound-guided vascular access. Ultrasound Clin. 2012;7:283–97. https://doi.org/10.1016/j.cult.2012.04.001.

Song YG, Byun JH, Hwang SY, Kim CW, Shim SG. Use of vertebral body units to locate the cavoatrial junction for optimum central venous catheter tip positioning. Br J Anaesth. 2015;115(2):252–7. https://doi.org/10.1093/bja/aev218.

Spentzouris G, Scriven RJ, Lee TK, Labropoulos N. Pediatric venous thromboembolism in relation to adults. J Vasc Surg. 2012;55(6):1785–93. https://doi.org/10.1016/j.jvs.2011.07.047.

Stolz LA, Stolz U, Howe C, Farrell IJ, Adhikari S. Ultrasound-guided peripheral venous access: a meta-analysis and systematic review. J Vasc Access. 2015;16(4):321–6. https://doi.org/10.5301/jva.5000346.

16

Post-Insertion Care Strategies in Pediatrics

Amanda Ullman and Tricia Kleidon

Abstract

Maintaining function throughout the VADs therapeutic dwell requires the use of effective post-insertion care strategies. Some aspects of post-insertion VAD management can be appropriately generalized from adult literature, and this has already been summarized in Chaps. 10–12. This includes the importance of regular assessment of the entire VAD and patients, including the administration set, for signs of complications and device malfunction. Also, previously summarized in Chaps. 2 and 10 is the use of bundles of care, to ensure the practical application of high-quality evidence to the bedside. These bundles are of great importance during the post-insertion phase, when considering the use of skin antisepsis, dressings, securement, and patency procedures. However, the focus of this chapter is on elements of post-insertion care that are specific to the pediatric population and their VAD.

Keywords

Pediatric VAD management · Pediatric catheter flushing · Pediatric skin considerations · Pediatric complications · Pediatric dressing considerations · Pediatric securement

A. Ullman (✉)
Alliance for Vascular Access Teaching and Research (AVATAR) Group, Menzies Health Institute Queensland, School of Nursing and Midwifery, Griffith University, Brisbane, QLD, Australia
e-mail: a.ullman@griffith.edu.au

T. Kleidon
Alliance for Vascular Access Teaching and Research (AVATAR), Queensland Children's Hospital, Brisbane, QLD, Australia
e-mail: tricia.kleidon@health.qld.gov.au

16.1 Introduction

As with vascular access devices (VADs) in other populations, insertion day is only the beginning of the pediatric vascular access journey. Reliability in pediatric VAD is of upmost importance. Infants and children need to be able to receive their vascular access-dependent treatments as prescribed. However, a recent meta-analysis demonstrated that after successful insertion, 25% of pediatric central venous access devices (CVAD) fail prior to completion of treatment due to complications including bloodstream infection, local site infection, phlebitis, thrombosis, dislodgement, and fracture (Ullman et al. 2015c). Single studies have reported pediatric peripheral VAD failure rates of between 25 and 35%, most commonly from infiltration, phlebitis, occlusion, and extravasation (Malyon et al. 2014; Rozsa et al. 2015).

16.2 Pediatric Skin Health, Antisepsis, Dressing, and Securement

16.2.1 Pediatric Skin Health

The skin is the largest organ in the body. Among other functions, the skin plays an important role in the prevention of infection, providing a barrier to environmental pathogens. Impaired skin integrity is common in pediatrics due to age-related skin pathologies and the sequelae of pediatric conditions. As described in Chap. 13, premature neonatal skin can be extremely fragile, with less developed epidermal layers. Inflammatory skin conditions, such as eczema and other forms of dermatitis, are common during childhood. Health conditions that commonly present during childhood, such as cystic fibrosis (CF) and acute lymphoblastic leukemia (ALL), involve treatment with medications that result in altered skin conditions and altered wound healing.

Children with these complex health conditions rely on the administration of vital medical treatment via their VAD despite loss of skin integrity. Their underlying impaired skin, coupled with the application and removal of adhesive and antiseptic products, results in skin complications surrounding their VAD. Skin complications that present around pediatric VAD include irritant and allergic contact dermatitis, skin tears and blistering, pressure injuries, maceration, and local site infections (Broadhurst et al. 2017) (see Fig. 16.1).

The promotion of pediatric skin health surrounding VAD plays an important role in maintaining VAD function. This can be achieved through the systematic monitoring, prevention, and treatment of VAD-associated skin complications. VAD assessment must include contemporaneous documentation of skin health progression within the patients' medical records, including photos. As presented in Chap. 9: Securement, the prevention of many VAD-associated skin complications is possible with the use of skin barrier films and the correct application of antisepsis, dressing, and securement products. The treatment of skin complications depends upon the diagnosis and severity. Broadhurst et al. (2017) published a consensus and evidence-based algorithm regarding CVAD-associated skin impairment (CASI) relevant to pediatrics. Shown in Fig. 16.2, the CASI algorithm provides direction surrounding the identification and treatment of exit site infection, skin injury (stripping, skin tear), skin irritation/contact dermatitis, and non-infectious weeping.

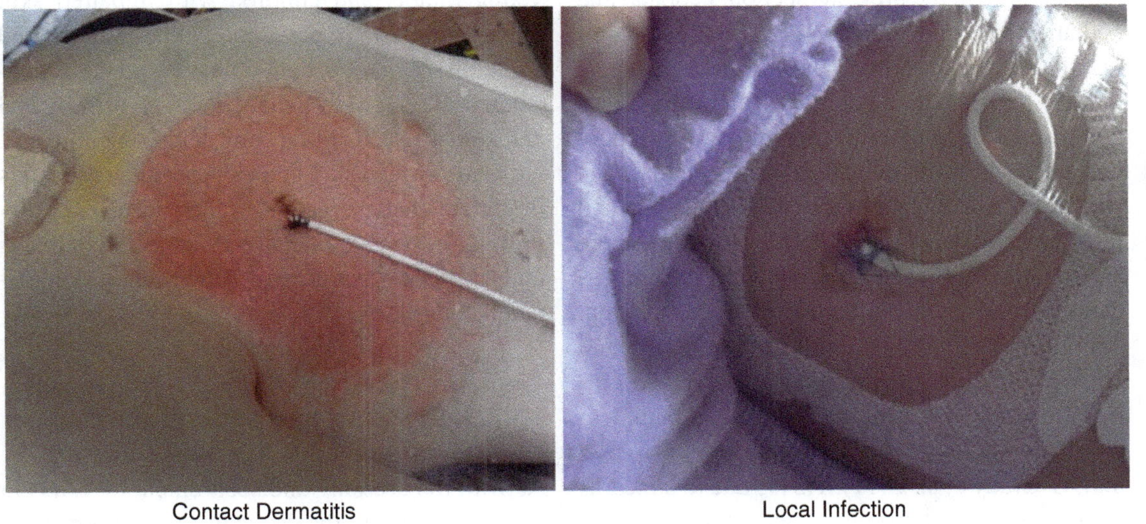

Contact Dermatitis | Local Infection

Fig. 16.1 Example of skin complications surrounding pediatric central VADs (used with permission A. Ullman and T. Kleidon)

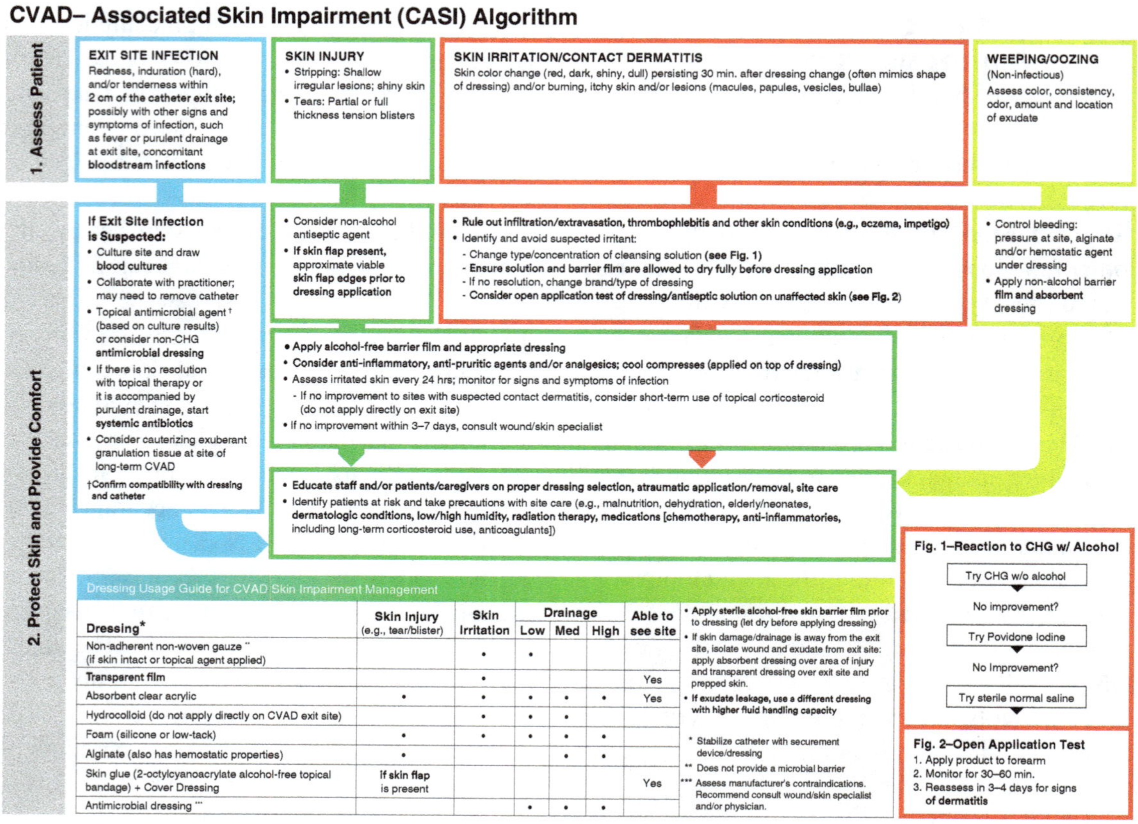

Fig. 16.2 CVAD-associated skin impairment (CASI) algorithm (Broadhurst et al. 2017) (open access, used with permission Broadhurst, Moureau and Ullman)

16.2.2 Skin Antisepsis

As described in the previous section, neonatal and pediatric skin have fundamental differences compared to matured skin. Chlorhexidine gluconate (CHG; ≥0.5%) in alcohol is demonstrated as being superior to other decontaminants at reducing microbial contamination of VAD insertion sites and thereby preventing VAD-associated infections (Mimoz et al. 2015). However, there are complexities when applying these recommendations to the neonatal and pediatric population. The US Federal Drug Administration (FDA) and clinical guidelines do not recommend, or recommend caution, when using CHG for infants less than 2 months of age (Federal Drug Administration n.d.; O'Grady et al. 2011). This is due to concerns regarding CHG absorption and skin irritation. Additionally, skin irritation, including contact dermatitis, has also been frequently reported when using alcohol-based solutions in the neonatal and young infant population. For neonates, young infants and children with impaired skin integrity, the use of povidone iodine, water-based solutions, or other decontaminants should be considered. The risk-to-benefit ratio of using CHG and alcohol needs to be considered by clinicians. No matter which skin antiseptic agent is used, it is important that the agent is allowed to dry fully prior to dressing application. Wet decontaminants under VAD dressings frequently result in skin irritation and injury.

16.2.3 Dressing and Securement

As with the dressing and securement of VADs in other populations, the dressing and securement of pediatric VADs has multiple functions to promote device patency and prevent complication.

Dressing products cover the VAD wound, providing a protective barrier from contamination from the environment, preventing extra-luminal contamination of the VAD insertion site (Ullman et al. 2015a). Securement products stabilize the VAD, ensuring stability of the device tip location either in a central or peripheral position. Securement products also aim to prevent micromotion of the VAD within the vessel (preventing vessel irritation and thereby thrombosis) and within the wound (preventing wound irritation and thereby local site infection) (Ullman et al. 2015a). The overarching literature regarding the range of products that are available to support VAD security has been presented in Chap. 9: Securement.

Within pediatrics, there are some unique features of VAD dressing and securement that must be considered. Infants and small children are rarely compliant in their dressing and securement application and may intentionally attempt to remove the device. The products need to withstand the mechanics of a crawling infant and a bored, non-compliant toddler. This means additional security and coverage, through splints and devices, are often necessary. Consider anchoring the device in an area that is difficult to reach such as over the infant or toddler shoulder. However, the composite of dressing and securement products in use must facilitate regular assessment of the VAD site to monitor for early signs of infiltration, extravasation, phlebitis, and local site irritation. Dressing and securement products must be easy to apply and remove by a variety of clinicians in challenging circumstances. VAD security and dressing products also need to be appropriately sized, with many of the modern non-suture securement products requiring a large footplate, making them difficult to apply in situations such as a jugular non-tunneled central VAD.

Medication-impregnated dressing products involve a slow release of antiseptic solutions onto the VAD insertion site. CHG-impregnated dressing products, either by disk or gel or built into the dressing, have been demonstrated to significantly reduce the rate of central VAD-related bloodstream infections (Ullman et al. 2015b). However, the effectiveness of CHG-impregnated products to prevent infection has not been comprehensively studied in the pediatric population or in devices outside of the critical care setting. While clinical practice guidelines (Loveday et al. 2014; O'Grady et al. 2011) and pragmatism recommend their suitability in most pediatric settings with a high rate of bloodstream infection, caution should again be employed. It is not currently recommended to use CHG-impregnated dressing products in neonates and small infants less than 2 months of age and those with significantly impaired skin integrity surrounding central VAD sites, due to risk of significant skin injuries and irritation. Silver-impregnated dressing products have been successfully used in a single-center neonatal pilot randomized controlled trial without evidence of systemic silver absorption and no evidence of skin damage (Hill et al. 2010). However, the effectiveness of silver-impregnated dressing products for infection prevention has not been demonstrated.

16.3 Pediatric Vessel Size and Patency

Typically, the smaller the patient, the smaller the vessels. As detailed in Chap. 14: The Right Device Assessment, for younger children, smaller gauge catheters are used to prevent complications of thrombosis and phlebitis. However, the use of smaller gauge catheters results in higher risk of intraluminal occlusion due to medication precipitate and thrombosis.

16.4 Flushing

As detailed in Chap. 19: Flushing, there are a variety of strategies that can be used to promote VAD patency including pulsatile flushing using normal saline and heparin, continuous infusion, and locking. Flushing is commonly used to verify VAD patency and theoretically clear the device between medications that could result in occlusion (Doellman et al. 2015). VADs are generally flushed with normal saline before and after medication administration and blood sampling and after an infusion is ceased (Doellman et al. 2015). Routine, pulsatile flushing with normal or heparinized saline is also used between medication administration to create turbulent flow, thereby promoting patency and reducing bacterial catheter colonization. Debate continues regarding the value of heparin flush when a VAD is not in use. Unfortunately, there is limited evidence regarding the optimal flushing frequency and solutions across all populations and even less in pediatrics. The most recent Cochrane systematic review concluded that there was not enough evidence to determine the effects of heparin versus normal saline to prevent occlusion in pediatric CVADs (Bradford et al. 2015), yet it remains the most commonly used flushing and locking solution (Doellman et al. 2015). The additional fluid administered during VAD flushing is an issue of concern for pediatric patients who may be fluid restricted because of their age (e.g., neonates) or medical conditions (e.g., renal disease) (Doellman et al. 2015).

16.5 Locking

VAD locking is most commonly used for CVADs and aims to prevent blood reflux during periods of disuse. A variety of heparin doses are used depending upon the device type, length, and the perceived risk of occlusion (see Table 16.1). To prevent occlusion in small-gauge devices (e.g., 1.9Fr PICC), pediatric vascular access specialists may choose to initiate a low-volume continuous infusion of crystalloid solution. While evidence of its effectiveness is poor, it is theorized that the continuous infusion promotes patency by preventing thrombus formation.

Additional lock solutions should be initiated based upon clinical indication. These include fibrinolytic agents, ethanol, antibiotics (e.g., vancomycin), antibiotic-heparin mixes, and taurolidine. There is limited evidence to support the routine prophylactic use of these lock solutions; however, a growing evidence base supports the use of ethanol and taurolidine lock solutions as either prophylaxis or as catheter salvage in pediatric patients at high risk of CVAD-associated bloodstream infection (Liu et al. 2013; Mokha et al. 2017; Raad et al. 2016).

16.6 Blood Sampling

Pediatric VADs are frequently used for blood sampling during chronic, acute, and critical illness. While blood sampling from peripheral VAD can be troublesome, and frequently results in device malfunction, blood sampling from CVAD is a common procedure. Despite the ubiquity of blood sampling from pediatric CVADs, there is substantial variation in technique and poor evidence to support good practice. Blood sampling from pediatric VAD is of common practice due to difficulty associated with peripheral phlebotomy, risks associated with iatrogenic anemia, volume depletion,

Table 16.1 Locking guidelines for pediatric CVAD (modified from (Doellman et al. 2015))

CVAD type and priming volumes	*Locked device (volume, solution, and frequency)* Add volume for add-on devices to priming volume
PICCs Device priming volume ranges from 0.06 to 0.6 mL. *Check manufacturer guidelines*	*2Fr and smaller*: continuous infusion preferred or 1 mL heparinized saline (10 U/mL) every 6 h *2.6Fr and larger*: 1–2 mL heparinized saline (10 U/mL) every 12 h
Tunneled and non-tunneled Device priming volume ranges from 0.12 to 1.3 mL. *Check manufacturer guidelines*	1–3 mL heparinized saline (10–100 U/mL) every 24 h
Totally implanted device Device priming volume ranges from 0.8 to 2 mL *Check manufacturer guidelines*	*If used for more than one medication daily*: 3–5 mL heparinized saline (10 U/mL) *Monthly maintenance flush*: 3–5 mL heparinized saline (100 U/mL)

catheter occlusion, and CVAD-associated bloodstream infections (Doellman et al. 2015; Ullman et al. 2016).

The three most common techniques for blood sampling from pediatric CVADs are the discard, reinfusion, and push-pull methods. The discard method is common in adult populations and involves the aspiration and then disposal of clearance blood (volume dependent upon line volume), prior to blood sampling. Within pediatrics, this technique can result in significant fluid loss and preventable anemia especially during times of frequent blood sampling (e.g., sepsis). Comparatively, the reinfusion method involves the aspiration of clearance blood sampling and then reinfusion of clearance blood. This technique potentially increases the risk of microbial colonization and thrombosis formation within the clearance volume. The push-pull method involves the multiple rapid infusion and aspiration of first saline, and then blood, through into the syringe, theoretically clearing the line of infusion fluid prior to sampling. This minimizes potential contamination, thrombosis formation, and fluid loss but increases the risk of inaccurate results. Previous clinical trials in pediatrics have demonstrated statistically, but not clinically different results using the push-pull method (Adlard 2008; Barton et al. 2004).

16.7 Pediatric Vascular Access Skills and Training

16.7.1 Clinicians

As described in Chap. 5: Vascular Access Teams, healthcare institutions must ensure development of vascular access qualified and competent staff, including a central core of vascular access specialists. All clinicians caring for children with VADs must be knowledgeable and skilled in the day-to-day management of the variety of VAD types, the prevention of complications, and post-insertion management strategies. Educational programs must be dynamic and completed by clinicians regularly (not just once). Successful clinician educational programs may include a combination of didactic lectures, web-based modules, and high- and low-fidelity simulation, including competency assessment with feedback. Educational programs must incorporate pediatric focused vascular access interventions including the use of child life specialists to promote compliance during procedures such as dressing changes and pain relief. Interdisciplinary clinician training plays a key role in the provision of quality post-insertion VAD care.

Within pediatrics, it is necessary to consider the higher level of advanced skills that are required to manage and problem-solve complex vascular access conditions. Institutions should be supported by a cohort of expert vascular access clinicians who are able to educate and lead high-quality post-insertion management of pediatric VADs. These clinicians may also be involved in the leadership of local clinical practice guideline review and implementation.

16.7.2 Family and Caregivers

Family and primary caregivers must also be comprehensively educated to manage VADs in the home environment. Home-based healthcare is growing across all specialties, with peripheral and central VADs the cornerstone of many home-based therapies, such as antibiotic and parenteral nutrition administration. These therapies range from short term to lifelong administration. Education and resources need to be provided so that the primary caregivers can manage and problem-solve potentially problematic pediatric VADs.

Family members are a significant resource in the prevention of post-insertion VAD complications in the acute care environment. Primary caregivers are intimately familiar with the complexities of their child and their VAD. Whether a short- or long-term device, they understand their child's reaction to pain, compliance with procedures, and, for those with a long-term vascular access dependency, the distinct tricks that may help promote device patency. Never, never ignore the parents and caregivers.

16.8 Conclusion

The management of pediatric VADs after insertion requires specialist focus. The prevention of post-insertion complications in pediatric VAD must be led by comprehensively trained staff, with easily accessible support from vascular access experts. Evidence-based strategies must be used to prevent complications including infection, occlusion, and site irritation. Parents and caregivers are an important resource to be utilized in the post-insertion phase.

Case Study

Rosie is a 4-year-old girl, undergoing treatment for relapsed acute myeloid leukemia (AML) including an allogenic bone marrow transplant. Rosie has a tunneled cuffed CVAD that exits through her right chest wall. Rosie developed symptoms of graft versus host disease 2 days ago, with initial symptoms of poor gut absorption. As her vascular access expert, consider:

1. What types of VAD-associated skin complications is Rosie at risk of developing?
2. What products and procedures could be initiated to reduce the risk of Rosie developing a VAD-associated skin complication?

Case Study

Jacob (18 months) is recovering in pediatric intensive care after cardiac surgery. He is lightly sedated but highly reliant upon his jugular central VAD for inotropes and other medicines. As his vascular access expert, consider:

1. Would you use a CHG-impregnated dressing product?
2. How would you secure his central VAD considering his risk of removal?

Summary of Key Points

1. Post-insertion complications are common in pediatrics with 25% of CVAD and 25–35% of peripheral VAD failing prior to completion of treatment.
2. Young age and common pediatric conditions impair skin integrity, rendering the promotion of skin health and regular assessment of skin complications surrounding VAD necessary.
3. Skin antisepsis in pediatrics can be challenging. Chlorhexidine use is restricted in infants <2 months, and alcohol may also be associated with inflammatory skin conditions. Other decontaminants should be considered, and the risk-to-benefit ratio must be evaluated by clinicians.
4. Young children are at increased risk for accidental and intentional VAD dislodgement. However, products used to promote device security must facilitate regular site assessment and easy application/removal.
5. VAD patency can be challenging, due to small lumen size. Consider the use of continuous infusion to maintain patency for very small lumen devices.
6. Healthcare institutions need to invest in high-quality, dynamic pediatric VAD education, to develop VAD competent interdisciplinary staff.
7. Parents and caregivers are an important resource to prevent VAD complications.

References

Adlard K. Examining the push-pull method of blood sampling from central venous access devices. J Pediatr Oncol Nurs. 2008;25(4):200–7. https://doi.org/10.1177/1043454208320975.

Barton SJ, Chase T, Latham B, Rayens MK. Comparing two methods to obtain blood specimens from pediatric central venous catheters. J Pediatr Oncol Nurs. 2004;21(6):320–6. https://doi.org/10.1177/1043454204269604.

Bradford NK, Edwards RM, Chan RJ. Heparin versus 0.9% sodium chloride intermittent flushing for the prevention of occlusion in long term central venous catheters in infants and children. Cochrane Database Syst Rev. 2015;11:Cd010996. https://doi.org/10.1002/14651858.CD010996.pub2.

Broadhurst D, Moureau N, Ullman AJ. Management of central venous access device-associated skin impairment: an evidence-based algorithm. J Wound Ostomy Continence Nurs. 2017;44(3):211.

Doellman D, Buckner JK, Hudson Garrett J Jr, Catudal JP, Frey AM, Lamagna P, et al. Best practice guidelines in the care and maintenance of pediatric central venous catheters. 2nd ed. Herriman, UT: Association for Vascular Access; 2015.

Federal Drug Administration. Medical devices. https://www.fda.gov/MedicalDevices/

Hill ML, Baldwin L, Slaughter JC, Walsh WF, Weitkamp JH. A silver-alginate-coated dressing to reduce peripherally inserted central catheter (PICC) infections in NICU patients: a pilot randomized controlled trial. J Perinatol. 2010;30(7):469–73. https://doi.org/10.1038/jp.2009.190.

Liu Y, Zhang AQ, Cao L, Xia HT, Ma JJ. Taurolidine lock solutions for the prevention of catheter-related bloodstream infections: a systematic review and meta-analysis of randomized controlled trials. PLoS One. 2013;8(11):e79417. https://doi.org/10.1371/journal.pone.0079417.

Loveday H, Wilson J, Pratt R, Golsorkhi M, Tingle A, Bak A, et al. EPIC3: national evidence-based guidelines for preventing healthcare-associated infections in NHS hospitals in England. J Hosp Infect. 2014;86(Suppl 1):S1–70. https://doi.org/10.1016/s0195-6701(13)60012-2.

Malyon L, Ullman AJ, Phillips N, Young J, Kleidon T, Murfield J, Rickard CM. Peripheral intravenous catheter duration and failure in paediatric acute care: a prospective cohort study. Emerg Med Australas. 2014;26(6):602–8. https://doi.org/10.1111/1742-6723.12305.

Mimoz O, Lucet JC, Kerforne T, Pascal J, Souweine B, Goudet V, et al. Skin antisepsis with chlorhexidine-alcohol versus povidone iodine-alcohol, with and without skin scrubbing, for prevention of intravascular-catheter-related infection (CLEAN): an open-label, multicentre, randomised, controlled, two-by-two factorial trial. Lancet. 2015;386(10008):2069–77. https://doi.org/10.1016/s0140-6736(15)00244-5.

Mokha JS, Davidovics ZH, Samela K, Emerick K. Effects of ethanol lock therapy on central line infections and mechanical problems in children with intestinal failure. JPEN J Parenter Enteral Nutr. 2017;41(4):625–31. https://doi.org/10.1177/0148607115625057.

O'Grady NP, Alexander M, Burns LA, Dellinger EP, Garland J, O'Heard S, et al. Guidelines for the prevention of intravascular catheter-related infections. Clin Infect Dis. 2011;52(9):e162–93.

Raad I, Chaftari AM, Zakhour R, Jordan M, Al Hamal Z, Jiang Y, et al. Successful salvage of central venous catheters in patients with catheter-related or central line-associated bloodstream infections by using a catheter lock solution consisting of minocycline, EDTA, and 25% ethanol. Antimicrob Agents Chemother. 2016;60(6):3426–32. https://doi.org/10.1128/aac.02565-15.

Rozsa AP, Bell AJ, Tiitinen MT, Richards S, Newall F. Peripheral intravenous catheters in a paediatric population: circumstances of removal and time in situ. Neonatal Paediatr Child Health Nurs. 2015;18(3):18–24.

Ullman AJ, Cooke M, Rickard C. Examining the role of securement and dressing products to prevent central venous access device failure: a narrative review. J Assoc Vasc Access. 2015a;20(2):99–110.

Ullman AJ, Cooke ML, Mitchell M, Lin F, New K, Long DA, et al. Dressings and securement devices for central venous catheters (CVC). Cochrane Database Syst Rev. 2015b;9:Cd010367. https://doi.org/10.1002/14651858.CD010367.pub2.

Ullman AJ, Marsh N, Mihala G, Cooke M, Rickard CM. Complications of central venous access devices: a systematic review. Pediatrics. 2015c;136(5):e1331–44. https://doi.org/10.1542/peds.2015-1507.

Ullman AJ, Keogh S, Coyer F, Long DA, New K, Rickard CM. 'True Blood' the critical care story: an audit of blood sampling practice across three adult, paediatric and neonatal intensive care settings. Aust Crit Care. 2016;29(2):90–5. https://doi.org/10.1016/j.aucc.2015.06.002.

Part VI

Efficient Management

17

PIVCs, PICCs and CVCs: Maintenance and Care

Val Weston

Abstract

Vascular access devices (VADs) such as peripheral intravenous vascular catheters (PIVCs), peripherally inserted central catheters (PICCs) and central venous catheters (CVCs) are essential and common components of modern healthcare practice. In the USA, over 1.4 billion vascular access device procedures are undertaken annually, whilst in the UK, one in three patients will have at least one cannula inserted during their hospital stay. Such devices deliver a myriad of treatments ranging from fluid replacement and delivery of medications to laboratory blood sampling. However, these devices are not without their unwanted complications including phlebitis, thrombosis, dislodgement and bloodstream infections, some of which have the potential to be life threatening. Great emphasis has been placed on the insertion of these devices in reducing their potential risks. However, the right maintenance and care of these devices is equally important and is the focus of this chapter.

Keywords

Site assessment · Catheter function · Catheter care and maintenance · Dressing change · Dressing adherence · Visual inspection · Site palpation · ANTT · Assessment for necessity

V. Weston (✉)
Alder Hey Children's NHS Foundation Trust, Liverpool, UK
e-mail: Valya.weston@alderhey.nhs.uk

17.1 Introduction

Management of vascular access devices represents the largest portion of time in the Vessel Health and Preservation (VHP) cycle. Right management includes assessment of the insertion site, dressing and device function prior to each infusion. Care and management using right infection prevention methods including Aseptic Non Touch Technique (ANTT) for device handling, disinfection of access site, pulsatile flushing the device before and after infusions, performing dressing changes consistent with policies and evaluation of device necessity with prompt removal when the VAD is no longer needed are cornerstones to safe patient care. Incorporated into management are the right supplies and technology needed to ensure the right outcomes. Right management is a process that requires consistency established through commitment to education, policy development based on guidelines and research and consistent evaluation of outcomes.

Care and maintenance of peripheral or central venous devices represents the longest period of time in the life of a VAD. Complications are more prevalent during this period and require close assessment with device removal as soon as no longer needed. Management of VADs requires assessment of function, dressing integrity and evaluation of the insertion site integrated with consistent disinfection prior to infusion access, flushing and evaluation for device necessity. Each of these components represents a level of safety necessary to protect the patient receiving intravenous treatments.

17.2 Assessment

Assessment is the active process of inspecting, monitoring and evaluating a vascular access device (VAD) and includes assessing the entire infusion system, from the solution container to the VAD insertion site (Gorski et al. 2016). The objective of these assessments is to monitor the device for complications, patency, position, function and necessity. The aim is to prevent the interruption of treatment, to assess the patency of the device and to detect signs of infection or other complications at the earliest possible stage (Moureau 2013; Loveday et al. 2014; RCN 2016).

Moureau (2013) identifies the five main components of VAD assessment as cannulation site, dressing, tubing or giving set labelling, catheter function and device necessity. Additionally, the RCN (2016) recommends the documentation of the ongoing care and maintenance of the device to include:

1. Details of the catheter care (Loveday et al. 2014)
2. Site and device care—to include appearance using local assessment scales for phlebitis
3. Dressing changes
4. Methods to evaluate the functioning of the VAD prior to use (Bodenham et al. 2016)
5. Continued documentation of the external or exposed length of the CVC or PICC line to monitor migration
6. Flush solution used to include type, volume, frequency and difficulties encountered

The Vessel Health and Preservation tool and framework produced in the USA and in the UK advocates the inclusion of a section for the daily assessment and evaluation of the VAD to assess for complications to determine if the VAD remains the right choice and indeed whether it is still needed (Moureau et al. 2012; Hallam et al. 2016) (see Fig. 17.1).

17.3 How Often Should the VAD Be Assessed?

17.3.1 Peripheral Intravenous Vascular Catheters (PIVCs)

Gorski et al. (2016) recommend that PIVCs be assessed by staff at least once every 4 h, 1–2 hourly for patients who are critically ill or sedated or who have cognitive impairment. These assessments need to increase to hourly for neonate and paediatric patients and more often when dealing with patients who are receiving an infusion of a vesicant medication or chemotherapeutic agent.

Alternatively, Loveday et al. (2014), NICE (2014) and the RCN (2016) recommend that the PIVC should be assessed every shift at a minimum. However, Ray-Barruel et al. (2014) in their systematic review reported that the frequency for phlebitis assessments to highlight the risk of infection ranged from every time the device was accessed for medication or infusions to twice daily, daily or even every other day. Therefore, there is clearly a difference of opinion in the frequency and timing of recommendations for assessments, and as recommended by RCN (2016), the frequency for assessment should be set out in organisational policies and procedures based on good-quality clinical evidence.

17.3.1.1 CVC and PICCs

NICE (2014), Gorski et al. (2016) and Hallam et al. (2016) recommend that CVC, PICC and midline catheters be assessed on a daily basis, whilst Loveday et al. (2014) recommend that CVC and PICC catheters should be assessed at least once a shift for signs of inflammation, infiltration or blockage.

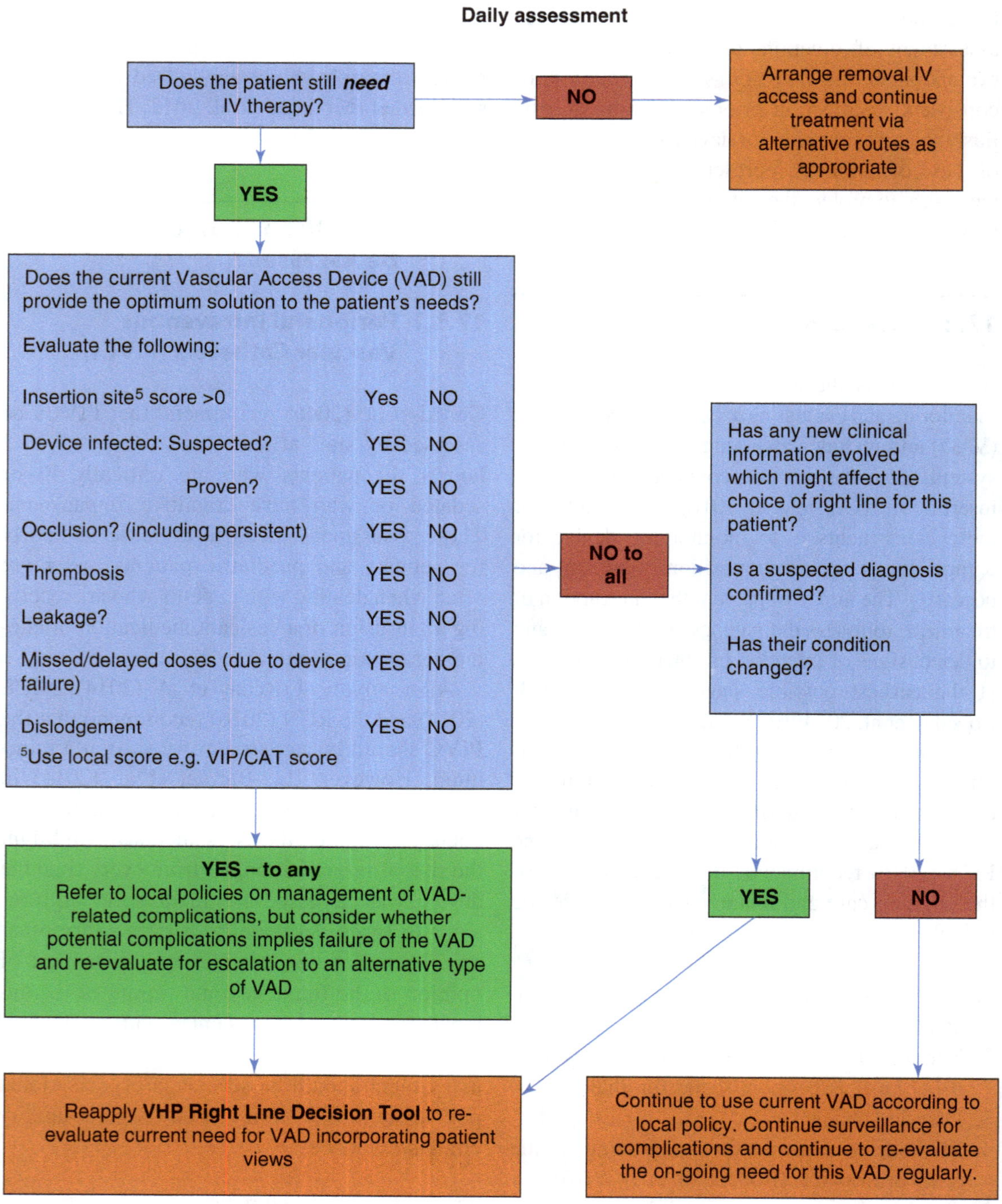

Fig. 17.1 Daily assessment chart (used with permission from Hallam et al. 2016)

17.3.1.2 Outpatients and Home Care

Tice et al. (2004) recommend that the VAD should be monitored daily, short and midlines twice weekly and CVCs at least once a week, whilst Chapman et al. (2012) and Gorski et al. (2016) advise that the patient and/or the care giver must have training to be able to check and assess the VAD at least once per day for signs of complications and report immediately any signs or symptoms of dressing dislodgement to their healthcare provider. Chapman et al. (2012) additionally recommend that the outpatient antibiotic therapy (OPAT) nurse specialists or other vascular nurse specialists must be satisfied of the patient/care giver competency in caring for and assessing the VAD and that this competency should be documented.

For paediatric care Chapman et al. (2012) recommend that the care giver or a family member must be capable of delivering/providing the necessary care for the patient.

17.4 Inspection of the VAD Insertion Site

The site inspection begins with a visual inspection of the VAD insertion site, assessing for redness, swelling or any signs of infection or other complications.

After the visual inspection, hands are decontaminated, and gloves are donned. The site is gently palpated through the dressing to determine if there are any signs of pain tenderness, firmness, blanching, moisture, oedema or oozing. All findings are noted and documented in the patient record (Moureau 2013). If possible, the patient is consulted to determine whether he or she is feeling pain or discomfort at the site or when medications are being administered. However, for patients with cognitive impairment and communication difficulties, this may not be possible; the practitioner will need to assess through body language if the patient is feeling discomfort or pain.

The catheter position is checked and measured to ensure it has not migrated in or out of the cannulation site. For central venous catheters (CVCs) and peripherally inserted central catheters (PICCs), this is verified by comparing the current external length of the catheter with the baseline measurement documented on the initial insertion of the cannula (Moureau 2013; Gorski et al. 2016). The upper arm circumference can be measured when clinically indicated to assess the presence of oedema and possible deep vein thrombosis (DVT). The measurement is taken 10 cm above the antecubital fossa and is compared to the baseline measurement to detect possible catheter-associated venous thrombosis. A 3 cm increase in arm circumference and the presence of oedema may be associated with an upper arm DVT.

17.5 Dressings and Dressing Changes

Next, the dressing is assessed. Remember, once the skin has been punctured for the insertion of the VAD, the dressing provides the only protective barrier keeping microorganisms from entering the body through the insertion site. The practitioner ensures that the dressing is completely intact, that all edges are adhering to the skin and that the dressing is clean and dry. The dressing should be replaced if its integrity has been compromised by moisture, drainage or blood under the dressing, if there are signs of sheering or dislodgement of the dressing or if there are signs and symptoms of infection such as redness, exudates or pain (Gorski et al. 2016; RCN 2016).

Following placement of a VAD, a dressing is used to protect the insertion site. The two most common types of dressings used for insertion sites are sterile, transparent, semipermeable polyurethane dressings with a layer of an acrylic adhesive (transparent dressings) and gauze and tape (Loveday et al. 2014). Transparent film dressings are used to cover VAD insertion sites whenever possible (Loveday et al. 2014; RCN 2016) to minimise the risk of extra luminal catheter contamination (Rupp et al. 2013). Transparent dressings are permeable to water, vapour and oxygen and impermeable to microorganisms.

After insertion the practitioner should ensure that the dressing is completely intact, that all edges are adhering to the skin and that the dressing is clean and dry. The dressing should be replaced if its integrity has been compromised by moisture, drainage or blood under the dressing, there are signs of sheering or dislodgement of the dressing or if there are signs or symptoms of infection such as redness, exudate or pain (Gorski et al. 2016; RCN 2016).

A gauze dressing is used if there is drainage of blood or fluid from the catheter exit site or if the patient has profuse perspiration (Loveday et al. 2014; Gorski et al. 2016; RCN 2016).

Ensure dressings are secure to reduce the risk of loosening or dislodgement of the catheter, as frequent dressing changes are associated with an increased risk of infection (Gorski et al. 2016)

Table 17.1 Current guidance available for the frequency of dressing changes

Dressing changes	Epic3—Loveday et al. (2014)	Infusion therapy standards of practice—Gorski et al. (2016)	Standards for infusion therapy (fourth edition)—RCN (2016)
Transparent semipermeable membrane dressing (TSM, transparent dressing)	Every 7 days or sooner if the integrity of the dressing is compromised	At least every 5–7 days or more frequently if the dressing becomes damp, loosened or visibly soiled	Every 7 days or sooner if the integrity of the dressing is compromised
Gauze or gauze under a transparent dressing	Change when inspection of the site is necessary or when the dressing becomes damp loosened or soiled Change the gauze to a transparent dressing as soon as possible	Every 2 days	Change when inspection of the site is necessary or when the dressing becomes damp loosened or soiled Change the gauze to a transparent dressing as soon as possible
Post insertion dressing	Changed after 24 h		Changed after 24 h

due to the risk of loosening or dislodging the catheter during dressing removal.

The practitioner should check to see if a dressing change is required according to standards and local protocols. A dressing is changed immediately, and the site is closely assessed, cleaned and disinfected if there is evidence of leakage, site tenderness and other signs of infection or if the dressing becomes loose or dislodged (see Table 17.1).

Compliance with recommended dressing change days is necessary to prevent endogenous patient flora/bacteria from infecting the catheter down the cannulation line.

It is recommended to use chlorhexidine gluconate-impregnated dressings over central VADs to reduce the risk of infection from an extra luminal source (Timsit et al. 2012; Loveday et al. 2014; Ullman et al. 2015; Gorski et al. 2016).

17.6 Securement

It is vitally important to secure VAD particularly PIVC, non-tunnelled central lines and PICC lines. Failure to adequately secure the VAD increases the risk of infection, malposition, treatment delays/failure and extravasation and can lead to premature removal of the VAD (Gorski et al. 2016). Dressings alone should not be relied on to stabilise the VAD, and a stabilisation device should be used.

There are two main types of stabilisation devices: adhesive-based devices or subcutaneous engineered stabilisation device. The choice of securement device should be based on a risk assessment considering the patients age, skin integrity, previous adhesive skin injury and any type of drainage from the insertion site (Gorski et al. 2016). Securement devices are covered in more detail in Chap. 9.

Assess the integrity of the stabilisation device at each dressing change, and change the device according to the manufacturer's directions for use. Remove adhesive devices during dressing change to allow for appropriate skin antisepsis, and then apply a new device (Gorski et al. 2016). Usually, subcutaneous engineered stabilisation devices can stay in place for the duration of the device and can be lifted to achieve skin antisepsis at each dressing change.

17.7 Tubing/Giving Set Labelling

Infusion tubing/giving sets aid in the administration of medications and fluids and are connected to the VAD. Standards and subsequent local policies and procedures establish the correct length of time that the tubing/giving set can be used based on the types of solutions being administered through them.

During the assessment of the VAD, ensure that the tubing/giving set change dates are checked, including additional equipment used for the administration of intravenous medications and solutions (Moureau 2013; Gorski et al. 2016; RCN 2016).

17.8 Catheter Function

Catheter function is addressed during each site assessment and with each use to check the flow and patency of the catheter.

Firstly, the practitioner checks to see if the catheter flushes easily without sluggishness as this is generally the first sign of a partial occlusion in the catheter. Ideally, flow should be easy and smooth without resistance. Once flow has been assessed, aspiration can be performed to check for a brisk blood return. The catheter should then be flushed again to clear the blood from the lumen. An inability to aspirate blood or flush the catheter may be resolved through flushing if identified early enough. (This is covered in more detail in the following chapters).

If sluggishness with blood flow or flushing is present in a CVAD, blood buildup may have formed within the walls of the catheter making it necessary to instil a thrombolytic solution to clear the catheter. Any problems regarding catheter function should be addressed and remedied promptly to avoid a delay in treatment, complete loss of function of the catheter and increased risk of infection (Moureau 2013).

17.9 Complication Prevention During Site Assessment and Management

17.9.1 Infection

All invasive devices are a known source of infection with VADs having a greater risk for bloodstream infections. Although evidence demonstrates that some cannulation sites such as the femoral vein carry a higher risk of infection (CDC 2011; RCN 2016), all devices have a risk regardless of where they are placed.

Sources of bacterial contamination and subsequent infection for any VAD include:

1. Practitioner hands—direct contact
2. Patient skin
3. Catheter hubs
4. Catheter tubing/giving sets
5. Infusates
6. Contamination of equipment—indirect contact

To prevent infection, specific steps must be taken to prevent the bacteria from entering the body through a portal of entry. It is the practitioner's duty to ensure the patient is kept safe by employing simple and timely management strategies to minimise the risk of infection. Examples of infection prevention strategies include the use of gloves during site assessment, disinfection of patient's skin during dressing changes and disinfection of the catheter hub prior to each access, all of which are discussed thoroughly in later chapters.

17.9.2 Phlebitis

Phlebitis, or inflammation of the vein, is one of the complications the clinician is looking for during a site assessment. Phlebitis has four main root causes and is classified and treated based on its origin. The four classifications of phlebitis are as follows:

- *Chemical Phlebitis:* associated with infusates administered to the patient or with skin antiseptics that have not fully dried and are pulled into the vein during device insertion
- *Mechanical Phlebitis:* associated with vein wall irritation caused by the catheter being too large for the vasculature, catheter movement, insertion trauma or catheter material and stiffness
- *Bacterial Phlebitis:* associated with bacterial contamination or colonisation of the VAD or the intravenous site
- *Post-Infusion Phlebitis:* may occur up to 48 h after removal of the device, necessitating continued assessment of the site

Phlebitis can cause a patient severe discomfort and interrupt therapy resulting in delayed treatment and, in the case of a PIVC, the need for the device to be resited. Repeated incidences of phlebitis may lead to difficulty with venous access and a possible need for more advanced venous access (Marsh et al. 2015). Phlebitis is treated based on its cause. See Table 17.2 for phlebitis interventions.

Table 17.2 Summary of phlebitis interventions recommended by Gorski et al. (2016)

Type of phlebitis	Intervention
Chemical	Evaluate infusion therapy and need for different vascular access, different medication or slower rate of infusion. Determine if catheter removal is needed
Mechanical	Stabilise catheter, apply heat, elevate limb, provide analgesia, monitor for 24–48 h, and if symptoms persist consider removal of the catheter
Bacterial	If suspected, remove catheter. Discuss with physician the need for further vascular access
Post-infusion	If bacterial source, monitor for signs of systemic infection If nonbacterial, apply warm compress, elevate limb, and provide analgesia

Phlebitis is diagnosed by observation of clinical signs or when a patient reports various symptoms. The insertion site should be visually assessed and documented during every shift at a minimum, and in the case of a PIVC, a visual infusion phlebitis score (Figs. 17.2, 17.3, and 17.4) (Jackson 1998) or other standardised phlebitis scale should be recorded (Loveday et al. 2014; Gorski et al. 2016; RCN 2016).

Gorski et al. (2016) recommend that phlebitis incidents causing harm or injury should be reviewed for quality improvement opportunities.

17.10 Keeping the Patient Safe During Site Assessment and Catheter Maintenance

Up to 99% of the catheter life happens after initial placement of a vascular access device. It is estimated that 71.7% of CVAD infection occur 5 days or more after insertion, during

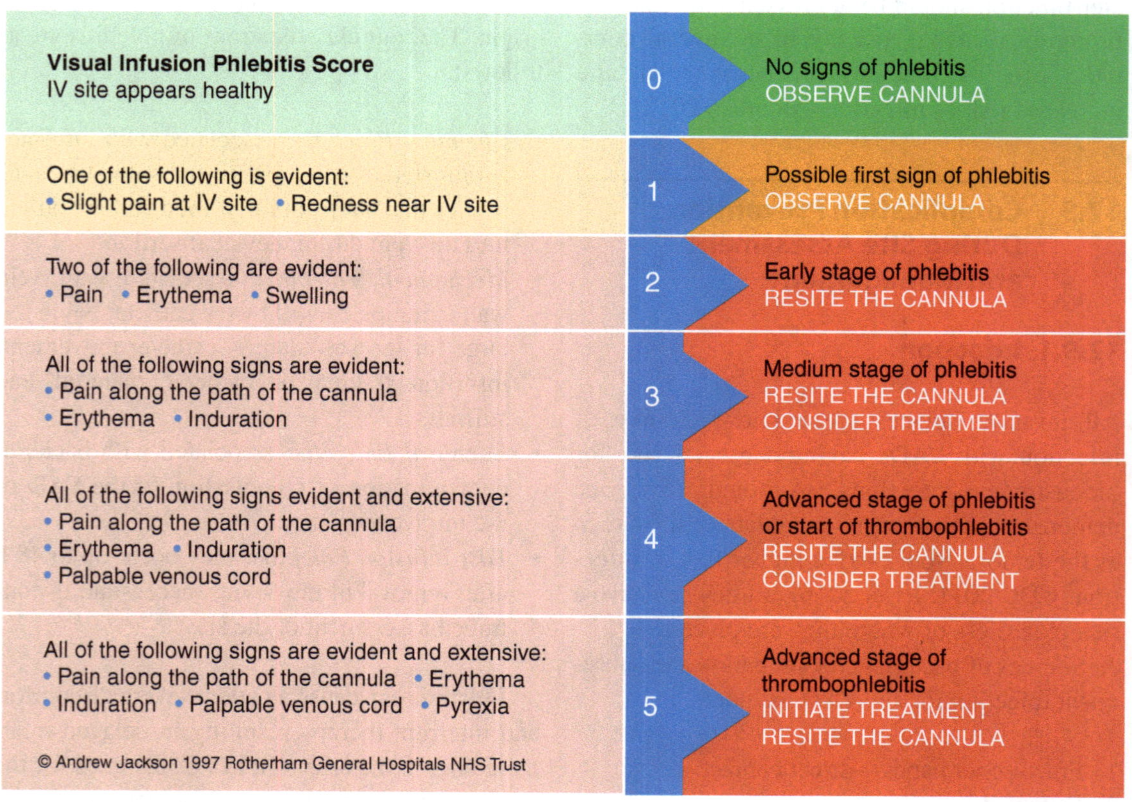

Fig. 17.2 Visual phlebitis score (used with permission from A. Jackson, www.IVTeam.com)

Daily Vessel Health Assessment Tool

Patient Medical ID #: ____________ **Date:** ____ / ____ / ______ (dd mm yyyy)

Nursing Information

1. How comfortable is the patient with their vascular access device? (ask the patient)
   ☐ 5 - Extremely comfortable ☐ 2 - Somewhat uncomfortable
   ☐ 4 - Somewhat comfortable ☐ 1 - Very uncomfortable
   ☐ 3 - Comfortable ☐ N/A due to confusion /sedation or other ________
   If #2 or #1 checked, please explain the reason for discomfort: ________

2. What is the current device(s)? (check all that apply)

Type:	☐ PIV	☐ Midline	☐ PICC	☐ CVC	☐ Port	☐ Dialysis		
Number of Lumens		☐ 1	☐ 2	☐ 3	Which Device?		☐ PICC	☐ CVC
No. of Lumens in Use		☐ 1	☐ 2	☐ 3	Which Device?		☐ PICC	☐ CVC

3. What complications, if any occurred within the last 24 hours (PIV)? (check all that apply)
   ☐ Infiltration ☐ Multiple restarts in 24 hrs
   ☐ Phlebitis/thrombophlebitis ☐ Infection ☐ Other ________

4. Did any complications occur within the last 24 hours with Central Venous Access Device(s)? ☐ Yes ☐ No
   If Yes, check all that apply. Which Device? ☐ PIV ☐ Midline ☐ PICC ☐ CVC ☐ Port ☐ Dialysis
   ☐ Infection ☐ Phlebitis ☐ Occlusion
   ☐ Partial Withdrawal Occlusion ☐ Thrombosis ☐ Other ________

5. Is this patient having any difficulty with eating and drinking? ☐ Yes ☐ No
6. Are there IV medications ordered other than PRN? ☐ Yes ☐ No
7. Is the VAD absolutely neccessary for blood draws with this patient? ☐ Yes ☐ No

Nursing Recommendation: **Print Name:** ________ RN/NP/PA/IVRN (circle)

8. Referring to the VHP Right Line Tool is the Venous access device(s) most appropriate for the current treatment plan? ☐ Yes ☐ No
   If No, What device would apply based on Right Line Tool Selection? ________
9. Is there any reason to maintain the current device(s)? ☐ Yes ☐ No
   If Yes, (other than the above reason) Why? ________

RECOMMENDATIONS:
☐ Discontinue device(s) ☐ Maintain device(s)
☐ Consider new device(s) from VHP Assessment Trifold Recommended new device(s) ________

Physician/Pharmacist Info: **Print Name:** ________ MD/PharmD (circle)
(Information can be obtained by interview or by phone)

10. would switch to all oral medications be contraindicated at this time for this patient? ☐ Yes ☐ No
11. Is there an active blood stream infection? ☐ Yes ☐ No
12. Will access be required once the patient is released? ☐ Yes ☐ No
13. What is the current discharge plan? # of days left ____
14. Is the current IV device still necessary for this treatment plan and this patient? ☐ Yes ☐ No
    If Yes, please explain:
    ☐ IV needed additional days Number of additional day(s) ________
    ☐ Critical condition ☐ Other ________

MD Action Plan:
See nursing recommendation(s). If two or more NO answers, consider discontinuation of all IV devices to reduce risk to patient.

FINAL ACTION:
☐ Discontinue device(s) ☐ Maintain device(s) ________ # day(s)

For internal review: ☐ 25% ☐ 50% ☐ 75% ☐ 100%

Fig. 17.3 Daily assessment (used with permission from the Teleflex)

maintenance of these devices (Davis 2011). Protocols have been established to promote patient safety during maintenance and manipulation of vascular access devices; these protocols include proper hand hygiene, the use of personal protective equipment, proper patient skin antisepsis during dressing changes and the use of aseptic technique throughout the maintenance and manipulation of all vascular access devices. It is the clinician's responsibility to adhere to the established protocols to ensure patient safety.

SAMPLE DAILY MONITORING TOOL

Clinical assessment due between 7A and 7p shift each day for each patient

Patient Name and Room Number: Date:

Clinician Name:

Please notify PICC/VAS Team if advanced assessment of device is needed.

Daily Assessment for Site Necessity:

Current Intravenous Devices (list all with quantity):

PIV **#1** Location: R / L; describe location size length of time in place (hrs/days)

Describe usage:

PIV **#2** Location: R / L; describe location size length of time in place (hrs/days)

Describe usage:

PICC Location: R / L; describe location size lumens **Describe usage:**

CVC Location (Chest /Neck): R / L; describe location lumens **Describe usage:**

Port Location: R / L; describe location **Describe usage:**

Current Infusions:

☐ Fluid Infusion - Type ☐ Intravenous Medications Check all that apply: ☐ Antibiotics ☐ Pain Meds ☐ TPN/PPN ☐ Chemotherapy ☐ Inotropes ☐ Other types

☐ Blood Draws from CVC, frequency _____

Venous Access Requirements:

☐ Peripheral sites adequate for prescribed therapy currently

☐ Peripheral vein sites available (prescriptive medications include known vein irritants)

Consider: ☐ Temporary Antimicrobial CVC ☐ PICC ☐ Tunneled CVC ☐ Port

☐ Limited peripheral sites – Central Venous Catheter needed

Consider: ☐ Temporary Antimicrobial CVC ☐ PICC ☐ Tunneled CVC ☐ Port

☐ Refer to Advanced Inserter under Vein Sparing Protocol -assessment related to patient diagnosis, complications as an inpatient and infusion history

Fig. 17.4 Monitoring tool (used with permission from the Teleflex)

17.11 Extravasation and Infiltration

Extravasation and infiltration are the result of fluids and medication inadvertently being infused into the surrounding tissues of the vessel in which the VAD is located (RCN 2016) and may occur in over a third of patients receiving IV therapy (Al-Benna et al. 2013). The term infiltration is used when a non-vesicant solution has been used and often doesn't cause long lasting damage compared to extravasation which is caused by vesicant solutions and can cause major tissue damage which may require plastic surgical interventions.

The risk of both extravasation and infiltration complications is more common in PIVC than central lines and can be prevented by choosing the appropriate IV gauge, care site selection, effective securement of the device and the frequent assessment of insertion site (Dwyer and Rutkowski 2016; Gorski et al. 2016).

The early detection and response to extravasation injuries can minimise the long-term damage. Extravasation of vesicant solutions is firstly noted by pain and swelling around the insertion site followed by blanching, blistering and discoloration of the skin, but it is usually pain that alerts the patient of the problem (Al-Benna et al. 2013).

Each medical facility or hospital should have a policy in place for the prevention, recognition, management and reporting of extravasation injuries (Gorski et al. 2016; RCN 2016). As a standard, the infusion should be stopped as soon as an extravasation injury is identified and the medical team informed. The device should not be removed, and an attempt to aspirate the extravasated drug should be made until the treatment plan has been determined (Al-Benna et al. 2013; RCN 2016).

17.11.1 Hand Hygiene

Hand hygiene is a key component of a group of evidence-based interventions to promote better outcomes for patients with a VAD (Gorski et al. 2016).

Hand hygiene prior to catheter maintenance combined with the correct aseptic technique during catheter manipulation provides protection against infection (WHO 2009; Loveday et al. 2014). Both patients and practitioners need to have a clear understanding of the importance of hand hygiene and the role that it plays in preventing the transmission of infection.

Hands should always be considered a source of infection. WHO (2009), Loveday et al. (2014), Gorski et al. (2016) and RCN (2016) recommend that hands are decontaminated with either soap and water or an alcohol sanitiser at these particular times:

1. When entering a patient's room or cubicle
2. Before patient contact
3. Before and after any procedure—such as putting on gloves
4. After patient contact
5. After leaving the patient's environment

Poor hand hygiene can result in the spread of microorganisms between patients and poses a direct risk factor for VAD infections (Zhang et al. 2016). Improving hand hygiene requires a multimodal approach (WHO 2009), and programmes should include focus on behavioural changes such as empowering healthcare workers to be able to stop unsafe practices where physicians or other colleagues have breached hand hygiene protocols (Chopra and Saint 2015).

17.11.2 Personal Protective Equipment (PPE)

The selection of PPE is based on the assessment of the risk of transmission of microorganisms to the patient and the risk of contamination of practitioner's skin and clothing by the patient's blood or bodily fluids (Loveday et al. 2014).

Gloves should be worn for all invasive procedures, contact with sterile sites and non-intact skin, including when changing the dressing of a VAD (CDC 2011; Loveday et al. 2014).

Gloves should be single use and are put on immediately before an episode of patient care. Equally, gloves need to be removed as soon as the episode of care has been completed. Upon glove removal, hands are decontaminated with either soap and water or an alcohol-based sanitiser to prevent the spread of microorganisms from the hands (Moureau 2013; Loveday et al. 2014).

Additionally, the use of single-use disposable plastic aprons is recommended when there is a risk of blood or bodily fluid exposure (Loveday et al. 2014).

17.11.3 Patient Skin Antisepsis

The skin acts as a protective barrier against bacteria and infection. When the skin is punctured or breeched in any way, this barrier is broken, creating a portal for bacteria to enter the body. When bacteria enter the body through this portal of entry, they have the potential to migrate into the bloodstream and cause infection.

The skin is punctured during VAD insertion, creating a direct entry for bacteria to ingress into the bloodstream. Therefore, it is vitally important that the skin is disinfected at each dressing change and at any time that the skin puncture site is exposed.

Chlorhexidine is considered the antiseptic of choice when cleaning the skin before VAD dressing changes and is consistently recommended by current guidelines (Moureau 2013; Loveday et al. 2014; Gorski et al. 2016; RCN 2016). However, in a recent systematic review by Lai et al. (2016), the conclusion was that there is a low quality of evidence to suggest that antiseptic solutions containing chlorhexidine reduce catheter microbial colonisation and CLABSI compared to antiseptic solutions containing povidone iodine.

Although antiseptics have traditionally been applied in a circular motion, current more up-to-date products such as SoluPrep™ (3M) and ChloraPrep™ (CareFusion) now recommend applying antiseptic solutions in a back and forth grid-like pattern with friction to agitate the surface layers of the skin (Broadhurst et al. 2016).

It is crucially important that the antiseptic used is allowed to dry completely prior to the application of the dressing, as inadequate drying may cause contact dermatitis, inactivate the adhesion of the dressing or, in certain circumstances, increase the risk of infection due to moisture being trapped underneath the dressing. Current guidance on the antiseptics to be used and drying times is given below in Table 17.3.

Assessment of the skin underneath the dressing should be performed regularly as there is potential risk for skin injury due to age, underlying skin condition, joint movement and the presence of oedema. There is also a potential risk which needs to be assessed from medical adhesive-related skin injury (MARSI) associated with the use of adhesive-based engineered stabilisation devices (ESDs). The use of a skin barrier solution helps to reduce the risk of MARSI (Gorski et al. 2016).

17.11.4 Aseptic Technique

Asepsis is defined as the absence of pathogenic (harmful) organisms. Aseptic technique is a set of

Table 17.3 Current guidance regarding antiseptic drying times

Guidance for antiseptic cleaning solutions	Epic3—Loveday et al. (2014)	Infusion therapy standards of practice—Gorski et al. (2016)	Standards for infusion therapy (fourth edition)—RCN (2016)
Chlorhexidine in alcohol	2% chlorhexidine in 70% alcohol	>0.5% chlorhexidine in 70% alcohol	2% chlorhexidine in 70% alcohol
Contraindications or allergy to chlorhexidine	Povidone iodine in alcohol	Tincture of iodine—idopher Povidone iodine	Povidone iodine in alcohol
Drying times	No exact timings given—but emphasises that the antiseptic solution should be dry	Chlorhexidine in alcohol—30 s Povidone iodine—90–120 s	No exact timings given—but emphasises that the antiseptic solution should be dry

specific practices and procedures performed under carefully controlled conditions with the goal of minimising contamination by pathogens. During invasive procedures or maintenance of invasive devices, patients rely on staff to protect them from infection.

Aseptic technique should be followed when accessing any component of the intravenous device, site or line or when dressing changes are required (Loveday et al. 2014; Gorski et al. 2016; RCN 2016). However, despite clear guidance for the use of an aseptic technique when caring for the VAD, there is evidence of poor compliance (Moureau 2014). One of the biggest challenges in aseptic technique is convincing healthcare workers of the danger they pose to patients of microorganism transference during any invasive procedure.

To achieve safe aseptic practice, practitioners must have the ability to perform effective aseptic technique consistently. The concept of Aseptic Non Touch Technique (ANTT), which originated in the UK, provides a standardised approach to aseptic technique by providing clear, uncomplicated steps to encourage compliance (Rowley and Clare 2009; Loveday et al. 2014). The essential components of an aseptic technique include hand hygiene, use of personal protective equipment and the promotion of a practice technique to minimise contamination from bacteria (Rowley and Clare 2009; O'Grady et al. 2011; Loveday et al. 2014).

17.12 Device Necessity

Check the catheter daily to ensure that the VAD is still required based on the patient's medical condition and treatment plan (Pronovost et al. 2006; CDC 2011; Moureau 2013; Gorski et al. 2016).

The practitioner should:

- Check the patient's prescribed therapy to see if the catheter is still necessary.
- Check to see if the intravenous treatment is complete or if the treatment can be switched to an oral form of the medication.
- Check if the VAD is being used for blood sampling only.

Since VADs are a proven source of infection, they should be removed as soon as they are no longer medically necessary to reduce the risk of infection (Pronovost et al. 2006; Gorski et al. 2016). This includes checking to see if the treatment can be switched to an oral form of the medication rather than intravenous treatment. As an infection prevention measure, change to an oral medication if possible. The best way to eliminate catheter infections is to eliminate the catheter as soon as possible.

Gorski et al. (2016) and RCN (2016) standards state that the VAD should be removed if there is an unresolved complication, if therapy has been discontinued or if it is no longer deemed medically necessary. Additionally, a catheter that is no longer necessary should not be kept in place just in case it may be needed in a few days, and consideration should be made to switch to oral medication as soon as a patient's condition allows to aid in the prompt removal of the VAD at the earliest possible time. This timely removal of the VAD when it is no longer necessary will assist in the minimisation of the infection risk.

17.13 Care Bundles/Compliance and Education

There is a plethora of evidence from Pronovost et al. (2006) onwards to demonstrate that the implementation of care bundles and ongoing maintenance for VAD care has a significant effect on reducing the risks of complications including infections (Pronovost et al. 2006; New et al. 2014; Duffy et al. 2015; Matthias Walz et al. 2015).

Components of the care bundle/maintenance programme should include procedural guidelines for hygiene, aseptic technique, dressing changes and a daily or more frequent assessment of the device for function, complications and signs and symptoms of infection. Failure to complete one of these components predisposes the patient to a bloodstream infection or other complications (Duffy et al. 2015).

It is essential that everyone involved in the care of the patient with a VAD is trained through structured and well-organised educational programmes that enable practitioners to provide, monitor and evaluate care and continually increase their competence which are crucial to the success of any strategy designed to reduce the risk of infection (Bianco et al. 2013; Loveday et al. 2014). Written policies, formal training and years of experience all contribute to an increase in knowledge, practice, positive attitudes towards CLABSI prevention and improved patient outcomes.

17.14 Summary

Practitioners need to be confident and proficient in VAD care practices and be aware of the signs and symptoms of clinical infection or complications affecting a VAD. It is essential that everyone involved in the care of the patient with a VAD has adequate training to identify complications, understand interventions and be aware of the need for documentation in the medical record. An in-depth assessment of each VAD performed daily or with each shift should evaluate the insertion site, the adherence of the dressing, the function of the device and the response of the patient to any associated pain. Structured and well-organised educational programmes that enable practitioners to provide, monitor and evaluate care and continually increase competence are crucial to the success of any strategy designed to reduce the risk of infection and other complications (Bianco et al. 2013; Loveday et al. 2014). Written policies, formal training and years of experience all contribute to an increase in knowledge, practice, positive attitudes towards CLABSI prevention and improved patient outcomes. The most important single action that can be performed by clinicians to reduce risk is the removal of unnecessary VAD, those that are not being used, where treatment is complete and when oral medications have been instituted.

Case Study

Kelly is a newly qualified nurse responsible for performing an assessment on Mr. Smith a 72-year-old stroke patient with a urinary tract infection. Mr. Smith is receiving IV antibiotics through a peripheral catheter in his left hand. Kelly performs a site assessment of the PIVC and notes it is placed in the hand with limited mobility. No drainage or redness is present, but Kelly identifies swelling surrounding the insertion site, in the hand and up the arm.

Kelly speaks with her preceptor who states if a complication is present, the PIVC needs to be discontinued and another restarted in a different location. Kelly discontinues the PIVC by loosening the dressing gently, applying pressure with a sterile gauze, and removes the catheter. A dry sterile dressing is applied. Kelly then seeks the assistance of a more experienced nurse to assist her with locating a suitable site for insertion of a new PIVC.

Summary of Key Points

1. The care and maintenance of a vascular access device (VAD) is equally as important as the insertion procedure in preventing complications and infection.
2. Assessments of the VAD should be carried out daily or more frequently depending on the type of VAD and the category of patient.
3. An assessment should include:
   (a) The cannula site
   (b) The integrity of the patient's skin, the type of dressing and how frequently the dressing needs to be changed
   (c) Catheter function
   (d) Tubing/giving set
   (e) Assessment for signs of complications or infection
   (f) Necessity for the device
   (g) Documentation

4. Hand hygiene must be performed prior to any VAD assessment or procedure.
5. An aseptic technique should be used for any VAD procedure.
6. A VAD should be removed as soon as it is deemed no longer medically necessary.

References

Al-Benna S, O'Boyle C, Holley J. Extravasation injuries in adults. ISRN Dermatol. 2013;2013:856541.

Bianco A, Coscarelli P, Nobile CGA, Pileggi C, Pavia M. The reduction of risk in central line—associated bloodstream infections: knowledge, attitudes and evidence-based practices in health care workers. Am J Infect Control. 2013;41:107–12.

Bodenham A, Babu S, Bennett J, Binks R, Fee P, Fox B, Johnston AJ, Klein AA, Langton JA, McLure H, Tighe SQM. Association of anaesthetists of great Britain and Ireland: safe vascular access 2016. Anaesthesia. 2016;71:573–585. www.aagbi.org/sites/default/files/safe20%vascular%access%202016.pdf. Accessed 2 April 2017.

Broadhurst D, Moureau N, Ullman AJ. Central venous access devices site care practices: an international survey of 34 countries. J Vasc Access. 2016;17(1):78–86.

Center for Disease Control and Prevention. 2011 guidelines for the prevention of intravascular catheter—related infection. Atlanta: CDC; 2011. p. 1–83. www.cdc.gov/hicpac.BSI/BSI-guidelines-2011.html. Accessed 17 March 2017.

Chapman AL, Seaton RA, Cooper MA, Hedderwick S, Goodall V, Reed C, Sanderson F, Nathwani D. Good practice recommendations for outpatient parenteral antimicrobial therapy (OPAT) in adults in the UK: a consensus statement. J Antimicrob Chemother. 2012;67:1053–62.

Chopra V, Saint S. Vascular catheter infections: time to get technical. Lancet. 2015;386:2034–6.

Davis J. Central line associated bloodstream infection: comprehensive, data-driven prevention. PA Patient Saf Advis. 2011;8(3):100–5.

Duffy EA, Rodgers CC, Shever LL, Hockenberry MJ. Implementing a daily maintenance care bundle to prevent central line-associated bloodstream infections in pediatric oncolgy patients. J Pediatr Oncol Nurs. 2015;32(6):394–400.

Dwyer V, Rutkowski B. IV infiltration and extravasation: prevention, recognition, and intervention. J Assoc Vasc Access. 2016;21(4):253.

Gorski L, Hadaway L, Hagle M, McGoldrick M, Orr M, Doellman D. Infusion therapy: standards of practice (supplement 1). J Infus Nurs. 2016;39(1S):S1–S159.

Hallam C, Weston V, Denton A, Hill S, Bodenham A, Dunn H, Jackson T. Development of the UK vessel health and preservation (VHP) framework: a multi-organisational collaborative. J Infect Prev. 2016;17(2):65–72.

Jackson A. Infection control: a battle in vein infusion phlebitis. Nurs Times. 1998;94(4):68–71.

Lai NM, Lai NA, O'Riordan E, Chaiyakunapruk N, Taylor JE, Tan K. Skin antisepsis for reducing central venous catheter-related infections. Cochrane Database Syst Rev. 2016;7:CD010140. https://doi.org/10.1002/14651858.CD010140.pub2.

Loveday HP, Wilson JA, Pratt RJ, Golsorkhi M, Tingle A, Bak A, Browne J, Prieto J, Wilcox M. Epic3: National evidence–based guidelines for preventing healthcare-associated infections in NHS hospitals. J Hosp Infect. 2014;86(Suppl 1):S1–S70.

Marsh N, Mihala G, Ray-Barruel G, Webster J, Wallis MC, Rickard CM. Inter-rater agreement on PIVC-associated phlebitis signs, symptoms and scales. J Eval Clin Pract. 2015;21:893–9.

Matthias Walz J, Ellison RT, Mack DA, Flaherty HM, McIlwaine JK, Whyte KG, Landry KE, Baker SP, Heard SO, CCoc Research Group. The bundle 'plus': the effect of a multi-disciplinary team approach to eradicate central line-associated bloodstream infections. Anesth Analg. 2015;120(4):868–76.

Moureau N. Safe patient care when using vascular access devices. Br J Nurs. 2013;22(2):S14–21.

Moureau NL. Catheter associated bloodstream infection prevention: what is missing? Br J Healthc Manag. 2014;20(11):502–10.

Moureau NL, Trick N, Nifong T, Perry C, Kelley C, Leavett M, Gordon SM, Wallace J, Harvill M, Biggar C, Doll M, Papke L, Benton L, Phelan DA. Vessel health and preservation (part 1): a new evidence—based approach to vascular access selection and management. J Vasc Access. 2012;13:351–6.

National Institute for Health. Infection prevention and control. Quality standard [QS61]. Quality standard 5: vascualr access devices. [online] available: www.nice.org.uk/guidance/qs61/chapter/Quality-statement-5-vascular-access-devices [accessed: January 2018] (Regulatory); 2014.

New KA, Webster J, Marsh NM, Hewer B. Intravascular device use, management, documentation and complications; a point prevalence survey. Aust Health Rev. 2014;38:345–9.

O'Grady NP, Alexander M, Burns LA, Dellinger EP, Garland J, Heard SO, Lipsett PA, Masur H, Mermel LA, Pearson ML, Raad II, Randolph AG, Rupp ME, Saint S, the Healthcare Infection Control Practices Advisory Committee (HICPAC). Guidelines for the prevention of intravascular catheter-related infections. Clin Infect Dis. 2011;52:e162–93.

Pronovost P, Needham D, Berenholtz S, et al. An intervention to decrease catheter—related bloodstream infections in the ICU. N Engl J Med. 2006;355(26):2725–32.

Ray-Barruel G, Polit D, Murfield J, Rickard C. Infusion phlebitis assessment measures: a systmatic review. J Eval Clin Pract. 2014;20(2):191–202.

Rowley S, Clare S. Improving standards of aseptic practice through ANTT trust-wide implementation process: a matter of prioritisation and care. J Infect Prev. 2009;10(1 Supplement):S18–23.

Royal College of Nursing. Standards for infusion therapy. 4th ed. London: RCN; 2016.

Rupp ME, Cassling K, Faber H, Lyden E, Tyner K, Marion N, Van Schooneveld T. Hospital—wide assessment of compliance with central venous catheter dressing recommendations. Am J Infect Control. 2013;41:89–91.

Tice AD, Rehm SJ, Dalovisio JR, Bradley JS, Martinelli LP, Graham DR, Brooks Gainer R, Kunkkel MJ, Yancey RW, Williams DN. Practice guidelines for outpatient parenteral antimocrobial therapy. Clin Infect Dis. 2004;38(12):1651–71.

Timsit JF, Mimoz O, Mourvillier B, Souweine B, Garrouste-Orgeas M, Alfandari S, Plantefeve G, Bronchard R, Trche G, Gauzit R, Antona M, Canet E, Bohe J, Lepape A, Vesin A, Arrault X, Schwebel C, Adrie C, Zahar JR, Ruckly S, Touregros C, Lucet JC. Randomised controlled trial of chlorhexidine dressing and highly adhesive dressing for preventing catheter-related infections in critically ill adults. Am J Respir Crit Care Med. 2012;186(12):1272–8.

Ullman AJ, Cooke ML, Mitchell M, Lin F, New K, Long DA, Mihala G, Rickard CM. Dressings and securement devices for central venous catheters (CVC) (review). Cochrane Database Syst Rev. 2015;(9):CD010367. https://doi.org/10.1002/14651858.CD010367.pub2.

World Health Organisation. A guide to the implementation of the WHO multimodal hand hygiene improvement strategy. 2009. http://apps.who.int/iris/bitstream/10665/70030/1/WHO_IER_PSP_2009.02_eng.pdf.

Zhang L, Cao S, Marsh N, Ray-Barruel G, Flynn J, Larsen E, Richard CM. Infection risks associated with peripheral vascular catheters. J Infect Prev. 2016;17(5):207–13.

18

Disinfection of the Catheter Hub

Carole Hallam

Abstract
The two most common causes of catheter-related bloodstream infections (CRBSI) are contamination of the external surface of the vascular device from the patient skin (extraluminal) and contamination of the internal lumen of the catheter via the catheter hub (intraluminal). This chapter focuses on disinfection of the catheter hub, allowing the reader to consider issues relating to contamination of the catheter hubs and connectors as well as what evidence and guidance are provided to prevent intraluminal colonisation.

Keywords
Hub disinfection · Passive disinfection caps
Active disinfection · Drying time
Disinfectants · Methods for disinfecting catheter hubs

18.1 Introduction

Needle-free connectors (NFC) are widely used on vascular access devices to provide easy access for infusion connection while eliminating the need to use a needle, thus reducing needle-stick injuries (Moureau and Flynn 2015). NFC are used to cap the hubs and should allow easy and effective decontamination between uses due to their flat surface design (Curran 2016). Results of a randomised clinical trial suggested that the use of NFC may reduce contamination compared to standard caps (Casey et al. 2003). However, results from a systematic review found that 33–45% of NFC were found to be contaminated (Moureau and Flynn 2015), suggesting the importance of disinfection of the needle-free connector prior to access of these devices.

18.2 Potential Microbial Contamination and Risk of CRBSI

Microorganisms found on the patient's skin easily contaminate the catheter hubs and are often the same organisms implicated in CRBSI such as coagulase-negative *Staphylococcus* and *Staphylococcus aureus*, enterococci, and *Candida* species (Loveday et al. 2014). As most vascular access devices are accessed frequently, often several times a day, there is great risk of microorganisms entering into the lumen of the catheter, therefore increasing the risk of CRBSI (Merrill et al. 2014; Loveday et al. 2014). High incidence of catheter hub colonisation has been shown to correlate with positive blood cultures (Holroyd et al. 2017).

C. Hallam (✉)
Calderdale and Huddersfield NHS Foundation Trust, Huddersfield, UK

Once a vascular device is inserted into the blood vessel, biofilms develop rapidly from plasma proteins, platelets, and neutrophils (Donlan 2001). These biofilms form a sticky surface that allows microorganisms introduced via the catheter hub to adhere to the internal lumen of the catheter where they can multiply. Eventually, segments from the biofilm break off, and the microorganisms enter the patients' bloodstream causing a bloodstream infection (Curran 2016).

The Infusion Nurse Society (Gorski et al. 2016) Standards of Practice recognise needle-free connectors have different designs with different internal mechanisms and fluid pathways but state that there is no consensus on design of type of NFC to prevent or reduce vascular access device infections (Gorski et al. 2016). To achieve adequate disinfection of a needle-free connector, the following factors should be considered:

1. The device should not have gaps between the membrane and the housing.
2. The membrane should be smooth.
3. The membrane should return to its initial position following access (Kelly et al. 2017).

The design selection of NFC is covered in more detail in Chap. 19.

Importantly, guidance from INS (Gorski et al. 2016), Royal College of Nursing (RCN 2016), Healthcare Infection Control Practices Advisory Committee (HICPAC) of the Centers for Disease Control and Prevention (CDC) (O'Grady et al. 2011) and Epic3 (Loveday et al. 2014) are all clear about the need to disinfect the NFC prior to each access of the device. However, consideration needs to be given as to which solution to use to decontaminate the NFC, what technique provides sufficient decontamination and optimal time required to achieve effective disinfection. These points will be considered in the rest of this chapter.

18.3 Choice of Disinfectants

The choice of disinfection must always be compatible with the device and should not cause damage that could affect the integrity or performance of the device (RCN 2016). Although manufacturers' guidance should be followed (Loveday et al. 2014; RCN 2016), it would seem prudent to check the guidance from the manufacturers prior to purchase to ensure it meets the regulatory standard that may be imposed either at local or national level.

Isopropyl alcohol in concentrations above 60% is an effective disinfectant against a range of organisms. It is able to rapidly kill organisms, but its activity time is very limited because it evaporates quickly on surfaces (CDC 2008). Alcohol is deactivated by the presence of organic matter such as blood, pus, serum and faecal matter, as these interfere with the properties of the disinfectant (WHO 2014). Alcohol is known to damage some surfaces including plastics and rubber (CDC 2008), but most manufacturers have ensured that catheter hubs and NFC are chemically compatible with alcohol (Loveday et al. 2014).

Chlorhexidine and povidone-iodine are both recognised as effective skin disinfectants for vascular access device insertion and are known to have residual activity (Chopra and Saint 2015), allowing for continued killing effect after the alcohol has dried. Loveday et al. (2014) recognised the lack of good evidence supporting disinfection of hubs and connectors, and therefore the Epic3 guidance was based on expert consensus following review of experimental studies.

More recently Flynn et al. (2017) found chlorhexidine gluconate swabs (2% chlorhexidine gluconate and 70% alcohol) to be more effective than alcohol swabs at reducing the number of organisms on NFC. However, these authors did highlight that it is unknown if there is any residual disinfectant activity or damage to the material of the NFC or if any traces of the chlorhexidine would get injected into the bloodstream. Chlorhexidine sensitivity is a known risk in some patients, and therefore alternative disinfectants should be available such as povidone-iodine (Loveday et al. 2014; RCN 2016).

Guidance in various countries differs, for example, Health Protection Scotland states 70% alcohol in their guidance and states that the method of cleaning is more important than the disinfectant (Health Protection Scotland 2012). American guidance (O'Grady et al. 2011; Gorski et al. 2016) states that chlorhexidine, povidone-iodine, or alcohol 70% should be used for the disinfection of the hubs and NFC with the guidance in England (Loveday et al. 2014, RCN 2016) stating the use of 2% chlorhexidine gluconate in 70% alcohol.

Finally, prior to making any decisions of what disinfectants to use for decontaminating the catheter hub and NFC, determine whether there is any local or national regulatory guidance that should be followed.

18.4 Disinfection Methods

Once the disinfectant has been selected to decontaminate the hubs and NFC, the disinfection technique needs to be decided upon; currently there is no defined best method (Zhang et al. 2016). There are two methods to decontaminate the hubs and NFC: active disinfection and passive disinfection (Curran 2016; Kelly et al. 2017).

Active disinfection is performed using a wipe to mechanically loosen the microorganisms allowing the disinfectant to destroy the microorganisms (Curran 2016). This procedure is often referred to as 'scrubbing the hub' (O'Grady et al. 2011; Cameron-Watson 2016; Kelly et al. 2017). Regardless of the disinfectant solution, the time spent on disinfection of the hub or NFC is deemed the most important (Moureau and Flynn 2015).

The active method for decontaminating the hubs is open to variation in both the technique used by the individual and the actual time spent carrying out the procedure (Cameron-Watson 2016). Arguably, it could be suggested that busy healthcare workers don't have enough time to spend decontaminating these hubs for the length of time necessary to achieve effective disinfection (Merrill et al. 2014; Cameron-Watson 2016).

Passive disinfection is achieved using alcohol-impregnated catheter hub protection caps (Gorski et al. 2016). These disinfection caps contain a sponge impregnated with alcohol that can be attached to the NFC, thus protecting the access point from contamination as well as providing disinfection (Flynn et al. 2015; Cameron-Watson 2016; Curran 2016). These disinfection caps are single-use items and must be changed following each use (Sweet et al. 2012; Kelly et al. 2017).

There is some evidence that these disinfection caps can reduce contamination of the NFC and reduce rates of CRBSI (Sweet et al. 2012; Loveday et al. 2014; Cameron-Watson 2016). The advantage of the disinfection caps is that once screwed into place, the alcohol covers the entire surface of the NFC providing continuous decontamination (Flynn et al. 2015; Curran 2016). In one study, the use of disinfection caps was associated with a 40% decrease in central line-associated bloodstream infections (Merrill et al. 2014). In addition, the use of a disinfection cap provides a standardised approach to disinfection (Curran 2016; Kelly et al. 2017).

18.5 Optimal Time for Hub Disinfection

Although disinfecting time is deemed important, there is a lack of clarity for the specific time required to reach optimal disinfection (Merrill et al. 2014; Moureau and Flynn 2015). Some studies have suggested as little as 5 s to be effective in disinfection of the NFC (Rupp et al. 2012; Flynn et al. 2017) but specify only if not heavily contaminated or the latter authors found a reduction only with alcohol and chlorhexidine as opposed to any other disinfectants. The obvious difficulty in assessing whether or not the NFC was heavily contaminated would be the fact that microorganisms are not visible to the naked eye; therefore, this would almost be a best guess situation (Curran 2016).

In the Epic3 guidelines, the lack of clear evidence for optimal disinfection time was recognised; therefore, their choice of a minimum of 15 s for disinfection was selected using expert opinion based on evidence from skin cleansing prior to insertion studies and experimental studies (Loveday et al. 2014). More recent evidence in an experimental study suggests that 30 s is the

Table 18.1 Summary table of guidance for disinfection of hubs and NFC

Guidance	Specified disinfectant	Specified time	Type of action
Healthcare Infection Control Practices Advisory Committee (O'Grady et al. 2011)	Chlorhexidine, povidone-iodine or 70% alcohol	Not specified	Active
Health Protection Scotland (2012)	70% isopropyl alcohol	15 s	Active
Queensland Government (2015)	70% alcohol or 2% alcoholic chlorhexidine	15 s	Active
Epic3 (Loveday et al. 2014)	2% chlorhexidine gluconate in 70% isopropyl alcohol (or povidone-iodine in alcohol for patients with sensitivity to chlorhexidine)	15 s	Active
Society of Healthcare Epidemiology of America (Marschall et al. 2014)	Alcoholic chlorhexidine preparation, 70% alcohol, or povidone-iodine	5 s	Active
Association for Professional in Infection Control and Epidemiology (APIC 2015)	Chlorhexidine, povidone-iodine, or 70% alcohol	15 s	Active
International Federation of Infection Control (IFIC) (DeVries 2016)	70% isopropyl alcohol	Not specified	Active
Infusion Nurses Society (Gorski et al. 2016)	70% isopropyl alcohol, povidone-iodine or >0.5% chlorhexidine in alcohol	5–60 s	Active/passive
Royal College of Nursing (RCN 2016)	2% chlorhexidine gluconate in 70% isopropyl alcohol	Not specified	Active/passive

ideal disinfection time to adequately decontaminate the NFC (Flynn et al. 2017).

The INS (2016) guidance is the only guidance that specifically states the need to disinfect the NFC prior to each subsequent administration when multiple accesses are required via the vascular device. They suggest a 5–15 s disinfection time for each subsequent access (Gorski et al. 2016).

In addition to the time required to effectively disinfect the NFC, the drying time to allow for the full activity of the disinfectant must be considered (DeVries 2016). Most of the guidance states 'allow the disinfectant to dry' as opposed to stating a specified time (O'Grady et al. 2011; DeVries 2016; Gorski et al. 2016; RCN 2016). Other recommendations state that the disinfectant should be visibly dry, and drying time could exceed 30 seconds (Loveday et al. 2014).

Further research is required to provide the optimal time for disinfection of hubs and NFC prior to access (Loveday et al. 2014; Gorski et al. 2016). Local, national or manufacturer's guidance mandates the time required to disinfect the hubs and NFC and should always be followed (Moureau and Flynn 2015; RCN 2016).

A summary of the published national guidance for disinfection of hubs and NFC is provided in Table 18.1 below.

18.6 Changing Needle-Free Connectors

The interval for changing NFC should be in accordance with the manufacturer's guidance and can vary between 72 h and 7 days (RCN 2016; Gorski et al. 2016; Kelly et al. 2017). However, there is no evidence to suggest the need to change NFC more frequently than 96 h (Sandora et al. 2014). Most importantly, an aseptic technique should be adopted when changing the NFC (APIC 2015). This can be adequately achieved using Standard-ANTT (Flynn et al. 2015).

Additionally, the NFC should be replaced if disconnected for any reason, if there is visible blood or debris in the NFC, or prior to obtaining a blood sample for culture (Gorski et al. 2016). NFC can become more difficult to disinfect once contaminated with blood, suggesting the NFC be discarded following blood draws and transfusions (Flynn et al. 2017). However, as of yet, this has not been included in national guidance.

18.7 Compliance with Standards

It is clear from the evidence that there are two critical areas of practice to prevent microbial contamination via the catheter hub: use of an aseptic technique including hand hygiene and effective disinfection of the NFC prior to access of the vascular device (Warren et al. 2006; O'Grady et al. 2011; Loveday et al. 2014).

The use of Aseptic Non Touch Technique (ANTT) provides a standardised approach to aseptic technique by providing easy-to-follow steps making compliance easier (Rowley and Clare 2009; Loveday et al. 2014). The essential components of an aseptic technique include hand hygiene and use of personal protective equipment (Rowley and Clare 2009; O'Grady et al. 2011; Loveday et al. 2014).

Despite the clear guidance for use of an aseptic technique, compliance has been reported as poor (Moureau 2014; Flynn et al. 2015). Poor hand hygiene can result in the spread of microorganisms between patients and results in a direct risk factor for vascular access device infections (Zhang et al. 2016). Improving hand hygiene requires a multi-modal approach (WHO 2009) and includes behavioural changes such as empowering nurses to be able to halt practices where physicians or other colleagues have breached hand hygiene (Chopra and Saint 2015).

Disinfection of the catheter hubs is considered central to patient safety (Kelly et al. 2017), yet compliance has been noted to be unacceptably low, particularly with timing (Moureau 2014; Caspari et al. 2017). One study showed up to an 80% failure rate of disinfecting key parts such as NFC (Rowley and Clare 2009).

Human factors should be considered to improve compliance with hub disinfection. Ensuring that disinfection wipes or caps are readily available at the point of use prevents busy staff from wasting valuable time searching for the equipment (Gorski et al. 2016). Additionally, the use of disinfection caps can make the disinfection method easier as it removes the need to time the process. Additionally, observation of practice and audit of compliance could become easier (Merrill et al. 2014; Cameron-Watson 2016).

A recent study found that both education and introduction of timing devices increased the compliance of recommended timing for disinfection of vascular access devices. These authors concluded that timing devices such as a timer or musical button should be implemented when there is a requirement of time-based procedures to account for human factors (Caspari et al. 2017).

Performance and quality improvement processes are essential to improving and maintaining compliance with practice standards in vascular access care (O'Grady et al. 2011). These should include continuing professional education, accessible protocols, audit with feedback of compliance with practice guidelines and visual prompts and reminders (Loveday et al. 2014).

Case Study

You have just started a new job at your local hospital. Since you have never worked there before, what do you need to consider prior to disinfecting the needleless connector prior to administering IV drugs to a patient?

Case Study

Carly is a 29-year old female who has undergone major resection of her bowel due to Crohn's disease and is now preparing to go home. She has a tunnelled central venous catheter for parenteral nutrition (PN) which she will be administering herself following discharge. What advice will you give her about how to disinfect the needle connector prior to connecting the PN?

Summary of Key Points

1. Hands must be decontaminated prior to access and manipulation of catheter hubs and NC.
2. An aseptic technique should be used for accessing and changing needleless connectors.
3. All vascular access points should be disinfected prior to access with a disinfectant compatible with the device.
4. Use either a scrub the hub technique to disinfect the NC or use a passive technique with alcohol-impregnated protective cap.
5. Consider human factors to achieve high levels of compliance.
6. Check manufacturer's guidance for the management of NC, preferably before purchase.
7. Ensure local and national guidance is followed.
8. Provide regular audit with feedback of compliance with standards.

References

Association for Professional in Infection Control and Epidemiology. APIC implementation guide: guide to preventing central line associated blood stream infections. 2015. http://apic.org/Resource_/TinyMceFileManager/2015/APIC_CLABSI_WEB.pdf.

Cameron-Watson C. Port protectors in clinical practice: an audit. Br J Nurs. 2016;25(8):S25–31.

Casey AL, Worthington T, Lambert PA, Quinn D, Faroqui MH, Elliott TSJ. A randomized, prospective clinical trial to assess the potential infection risk associated with the PosiFlow® needleless connector. J Hosp Infect. 2003;54:288–93.

Caspari L, Epstein E, Blackman A, Jin L, Kaufman DA. Human factors related to time dependant infection control measures "scrub the hub" for venous catheters and feeding tubes. Am J Infect Control. 2017;45(6):648–51. https://doi.org/10.1016/j.ajic.2017.01.004. (Epub ahead of print).

Centers for Disease Control and Prevention (CDC) Healthcare Infection Control Practices Advisory Committee (HICPAC). Guideline for disinfection and sterilisation in healthcare facilities. 2008. https://www.cdc.gov/hicpac/disinfection_sterilization/6_0disinfection.html.

Chopra V, Saint S. Vascular catheter infections: time to get technical. Lancet. 2015;386:2034–6.

Curran E. Needleless connectors: the vascular access catheter's microbial gatekeeper. J Infect Prev. 2016;17(5):234–40.

DeVries C. Prevention of intravascular device-associated infections. Basic concepts. Chapter 17. International Federation of Infection Control. 2016. http://theific.org/wp-content/uploads/2016/04/17-IV_2016.pdf.

Donlan RM. Biofilms and device-associated infections. Emerg Infect Dis. 2001;7:277–81.

Flynn J, Keogh S, Gavin N. Sterile v aseptic non-touch technique for needle-less connector care on central venous access devices in a bone marrow transplant population: a comparative study. Eur J Oncol Nurs. 2015;19:694–700.

Flynn J, Richard C, Keogh S, Zhang L. Alcohol caps or alcohol with and without chlorhexidine: an in vitro study of 648 episodes of intravenous device needless connector decontamination. Infect Control Hosp Epidemiol. 2017;38(5):617–9.

Gorski L, Hadaway L, Hagle M, McGoldrick M, Orr M, Doellman D. Infusion therapy standards of practice. J Infus Ther. 2016;39:1S.

Health Protection Scotland. Targeted literature review: what are the key infection prevention and control recommendations to inform peripheral vascular catheter (PVC) maintenance care quality improvement tool? 2012.

Holroyd JL, Vasiloppoulos T, Rand K, Fahy B. Incidence of central venous catheter hub contamination. J Crit Care. 2017;39:162–8.

Kelly L, Jones T, Kirkham S. Needlefree devices: keeping the system closed. Br J Nurs. 2017;26(2):S14–9.

Loveday HP, Wilson JA, Pratt RJ, Golsorkhi M, Tingle A, Bak A, Browne J, Prieto J, Wilcox M. Epic3: national evidence–based guidelines for preventing healthcare-associated infections in NHS hospitals. J Hosp Infect. 2014;S86:S1–S70.

Marschall J, Mermel LA, Fakih M, Hadaway L, Kallen A, O'Grady N, Pettis A, Rupp ME, Sandora T, Maragakis LL, Yokoe D. Strategies to prevent central line-associated bloodstream infections in acute care hospitals: 2014 update. Infect Control Hosp Epidemiol. 2014;35(7):753–71. http://digitalcommons.wustl.edu/open_access_pubs/3453

Merrill KC, Sumner S, Linford L, Taylor C, Macintosh C. Impact of universal disinfectant cap implementation on central-line associated bloodstream infections. Am J Infect Control. 2014;42:1274–7.

Moureau NL. Catheter associated bloodstream infection prevention: what is missing? Br J Healthc Manag. 2014;20(11):502–10.

Moureau NL, Flynn J. Disinfection of needless connector hubs: clinical evidence systematic review. Nurs Res Pract. 2015;2015:796762.

O'Grady NP, Alexander M, Burns LA, Dellinger EP, Garland J, Heard SO, Lipsett PA, Masur H, Mermel LA, Pearson ML, Raad II, Randolph AG, Rupp ME,

Saint S, the Healthcare Infection Control Practices Advisory Committee (HICPAC). Guidelines for the prevention of intravascular catheter-related infections. Clin Infect Dis. 2011;52:e162–93.

Queensland Government. Guideline: peripheral intravenous catheter (PIVC). Queensland Government. 2015. https://www.health.qld.gov.au/__data/assets/pdf_file/0025/444490/icare-pivc-guideline.pdf.

Rowley S, Clare S. Improving standards of aseptic practice through ANTT trust-wide implementation process: a matter of prioritisation and care. J Infect Prev. 2009;10(1 Supplement):S18–23.

Royal College of Nursing. Standards for infusion therapy. 4th ed. London: RCN; 2016.

Rupp ME, Yu S, Huerta T, Cavaleri RJ, Alter F, Fey FD, Van Schooneveld T, Anderson JR. Adequate disinfection of a split-septum needleless intravascular connector with a 5-second alcohol scrub. Infect Control Hosp Epidemiol. 2012;33:661–5.

Sandora TJ, Graham DA, Conway M, Dobson B, Potter-Bynoe G, Margossain SP. Impact of needless connector change frequency on central line-associated. Am J Infect Control. 2014;42(5):485–9.

Sweet MA, Cumpston A, Briggs F, Craig M, Harmadini M. Impact of alcohol-impregnated port protectors and needleless neutral pressure connectors on central line-associated bloodstream infections and contamination of blood cultures in an inpatient oncology unit. Am J Infect Control. 2012;40:931–4.

Warren DK, Cosgrove SE, Diekema DJ, Zuccotti G, Climo MW, Bolon MK, Tokars JI, Noskin GA, Wong ES, Sepkowitz KA, Herwaldt LA, Perl TM, Solomon SL, Fraser VJ, Prevention Epicenter Program. A multicentre intervention to prevent catheter-associated bloodstream infections. Infect Control Hosp Epidemiol. 2006;27(7):662–9.

World Health Organisation. A guide to the implementation of the WHO multimodal hand hygiene improvement strategy. 2009. http://apps.who.int/iris/bitstream/10665/70030/1/WHO_IER_PSP_2009.02_eng.pdf.

World Health Organisation. Infection prevention and control of epidemic-and pandemic-prone acute respiratory infections in healthcare. Geneva: WHO; 2014.

Zhang L, Cao S, Marsh N, Ray-Barruel G, Flynn J, Larsen E, Richard CM. Infection risks associated with peripheral vascular catheters. J Infect Prev. 2016;17(5):207–13.

19

Vascular Devices and Flushing

Caroline Cullinane

Abstract

Peripheral and central vascular access devices are a fundamental and essential part of healthcare delivery, used extensively in hospital and community settings to meet the challenging and complex IV therapy requirements of the modern-day patient. For vascular access devices (VAD) to be a safe and effective tool for the administration of IV therapy, they must be reliable. Reliability in this context refers to optimal catheter function, demonstrated by the ease of flushing and aspirating, combined with an absence of associated complications. Proficient care and maintenance of these devices by healthcare professionals requires a high degree of knowledge, skill and understanding. In this section, we explore the details of flushing by examining how, why, when and with what solution vascular devices are to be flushed.

Keywords

Flushing · Flushing technique · Flushing and locking · Flushing solutions · Flushing volume

C. Cullinane (✉)
Health and Social Care (1st Class), Liverpool, UK
e-mail: caroline.cullinane@rlbuht.nhs.uk

19.1 Introduction

Flushing of a VAD is a crucial intervention that facilitates a proactive approach in relation to maintaining catheter patency and function. It also supports complication prevention, surveillance and early escalation to relevant multidisciplinary team (MDT) members when limitations are met. Absent, untimely or ineffective flushing can cause catheter malfunction and result in associated complications such as occlusion, thrombosis and infection, which can increase patient morbidity and mortality (Baskin et al. 2012). Consequences of inadequate flushing could include negative patient outcome and experience, treatment delays, costly thrombolytic therapy, antimicrobial therapy, device removal and reinsertion, increased hospital stay and organisational costs (Mitchell et al. 2009). Maintaining the function of VADS for patients is therefore an essential responsibility that should be carried out by skilled health professionals using the best available scientific evidence (Anderson et al. 2010; Moureau et al. 2013).

19.2 Flushing Rationale

Proper flushing techniques are effective, inexpensive and associated with good clinical practice (Ferroni et al. 2014). National and international guidelines include flushing recommendations in concurrence with manufacturer instructions for use (IFUs) to optimise VAD safety, function and durability, for all patients requiring short- to long-term IV therapy (RCN 2016; Gorski et al. 2016; Lyons 2012; Loveday et al. 2014).

The Royal College of Nursing (2016) advocates flushing to maintain catheter patency and prevent the mixing of incompatible medications that may precipitate and occlude the lumen (Baskin et al. 2012). This endorsement is echoed by the Infusion Standards of Practice (Gorski et al. 2016), which highlight the importance of flushing as a method of assessing catheter function, identifying malfunction and minimising the risk of occlusion, thrombus and catheter-related bloodstream infection (CRBSI).

Ideally, the lumen of a vascular device should flush freely without resistance (Hadaway 2009) and is classed as malfunctioning if flushing and/or aspiration becomes difficult or impossible (Goossens 2016). Sluggish infusion and aspiration are caused by the accumulation of blood, fibrin and/or drug deposits that adhere to the internal surface and the tip of the catheter, leading to total occlusion if not adequately rinsed away (Hadaway 2006b; Dougherty and Lister 2015).

Flushing in the context of rinsing a catheter, can be defined as a manual injection of 0.9% sodium chloride or normal saline (NS) for the purpose of cleaning the internal walls of the lumen (Goossens 2015). Compared to other forms of VAD management, the act of flushing, when performed correctly, represents a key procedure in maintaining patency by preventing occlusion (Royon et al. 2012) and minimising the potential for the adherence of harmful microorganisms that can lead to biofilm formation and catheter related blood stream infection [CRBSI] (Hadaway 2006b, 2009; Goossens 2013).

Flushing a vascular access device using the proper technique, at the right time, and with the correct solution and volume should not be underestimated (Goossens 2015). Flushing of catheters initially appears to be a straightforward concept. However, flushing is much more than just injecting fluid into a catheter lumen (Hadaway 2009); it requires knowledge of flushing techniques and needle-free connectors by the healthcare professional providing the hands-on care (Moureau 2013).

19.3 Flushing and Locking Principles

The basic principles that underpin an effective VAD flushing and locking technique, include adequate rinsing or flushing of the catheter, (Goossens 2015) followed by instillation of a solution lock, that will reside witin the inner lumen. This prevents blood reflux into the tip of the catheter, blood coagulating within the VAD lumen and maintains patency inbetween infusions (Gorski 2016). Locking an approved solution into a VAD, creates a column of fluid inside to help maintain lumen patency (Hadaway 2012). According to NICE (2017) guidelines, a sterile 0.9% sodium chloride injection should be used to flush and lock catheter lumens (NICE CS174, 2017). Antibiotic lock solutions should not be routinely used to prevent CRBSIs (NICE 2017), as low-level exposure of antibiotics may potentially increase the risk of resistance (Justo and Bookstaver 2014).

National guidelines recommend peripheral cannulas are flushed and locked with 0.9% sodium chloride only (Gorski et al. 2016). There is insufficient evidence to suggest heparin-saline solution is more effective than 0.9% sodium chloride, in maintaining lumen patency (Randolph et al. 1998), and heparin is known to cause serious adverse effects in susceptible patients (Alexander 2010). This topic will be discussed in greater depth later in the chapter. Studies have successfully demonstrated that flushing and locking technique is considered more important than the solution used, to adaquately clean and prevent blood reflux into the catheter, when maintaining VADs and to prevent VAD associated infection (Ferroni et al. 2014, Guiffant et al. 2012).

Central venous access devices (CVADs) can be locked with various solutions ranging from 0.9% sodium chloride, anticoagulation therapy (Heparin/hepsal) and thrombolytic therapy (urokinase/alteplase) to antibiotic treatment (Hadaway 2006a). The lock objective is to maintain lumen patency, restrict blood reflux and, depending on the solution instilled, prevent thrombus or fibrin formation in or around the catheter tip. Locking can also be used to break down an existing clot or treat an infection by penetrating and breaking apart any existing intraluminal biofilm (Goossens 2015).

19.4 Optimal Flushing

A combination of two flushing methods is recommended to facilitate effective VAD rinsing and locking objectives: use of a pulsatile flushing technique and the application of positive pressure at the end of the flush (RCN 2016). These methods are directly associated with specific flow dynamics, which impact the quality of the flush in terms of achieving the desired effect (Goossens 2015). Most non-infective VAD-associated complications can be minimised and even prevented by strict adherence to standardised flushing protocols (Pittiruti et al. 2009).

A pulsatile flush involves a rapid stop-start or push-pause technique as the solution is injected into the catheter. Studies have shown that the resulting turbulent flow created by the push-pause technique is considerably more effective at rinsing the lumen, in comparison to a continuous laminar flow (Vigier et al. 2005; Guiffant et al. 2012). This technique has also been found to significantly reduce catheter, bacterial attachment and growth in VADs, in comparison to a continuous flushing method without the turbulence (Ferroni et al. 2014). In addition, a time interval of 0.4 s between two boluses is a critical factor, to optimise effective flushing (Guiffant et al. 2012). These studies are suggestive that a manual pulsatile, positive pressure flush of 10 mL is administered immediately before and after any IV infusion.

Hydrodynamics coupled with an intermittent flushing method is an important contributing factor that effectively removes proteins and other adhering substances from the endoluminal wall of a vascular device (Ferroni et al. 2014). Pulsatile flushing must therefore be considered a key strategy in occlusion and infection prevention, as clearing the catheter lumen of all traces of blood and medications can reduce the potential for bacterial adhesion and colonisation, leading to CRBSI (Ferroni et al. 2014; Moureau 2013). VAD-associated infection is increasingly being regarded as a measure for quality of care within healthcare settings (Bodenham et al. 2016). There is currently zero tolerance for VAD-associated infections within health care organisations, as they are considered a preventable complication if the correct infection prevention techniques are adhered to.

19.5 Flushing Technology

In addition to good technique, effective flushing is enhanced by specifically designed technology and an understanding of how effective technology and flushing work together (Hadaway 2006b). Understanding is critical because optimum flush outcome relies heavily upon the knowledge and skills of the healthcare worker to perform the correct technique, whilst considering the assisting technology design and function (Goossens 2015). Evidence demonstrates that adequately trained and educated health professionals who adhere to practice guidelines when accessing and flushing VADS achieve the best patient outcomes (Moureau 2013). This knowledge must extend to the variety of medical devices available that aid flushing and optimisation of VAD management, such as integrated catheter valves, pre-filled syringes and neutral or positive displacement needle-free connectors (Goossens 2015). These innovations along with evidence-based clinical practices have led to advances in vascular access, improved safety and reduced complication rates (Krzywda and Andris 2005).

19.6 Pre-filled Syringes

One of the technological answers to help eliminate the 'rebound' problem and inadvertent blood reflux is to use a commercially prepared syringe, pre-filled with 0.9% sodium chloride (Fig. 19.1) (Hadaway 2009). Pre-filled syringes have a plunger rod design to maintain application of positive pressure whilst flushing (Goossens 2015). Pre-filled syringe flush volumes are available in 3, 5 and 10 mL options for various VAD type, length and size. The smaller volume pre-filled syringes are produced in diameters and dimensions consistent with a 10 mL syringe barrel (Keogh et al. 2016), generating significantly less pressure (Gorski et al. 2016) than standard 5 and 3 mL syringes. Flushing vascular access

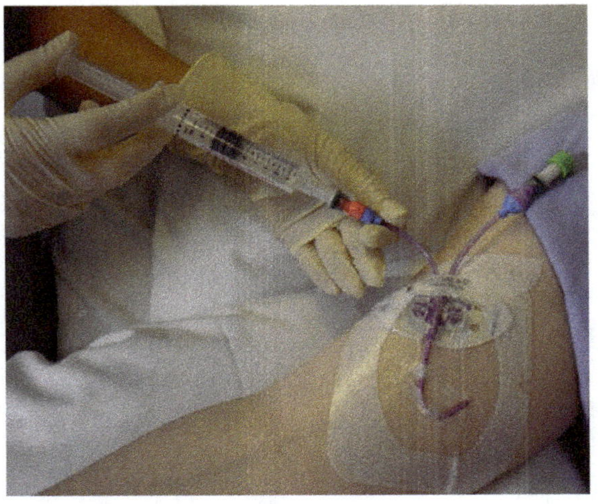

Fig. 19.1 Saline flushing with 10 mL pre-filled syringe (Used with permission of the Royal Liverpool University Hospital)

devices incorrectly, by exerting high pressures with smaller syringes than the manufacturer's recommendations, suggests that it may contribute to catheter rupture, especially if resistance is met on flushing the device (Bishop et al. 2007; Pittiruti et al. 2009; Goossens 2015; Hadaway 2006b; Miyagaki 2012). Pre-filled syringes are recommended for use in relevant guidelines (Gorski et al. 2016; RCN 2016) as they aid optimal flush objectives, by promoting zero blood reflux, reduce the amount of pressure exerted against the inner catheter wall and minimise vein injury (Keogh et al. 2016).

Silicone VADS such as non-powered peripherally inserted catheters (PICCS) and tunnelled central venous catheters are more prone to fracture than polyurethane devices that have superior strength and are power-injectable (Ong and Sudhakar 2010; Goossens 2015). Consequently, an increasing number of VADS, particularly peripherally inserted central catheters (PICCS) and totally implantable venous access devices (TIVADS), are using improved polyurethane, able to withstand higher pressures. This calls into question the strict use of 10 mL diameter standard syringes for flushing, which may eventually become redundant if VAD materials can withstand the high pressure of power injection (Goossens 2015). Currently, however, the RCN (2016) infusion guidelines and manufacturer's instructions for use continue to recommend a 10 mL syringe option to flush vascular access devices, including for use with powered devices.

A manual, positive pressure technique required for use with a standard syringe may not be necessary when flushing with pre-filled syringes designed to reduce syringe plunger reflux. The innovative design prohibits the rod plunger from rebounding at the end of the flush, allowing for total emptying of the solution from the barrel prior to disconnection (Data on file Excelsior Medical, LLC http://swabflush.excelsiormedical.com/zr-flush-syringes/). However, removal of the syringe tip from the needle free connector prior to clamping, will cause reflux related to tip volume displacement (Hadaway 2006b).

19.7 Positive Pressure Flushing

A correct, positive pressure technique when using a standard 10mL syringe, requires a constant, even force on the syringe plunger during flushing, to create an effective means of preventing backflow of blood or reflux into the catheter tip (Gorski et al. 2016; Goossens 2015). This form of flushing is recommended in combination with a pulsatile technique for maximum efficiency (RCN 2016), which depends more on technical practice than the flushing solution used (Royon et al. 2012; Pittiruti et al. 2009). Ineffective positive pressure results in a rebound effect that pulls blood into the catheter tip as the syringe is detached from the hub, also known as reflux (Hadaway 2009). This problem can be overcome by maintaining the forward positive flow of solution as the syringe is removed towards the end of the flush (0.5–1 mL remaining) whilst simultaneously applying pressure to the plunger (Bishop et al. 2007; Goossens 2015). This technique often results in an external spray of fluid (Hadaway 2009) indicating positive pressure has been applied correctly. This method can also be applied successfully by clamping the catheter just prior to injecting the last 1 mL of flushing solution, if external clamps are present (Goossens 2015). It is necessary to fasten external clamps when the catheter is not in use to prevent backflow of blood into the lumen.

When recommended by the manufacturer, implanted ports or non-valved, open ended catheter lumens should be flushed and locked with heparin sodium flush solutions. Positioning the Huber needle bevel towards the port body catheter connection increases flush efficacy within the port (Guiffant et al. 2012). Application of positive pressure (achieved by the injection of additional solution) during Huber needle withdrawal reduced the incidence of reflux by nearly 80% (Lapalu 2010). This study demonstrates the value of positive pressure to port patency and complication reduction and supports the use of applying positive pressure during port needle removal.

An experimental study designed to quantify the impact of positive pressure application during an implantable port needle removal has demonstrated statistically significant results, depending on whether or not positive pressure was used during the removal process (Lapalu 2010). The studies findings report the creation of negative pressure on the port septum during Huber needle removal when positive pressure was not applied. This negative pressure was found to cause a suction effect resulting in an upward movement of the septum at the distal catheter tip, followed by an unwanted influx of blood.

19.8 Blood Reflux

Despite optimal flushing and locking techniques, there are external influences that displace the internal locking volume causing blood to reflux into the catheter. Body or muscle movements, intrathoracic pressure changes caused by coughing or vomiting, arm abduction or adduction, application of blood pressure cuff, catheter mechanical changes of clamping and unclamping, syringe plunger rebound in certain syringes after flushing and connection and disconnection of syringes or needle free connectors, all cause pressure changes within a catheter that may pull blood into the catheter tip (Goossens 2015; Hadaway and Richardson 2010). Neutral or anti-reflux needle free connector technology should theoretically prevent blood reflux from occurring; however, it is suggested by Hadaway and Richardson (2010) that up to 0.02 mL of blood can still be drawn into the catheter tip depending on theneedle free connector design and clamping sequence followed by clinicians (Hadaway and Richardson 2010). Unwanted reflux volumes have also been demonstrated by other researchers (Elli et al. 2016; Hull et al. 2018). It is therefore rational to conclude that proper flushing techniques can only guarantee the prevention of blood reflux into the catheter tip at the very instant the catheter is being locked (Goossens 2015).

Different types of needle free connectors (positive, negative, neutral and anti-reflux), each with a recommended clamping sequence, create confusion among clinical users. Blood reflux occurs when needle free connectors are used with improper clamping sequences. This suggests a timely, manual flush with the correct technique or pre-filled syringe is advisable immediately post disconnection with an appropriate clamping sequence to follow. Without clamping or an anti-reflux valve, the flushing may provide a short-term solution to compensate for backflow of blood, which may later lead to patency problems and potentially other associated complications (Hadaway 2006b). Timely and efficient flushing of VADS using the correct technique for clamping and flushing the needle free connector is therefore critically important to ensure optimal removal of blood or other medications or infusions (Ferroni et al. 2014).

Investigative in vitro (Agharazii et al. 2005; Polaschegg and Shaht 2003; Sungur et al. 2007; Polaschegg 2005) and in vivo (Markota et al. 2009; Barbour et al. 2015) studies have demonstrated significant early- and late-stage leakage of locking solution into the systemic circulation during and after the administration process. The most significant losses occur during lock instillation (Agharazii et al. 2005; Markota et al. 2009; Polaschegg and Shaht 2003; Sungur et al. 2007; Barbour et al. 2015) which can account for up to 25–30% of the total lock volume (Barbour et al. 2015). Depending on fluid dynamics and catheter compliance and speed of instillation during the locking process, the lock volume and concentration at the catheter tip can be greatly reduced and replaced by an unwanted reflux of blood (Polaschegg and Shaht 2003).

Instillation leakage is a result of inertia due to flow velocity, that develops inside the catheter lumen as it is filled, transporting the locked solution out into the systemic circulation (Barbour et al. 2015), and is associated with the rate (or propulsion) at which administration occurs (Barbour et al. 2015; Agharazii et al. 2005). An in vitro study comparing a lock injection time of 2–3 and 23 s found this to have negligible influences upon the dynamics of the loss (Polaschegg 2005). Contrary to these findings, a subsequent in vivo study recommends a slower rate of lock instillation, as it may result in less initial leakage and should therefore be considered (Barbour et al. 2015).

In vitro studies use static flow and environmental conditions to study lock leakage rates; however, these models do not consider the numerous parameters that can affect the catheter leakage in vivo (Markota et al. 2009). Contrastingly, in vivo studies use experimental models of the SVC that mimic its internal, rhythmical flows that follow each heartbeat (Agharazii et al. 2005). In vivo experiments are thought to produce more accurate data as they simulate realistic, physiological conditions; however, they do have their limitations (Barbour et al. 2015; Markota et al. 2009).

Regardless of the care taken to instill a locking solution, both types of studies have demonstrated a secondary, more gradual leakage of the locked volume that occurs because of convective and diffusive transport (Barbour et al. 2015; Markota et al. 2009). In vitro studies have demonstrated secondary losses as high as 70–80%. However, this is not consistent with more reliable in vivo reports which show much smaller losses of 2% loss over a 24-h period, which are attributed to the low diffusivity of the lock solution (Barbour et al. 2015). Convective fluxes within the pulsatile, dynamic environment of the SVC surround the catheter and act to rapidly deplete the near-tip lock concentration. Diffusive fluxes draw more locking solution from the internal lumen back into the near-tip region, only to be transported immediately away by blood-driven convective currents (Barbour et al. 2015).

CVADs with distal side holes situated at the catheter tip (found on dialysis, apheresis and non-tunnelled catheters) are potentially more susceptible to convective fluxes than CVADs without side holes (Barbour et al. 2015). An in vivo study conducted by Markota et al. (2009) concludes that early and late leakages are significantly higher in non-tunnelled catheters compared to tunnelled catheters ($p = 0.05$) that do not have proximately situated holes (Markota et al. 2009). Catheters without side holes are likely to be less susceptible to convective fluxes and therefore more conducive to maintaining lock concentration (Barbour et al. 2015). Data collected from these studies have contributed to a greater understanding of lock depletion in and around the central venous catheter tip (Markota et al. 2009); however, more research is needed in this area.

19.9 Needle-Free Connectors

Since their introduction in the early 1990s, needle-free connectors (NFCs) have successfully achieved their original purpose of minimising the risk of needle stick injury posed to healthcare providers accessing vascular devices (Hadaway 2012; Moureau and Flynn 2015). This technology is now commonly used to facilitate needle-free connection between catheters, administration sets and syringes (Jarvis 2010), creating a closed system between the internal vasculature and the external environment, via a Luer connection to the catheter hub (Moureau and Flynn 2015).

Despite achieving the original objective, many published studies have raised concerns regarding an association between NFCs and increased risk of CRBSI and catheter occlusion (Hadaway 2012; Ryder 2010; Field 2007; Jarvis et al. 2009; Marschall et al. 2014). This association of increased risk of CRBSI with positive pressure NFCs (Ryder 2010) has prevented them from being actively recommended in certain guidelines (Pittiruti et al. 2009). Studies have demonstrated that during disconnection of a syringe or intravenous tubing from the NFC, pressure

Table 19.1 Needle-free connector displacement functions (Hull et al. 2018)

Types of NFCs	Negative displacement NFC	Neutral displacement NFC	Anti-reflux NFC	Positive displacement NFC
Fluid movement upon disconnection	Blood refluxes into the catheter	Blood refluxes into the catheter	Fluid restricted by diaphragm	Fluids moves towards patient
Fluid movement upon connection	Fluid moves towards patient	Fluid moves towards patient	Fluid restricted by diaphragm	Blood refluxes into catheter
Manufacturer recommended clamping sequence	Clamp before disconnection	No specified clamping	No specified clamping	Clamp after disconnection

changes within the catheter cause varying degrees of fluid movement or displacement resulting in unwanted blood reflux into the catheter tip (Hull 2018; Elli et al. 2016). Improving clinical outcomes for patients by reducing complications such as CRBSI and VAD occlusion has propelled modern NFC design to incorporate an internal mechanism that reduces fluid displacement within the intravascular device (Kelly et al. 2017; Hadaway 2012). Used correctly, NFCs are of great benefit to assist in the successful care and maintenance of VADs; however, they are only as safe and reliable as the individuals that use them (Hanchet 2005).

Confusingly there are four different types of NFC. Each has a complex mechanical valve design and are marketed as either negative, neutral, positive displacement or anti-reflux depending on the characteristics of the internal mechanism and action of fluid displacement upon connection and disconnection from a syringe or tubing (Btaiche et al. 2011; Elli et al. 2016; Hull et al. 2018). Hull et al. (2018) have published a clear and concise summary (Table 19.1), revealing the details associated with different fluid displacement mechanisms and recommended clamping sequence for each type of NFC.

Optimal management of NFCs depends upon an understanding of the type of NFC, the internal membrane and valve function and method of recommended flushing and clamping for each. INS (2016) acknowledge the sequence for flushing depends on the particular NFC used and warns of the potential for confusion and inconsistency within healthcare workers who are not aware of the differences (Gorski et al. 2016; Hadaway 2012; Kelly et al. 2017). Lack of knowledge, skill and understanding can result in VAD mismanagement, leading to an increased risk of reflux and VAD-associated complications (Kelly et al. 2017). Applying the same management to all NFCs can result in an increased occlusion rate due to blood reflux after flushing (Elli et al. 2016). There is still much debate within the literature regarding the most effective NFC design and therefore a need for further research into the area of reflux, valves, NFC and the impact they have on device function (Kelly et al. 2017; Jarvis 2010). It is therefore recommended that healthcare organisations standardise the choice of NFC to one brand/style of needless connector, to help employees understand design characteristics and maximise proficiency in use (Jarvis 2010; Hadaway 2012). Used correctly, NFCs are of great benefit, functioning as a closed system to assist in the care and maintenance of VADS and are one of the main contributors to catheter patency (Elli et al. 2016). Proper care, maintenance and management of NFCs enhance patient safety and the durability of vascular access devices (Kelly et al. 2017).

19.9.1 Negative Displacement Connectors

A negative displacement connector is designed to allow a two-way flow of fluid for infusion and aspiration and will permit blood reflux into the catheter during connection and disconnection, including when the administration set, or syringe is attached and detached (Hadaway and Richardson 2010). This is caused by movement of the inner valve mechanism (Hadaway 2012) and is a potential contributing factor of thrombotic occlusion (Btaiche et al. 2011) and biofilm formation (Jarvis 2010) if a proper flushing technique or clamping sequence is absent or ineffective post disconnection from the hub (Hadaway and Richardson 2010).

19.9.2 Positive Displacement Connectors

Positive needle-free connectors are designed to compensate for an ineffective or absent flush (Hadaway 2006b). User knowledge and understanding is vital if complications are to be avoided with this type of NFC design (Hadaway and Richardson 2010). The internal mechanical valve has a fluid reservoir for withholding a small amount of solution, which is passively expelled upon disconnection, preventing a residual flow of blood into the lumen (Btaiche et al. 2011). The resulting positive displacement can only occur after disconnection has taken place (Btaiche et al. 2011). If disconnection fails to happen, negative pressure is created within the system followed by an influx of blood into the catheter lumen (Hadaway and Richardson 2010). This is a major contributing factor of preventable VAD occlusion and can happen regardless of NFC used. A time delay following disconnection is recommended by manufacturers to facilitate the positive fluid displacement effect (Hadaway 2006b).

19.9.3 Neutral Displacement Connector

A neutral displacement mechanism is designed to work by inhibiting movement of solution in either direction when connecting to and disconnecting from the device, preventing fluid displacement into the catheter lumen (Btaiche et al. 2011). A study comparing neutral with positive needle-free connectors demonstrated improved occlusion rates (26%) with the neutral connector option, but failed to show any difference in rates of infection. Findings were not statistically significant, but staff satisfaction was higher with the neutral device resulting in its implementation throughout the healthcare organisation (Logan 2013).

19.9.4 Anti-reflux Connectors

Anti-reflux NFC entered the market following concerns over increased infection and occlusion caused by NFC use (Jarvis et al. 2009; Macklin 2014). The design of the anti-reflux NFC is based on a pressure-sensitive valve that allows opening for infusion when pressure increases, closes when pressure drops or not in use and inverts when negative pressure is applied (Hull 2017; Elli et al. 2016). Jasinsky and Wuester (2009) demonstrated statistical significance with the reduction of occlusion of CVADs from 30% to 7.6% with use of an anti-reflux NFC; later the study was expanded to include peripheral intravenous catheters, resulting in lower phlebitis rates and longer dwell times (Jasinsky and Wuerster 2009).

Recent studies have found anti-reflux connectors are having a positive impact in maintaining patency and reducing occlusion rates and catheter malfunction (Jazinsky and Wuerster 2009, Elli et al. 2016, Hull 2018, County Durham and Darlington NHS Foundation trust). A quantitative, in vitro study conducted by Hull et al. (2018) demonstrates minimal fluid movement upon connection and disconnection of anti-reflux NFCs and suggests these devices should be considered for incorporation into clinical practice (Hull 2018). The study adds that more research is needed in this area.

19.10 Integrated Catheter Valves

Catheters which have an integrated valve were originally designed to maintain lumen patency and reduce catheter occlusion rates, by preventing retrograde blood flow (Hoffer et al. 1999, 2001). Multiple designs of these valves exist and are located at the distal or proximal end of the catheter (Gorski et al. 2016). Integral valves function as an automatic clamp (Hoffer et al. 1999), locking the instilled solution and theoretically minimising blood reflux into the catheter tip (Carlo et al. 2004). The recommended locking solution for valved devices is 0.9% sodium chloride (Gorski et al. 2016).

19.10.1 Other Factors Affecting Blood Reflux

Neutral or anti-reflux NFCs, non-rebounding syringes and other assisting technologies like integrated catheter valves are currently recommended, alongside timely effective flushing techniques and health professional knowledge, in national and international guidelines, to assist in VAD maintenance, facilitating optimal removal of blood or other intraluminal debris from medications and infusions (Ferroni et al. 2014). To maximise catheter lumen patency, neither technique nor technology can stand alone (Hadaway 2006b). Guidelines also always suggest adherence to local policy and manufacturer's instructions for use (RCN 2016; Lyons 2012; EPIC 3 2014; ESPEN 2009; Gorski et al. 2016). Short peripheral catheters, extended dwell catheters, midlines and PICCs may be particularly affected by blood reflux due to small lumen size and greater surface area.

19.11 Flushing and Locking Volumes

19.11.1 Flushing Volumes

The intraluminal volume capacity and required flushing volumes for venous catheters can vary considerably depending on the patient group, type of catheter, nature and type of infusion or medication used (RCN 2016). Flushing should continue until all blood, fluid and medication residue is cleared (Moureau 2013), and a larger volume may be required post blood sampling or post blood transfusion procedures (Gorski et al. 2016). Blood or medication residue can lead to partial or complete occlusion, which is linked to blood stream infection, as microorganisms introduced into the catheter over time develop into a biofilm-fibrin combination (Hadaway 2009). Adherence to evidence-based infection control practices (evidence-based hand washing standards and proficient ANTT) combined with effective flushing and locking techniques can sustain VAD patency and reduce complication risk such as CRBSI (Moureau 2013; Gorski et al. 2016).

Current guidelines suggest the quantity of solution needed to adequately flush a lumen should be equal to twice the internal volume of the catheter system, which includes the catheter extension set and/or needle-free injection system added to the catheter hub (Gorski et al. 2016; RCN 2016). This translates into 3–5 mL for a peripheral intravenous cannula (Keogh et al. 2016) and 10 mL for a central venous catheter (Bishop et al. 2007), increasing to 20 mL post blood sampling or when rinsing vesicant medications from CVADs (Goossens 2015; Guiffant et al. 2012). These volumes far exceed twice the internal volume (Goossens 2015) recommended in the INS (2016) and RCN guidelines (2016); however, this excess should guarantee sufficient rinsing of the lumen, especially for longer central venous catheters, and TIVADS in particular, that can accumulate debris or sludge in the port reservoir if inadequately flushed (Goossens 2015).

19.11.2 Locking Volumes

Locking refers to the installation of fluid into a catheter lumen after the completion of the last flush (Gorski et al. 2016) to maintain patency between infusions and/or reduce the risk of CRBSI (Gorski 2016). Types of locking solutions include saline, heparin, antibiotics, thrombolytics, citrate, ethanol and bicarbonate solutions. Catheter manufacturers specify precise intraluminal volume to assist the healthcare provider to instill the amount of lock solution required and reduce the risk of overspill into the patient's circulation (Polaschegg and Shaht 2003). Physiologic solutions, such as saline, are used as both flushing and locking solutions with the volume dictated by the judgement of the clinician. It is recommended that organisational locking policies and practice guidelines be in accordance with manufacturer's instructions for use and guidelines (Gorski et al. 2016).

Caution must be taken with lock solutions that can potentially cause adverse effects if excess amounts spill into the systemic circulation

(Polaschegg and Shaht 2003). Some thrombolytic agents used to restore catheter patency by resolving thrombotic occlusion (Cummings-Winfield and Mushani 2008) may be particularly dangerous (Bunce 2003). The most serious adverse reactions to this type of drug in clinical trials include sepsis, gastrointestinal bleeding and thromboembolism (Bunce 2003). Other thrombolytic agents indicated for clearance of catheter occlusions have demonstrated safety and efficacy when used according to the labelling instructions (Baskin et al. 2009; Deitcher et al. 2002; Ponec et al. 2001; Semba et al. 2002).

The Lyons guidelines (2012) advocate the use of the thrombolytic drug, human urokinase (10,000 U/mL), reconstituted with 4 mL 0.9% saline, using 2 mL of this solution to lock each lumen (Bishop et al. 2007). This recommendation is to ensure that the intraluminal volume or internal space only is filled (Bishop et al. 2007). Insufficient locking volumes or underfilling can have negative clinical implications, especially if the prescribed treatment or prophylactic dose is depleted further during the instillation process and again due to convective losses post administration (Barbour et al. 2015).

As mentioned previously in this chapter, in vitro and in vivo studies have demonstrated significant lock leakage from the distal catheter tip of central venous catheters during administration and then gradually over time (Agharazii et al. 2005; Markota et al. 2009; Polaschegg and Shaht 2003; Polaschegg 2005; Sungur et al. 2007; Barbour et al. 2015). Locking volumes need to be enough to fill the entire catheter plus any add-ons (Goossens 2015) and surround the external near-tip region for maximum effectiveness (Barbour et al. 2015).

To compensate for any leakage from the instilled lock over time, it is suggested that catheters should be overfilled by approximately 15–20%, plus up to 1 mL for any add-ons (Goossens 2015). However, this excess can only be recommended for physiologic locking solutions and not solutions with medications or substances that may cause adverse effects (Polaschegg and Shaht 2003; Polaschegg 2005; Goossens 2015).

Table 19.1 below provides guidance for lock solutions that do not cause adverse effects when injected into the bloodstream.

19.12 Frequency of Flushing

The expert consensus to date is that flushing should be carried out immediately before, in-between and immediately after the administration of IV medications (RCN 2016; Gorski et al. 2016). This allows the practitioner to confirm catheter patency and function prior to use, prevent the mixing of potentially incompatible infusions and clear the lumen of any residue that may lead to associated complication (Gorski et al. 2016). CVADS that are not in frequent use should be flushed and locked weekly, with the exception of implantable ports that require monthly maintenance (Bishop et al. 2007).

Similar to flush volumes, there are limited studies that evaluate the effect of flush frequency on patient outcomes (Keogh et al. 2016). A randomised control trial (RCT) published by Keogh et al. (2016) is one of the first RCTs to evaluate the impact of different flushing volumes and frequencies on peripheral intravenous catheter (PIVC) outcomes in adult patients. This research was conducted in response to a growing concern of high cannula failure rates and variations in flushing practice. Patients were randomised to one of four flushing groups, to receive a manually prepared 0.9% sodium chloride flush of 10 or 3 mL every 24 or 6 h. Results found that neither flushing volumes nor frequencies or their interaction together was significantly associated with cannula failure. Interestingly, however, cannula malfunction was demonstrated as being significantly associated with increased episodes of access. As a small pilot study, the author calls for larger, more definitive trials to provide more substantial data on the effect of flushing volume and flushing frequency on PIVC outcome (Keogh et al. 2016).

The following acronyms have been developed to assist healthcare professionals follow the correct flushing and locking regimes:

SAS flushing recommendation (post IV medication/IV fluids)

Saline (pre-flush)	0.9% sodium chloride
Administration of IV therapy	Medication or fluids
Saline (post-flush)	0.9% sodium chloride

SBS flushing recommendation (post blood sampling or blood product transfusions)

Saline (pre-flush)	0.9% sodium chloride
Blood sampling/blood product transfusion	Blood withdrawal or administration[a]
Saline (post-flush)	0.9% sodium chloride

[a]A 10–20 mL flush post blood transfusion is necessary because fibrin will develop with prolonged contact or blood reflux into the catheter and adhere onto the internal catheter wall (Goossens 2015)

SASH/SBSH flushing recommendation for implantable ports and open-ended central venous catheters (if recommended in the manufacturers instructions for use)

Saline (pre-flush)	0.9% sodium chloride
Administration of IV therapy	Medication or fluids
Saline (post-flush)	0.9% sodium chloride
Heparin lock	This varies depending on patient population, local policy and protocol and manufacturers information for use
OR	
Saline (pre-flush)	0.9% sodium chloride
Blood transfusion/ blood sampling	Blood withdrawal or administration
Saline (post-flush)	0.9% sodium chloride
Heparin lock	This varies depending on patient population, local policy and protocol and manufacturers information for use

Flushing and locking recommendations 'based on research and insights' have been summarised in a review article by Goossens (2015) (Tables 19.2 and 19.3):

19.13 Blood Return

Flushing techniques cannot be thoroughly discussed without mentioning the importance of a blood return check prior to the administration of IV therapy via a CVAD. The absence of a blood return should result in an investigation and evaluation of potential causes (Gorski et al. 2016).

Blood return check does not apply to peripheral catheters as their correct position within the vein is assessed according to ease of flush and absence of signs that indicate tissue infiltration, inflammation or blockage (Loveday et al. 2014). Blood return check is relevant when a peripheral cannula is newly inserted; if patency cannot be established, it may be necessary to remove the device (Gorski et al. 2016).

Obtaining a brisk blood return on aspiration prior to administering IV therapy via a central venous catheter is a vital safety measure, recommended in relevant guidelines, to verify optimum function and catheter tip position within the SVC

Table 19.2 Flushing and locking recommendations (Goossens 2015)

Technique	Use a pulsatile flow when flushing Use a 10 mL flush with 10 × 1 mL boluses with a time interval of 0.4 s between 2 boluses Use SAS and SBS order for the administration of medication/fluids and blood sampling
Volume	Use a 10 mL flush for all IV catheters (except peripheral cannulas, use 5 mL) Use a 20 mL flush after infusion of viscous products like blood components, parenteral nutrition and contrast media
Regimen	Flush with NS before and after administration of drugs and fluids (SAS) Flush with NS before and after blood sampling (SBS)

Table 19.3 Locking recommendations (Goossens 2015)

Technique	Use the positive pressure technique when disconnecting a syringe Close clamps and keep them closed when not in use
Volume	1.0 for peripheral cannulas 1.5 for midlines, PICCS, non-tunnelled CVADs and small-bore tunnelled catheters (<1 mm ID) 2.5 mL for large bore tunnelled catheters (>1 mm ID) and ports (reservoir volume up to 0.6 mL, Huber needle volume not included)
Regimen	q8h–q24h for short-term catheters Weekly in long-term catheters q6w–q8w in ports

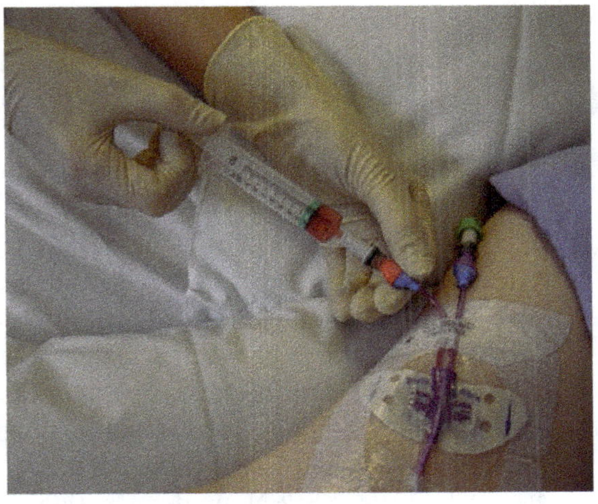

Fig. 19.2 Blood return aspiration and verification from PICC (Used with permission of the Royal Liverpool University Hospital)

(Fig. 19.2) (Gorski et al. 2016; RCN 2016; ESPEN 2009; Lyons 2012). The absence of blood return should prompt an attempt to flush the device (RCN 2016), and if this fails, action must be taken to investigate the potential root cause (RCN 2016; Gorski et al. 2016).

Absence of blood return on aspiration is more commonly due to thrombotic causes (Gorski 2016) such as fibrin sheath or tail formation (Pittiruti et al. 2009; Gabriel 2013). Fibrin is derived from fibroblastic tissue that gradually covers the intra- and extra-luminal surfaces of venous catheters and is associated with persistent withdrawal occlusion (ease of flushing but unable to withdraw blood) and occlusion (Pittiruti et al. 2009). Other potential causes can be attributed to the catheter tip abutting against the wall of the SVC, more common in left-sided placements (Rolden and Paniagua 2015), migration (Gabirel 2013; Bishop et al. 2007) and catheter tip malposition (Rolden and Paniagua 2015).

Undiagnosed CVAD malposition poses a serious but preventable risk to patient safety (Rolden and Paniagua 2015; Goossens 2016). Associated complications range from life-threatening, such as cardiac tamponade and intrathoracic infiltration (Gorski et al. 2016), to a debilitating thrombus or progressive tissue damage (Sauerland 2005). In addition to conventional radiography to confirm or rule out malpositioning, assessment and investigation into catheter dysfunction is a strongly recommended safety measure within the current literature to maximise patient outcome (Gorski et al. 2016; Goossens 2013, 2016; Rolden and Paniagua 2015; Pikwer et al. 2008; Bishop et al. 2007; Hackert et al. 2005). Ongoing re-evaluation of CVAD function (ease of flushing and aspirating) can assist early identification of malposition and may prevent serious, CVAD-related complications (Goossens 2016). For example, absent blood return on aspiration is frequently documented in published case studies as a warning sign (Rolden and Paniagua 2015) and an important clue into the identification of catheter tip malposition, or a misplaced/dislodged Huber needle. These situations can result in serious safety implications for patients (Goossens 2013; Hackert et al. 2005; Pereira et al. 2013; Breitling 2010).

Pereira et al. (2013) presents two cases of malpositioned CVADs whereby the only clinical feature that indicated a problem was the absence of free flowing blood return. The case studies conclude that this safety check should not be undervalued (Pereira et al. 2013). Blood return check is not 100% infallible, as demonstrated by two case studies that report CVAD malposition despite successful aspiration of blood return (Losert et al. 2000; Klockgether-Radke and Gaus 2004). Interestingly, the authors continue to advocate periodic checking of CVAD function before every infusion of fluid or drugs due to the rare and unusual nature of the case circumstances (Losert et al. 2000).

These case studies demonstrate that no one, preventive measure alone, should be relied upon to diagnose malposition. The Infusion Nursing Standards of Practice Guidelines (2016) and the RCN 2016) strongly recommend that health professionals assess catheter function prior to use and advise investigation into potential malposition for CVADs that fail a blood return check. The absence of blood return may provide an invaluable sign, that can alert the clinician in the diagnosis of CVAD malposition. This may prompt other investigative measures such as the use of radio-contrast, as reported in a case by Breitling (2010), where serious patient harm was avoided. The consensus amongst experts is that a malpositioned catheter should be repositioned or removed and replaced as a priority (Rolden and Paniagua 2015; Gorski et al. 2016).

19.14 Flushing and Locking Solutions: Heparin Versus Saline

The use of heparinised solution to maintain CVAD function has been an accepted practice for decades (Anderson et al. 2010) despite the lack of definitive, high-quality evidence to support its continued use (Lopez-Britz et al. 2014; Hadaway 2006a). More emphasis is being placed on risk associated with heparin use from contamination issues or other disorders, and newer guidelines are reflecting the change to saline only, with elimination of heparin as a flushing agent for general use (Gorji et al. 2015). Heparin can result in serious side effects (Lopez-Britz et al. 2014) such as heparin-induced thrombocytopenia (HIT), heparin-induced thrombosis and thrombocytopenia syndrome (HITTS), allergic reaction, drug incompatibility and possible iatrogenic haemorrhage (Jonker 2010). Despite heparin-induced disorders being uncommon (Anderson et al. 2010), it has been estimated that they can develop in up to 30% of patients with the possibility of occurrence 40 days after the cessation of heparin (Gorji et al. 2015). Even small concentrations of heparin can induce HIT in susceptible patients (Musliamani 2007), often with serious and life-threatening consequences (Anderson et al. 2010).

Given potential safety concerns with the use of heparin, 0.9% sodium chloride may be the preferred flushing and locking solution for short-term CVAD maintenance (RCN 2016; Loveday et al. 2014; NICE 2012). There is a growing body of evidence to suggest that flushing with 0.9% saline is equally as effective in preserving catheter patency (Pittiruti et al. 2009; Mitchell et al. 2009; Anderson et al. 2010; Jonker 2010; Shallom 2012; Lopez-Britz et al. 2014; NICE 2015; Gorji et al. 2015; Hoffer et al. 1999). Current guidelines recommend that short peripheral catheters be locked with preservative-free 0.9% sodium chloride following each catheter use in adults and children (Gorski et al. 2016). The ESPEN guidelines (2009) advocate sterile sodium chloride to flush and lock CVAD catheter lumens that are in frequent use for administration of parenteral nutrition (PN), warning that heparin may facilitate the precipitation of lipids within the catheter lumen (Pittiruti et al. 2009).

The current evidence reported in the literature is of poor to moderate quality (Lopez-Britz 2014); however, the most recent study by Gorji et al. (2015) is a high-quality double-blind RCT with a moderate cohort of 84 patients who were randomly assigned to two groups, to receive either heparin saline (3 mL) or 0.9% saline (10 mL). Results are consistent with an earlier, similar trial by Shallom (2012) demonstrating that heparinised saline did not have a statistically significant effect on improved patency and survival of CVADs compared with 0.9% sodium chloride (Gorji et al. 2015). More RCTs are needed to ensure National and International guidelines can be developed based on the best available scientific evidence (Anderson et al. 2010) to help organisations ensure the best possible experience and outcomes for patients.

A recent Cochrane Report (2014) comparing heparin with 0.9% saline flushes to prevent CVAD occlusion in adults analysed six studies with a combined total of 1433 participants. This systematic review found no compelling evidence to suggest that heparinised solutions were more effective than saline in reducing CVAD occlusion or associated complications such as thrombosis or infection (Lopez-Britz et al. 2014). The implications for practice section of the review acknowledge that heparin flushing and locking are currently a recommended practice in many guidelines and clinical settings. Lack of conclusive evidence combined with higher cost and potential side effects resulted in heparin not being recommended for use (Lopez-Britz et al. 2014).

NICE guidelines (2017) have developed this Cochrane Quality and Productivity topic and support its view that there is insufficient evidence to support heparin-based flushes. Recommendations are made to flush and lock CVAD catheter lumens with sterile 0.9% sodium chloride (NICE 2017). However, NICE guidelines also advise that when recommended by the manufacturer, implanted ports or open-ended catheter lumens should be flushed and locked with heparin sodium flush solutions (NICE 2017).

Guidelines such as EPIC 3 (Loveday et al. 2014), ESPEN (Pittiruti et al. 2009) and HICPAC (O'Grady et al. 2011) also recommend using sterile normal saline for injection to flush and lock catheter lumens that are accessed frequently, stating that manufacturers may recommend heparin flushes for implanted ports or open-ended CVADs that are accessed infrequently. Adherence to manufacturer's instructions is echoed in the guidelines published by NICE (2017), and the Infusion Standards of Practice (Gorski et al. 2016). Flushing with a heparin solution is recommended potentially useful for CVADs that are infrequently accessed or for patients receiving home PN or for ports (Pittiruti et al. 2009).

19.15 Education and Flushing

Effective VAD management starts with knowledge (Bunce 2003), which is why health professionals must have access to education and training, on how to effectively care for and maintain the wide variety of vascular access devices used in health care today (Moureau 2013). Clear, evidence-based guidelines should be available, easily accessible and, adhered to. This will standardise and facilitate best practice (Keogh et al. 2016; Sona et al. 2012), leading to improved patient satisfaction and outcome (Moureau 2013).

Epic 3 (2014) guidelines emphasise the importance of staff training, education and competency prior to caring for patients with intravascular catheters, whilst recommending healthcare workers have additional knowledge of manufacturer's advice relating to individual catheters, antiseptic solutions, dwell time and connections to ensure safe device use (Loveday et al. 2014).

19.16 Conclusion

Flushing is a fundamental clinical intervention, that will assist the maintenance and preservation of an optimally functioning vascular access device (Keogh et al. 2015). Flushing practices however, can vary, (Sona et al. 2012) relating to technique, frequency, volume and solution, which may be caused by conflicting recommendations and lack of education (Mitchel et al. 2009). Factors which influence proficient, clinical practice include practitioner compliance, knowledge and access to education (Moureau 2013; Loveday et al. 2014). Despite the current lack of concencous within the research literature (Keogh et al. 2015; Guiffant et al. 2012), there are studies that have generated enough evidence to inform current practice guidelines to support healthcare workers as they strive for and achieve the best possible outcome for patients.

Case Study

An interesting case study reported by Goossens (2013) was of a patient who received an implantable port for the administration of chemotherapy following a diagnosis of breast cancer. The first cycle of treatment was infused via the port following a satisfactory routine Huber needle insertion into the port. The port had a confirmed free-flowing blood return. The clinician administered saline with a pulsatile, positive pressure, nonresistant flush that was associated with no discomfort by the patient. During the second cycle of chemotherapy (28 days later), the port access was noted as difficult. A subsequent CXR failed to report any obvious device or catheter tip positioning problems. Access required six attempts to fix the Huber needle into the port septum. Flushing was without resistance; however, blood return was 'limited'. Despite these concerns chemotherapy treatment was administered. Within 30 min a painless red swelling was noted around the port, immediately prompting discontinuation of the infusion and port needle removal. The next day port assessment was conducted by an IV specialist nurse. During port needle insertion by the specialist, there was a notable absence of the needle tip abutting against the solid chamber bottom. More than 50 mL of NS was easily flushed; however, only 'pink-tinged' saline could be aspirated. Another attempt to access the port with a longer Huber needle was unsuccessful. A subsequent CXR revealed the implantable port chamber had rotated internally 180°. Root cause analysis of the study concluded that clinical warning signs of the needle tip not hitting the chamber bottom, absence of free-flowing blood return, despite the incorrect verification of port chamber position (on the initial CXR), should have prompted a corrective intervention prior to drug delivery. Risk factors for needle misplacement were noted as access by inexperienced clinicians and the absence of a brisk blood return. Recommendations are made for clinicians to have adequate skills and knowledge to be able to correctly choose needle length and be aware of what to expect during port (Huber) needle insertion. This case study demonstrated how a malpositioned, implantable port resulted in an extravasation injury and emphasises the importance of the need for skill and knowledge by health professionals when accessing vascular access devices to maximise patient safety, experience and outcome (Goossens G.A, Kerchaever I, Despierre E, Marguerite, S (2013) Access of a fully rotated implantable port leads to extravasation. J Vasc Access 14 (3): 299–300).

Summary of Key Points

1. Flushing is an integral clinical intervention to the maintenance and preservation of an optimally functioning vascular access device.
2. Flushing practices vary greatly regarding technique, frequency, volume and solution.
3. There are a variety of types of needleless connectors including:
   (a) Positive displacement connectors
   (b) Negative displacement connectors
   (c) Neutral displacement connectors
   (d) Anti-reflux connectors
4. Each style of needless connector requires a specific clamping technique to prevent blood reflux.
5. To eliminate confusion and ensure patient safety, facilities should use one type of connector to ensure proper flushing and clamping technique, training and adherence by all clinicians.
6. Proficient care and maintenance of VADS requires a good degree of knowledge, skill and understanding.
7. Effective flushing requires a pulsatile, positive pressure technique to adequately rinse and lock the catheter. In

addition to flow type, time interval between boluses is an important factor (Goossens 2015).

8. There is insufficient evidence to suggest heparinised solutions are more effective than 0.9% sodium chloride when locking VADS. Flushing technique is considered more important than solution used.
9. Pre-filled syringes are recommended for use in relevant guidelines (RCN 2016; INS 2016).
10. Needle-free connectors (NFCs) reduce needle stick injury risk but can contribute to catheter occlusion and central line blood stream infection if not used correctly.
11. NFCs when used according to manufacturer's instructions can be of great benefit in assisting successful VAD care and maintenance by promoting patency and reduced complications.
12. Recent studies have found anti-reflux NFCs have a positive impact of maintaining VAD patency by reducing blood reflux into the catheter.
13. Flushing volumes should be equal to twice the internal volume of the catheter system, which includes the catheter extension set, and/or needleless injection system added to the catheter hub (RCN 2016; Gorski et al. 2016). Locking volumes should be overfilled by approximately 15–20% plus 1 mL for extension; only for physiologic solutions without adverse effects, VADS should be flushed immediately pre and post administration of IV therapy/blood sampling with 10 mL 0.9% sodium chloride. Increase to 20 mL post blood transfusion.
14. Blood return check post flush via a central venous access device (CVAD) may identify CVAD tip malposition. Absent blood return should prompt investigation into the root cause.

References

Agharazii M, Plamondon I, Lebel M, Douville P, Desmeules S. Estimation of heparin leak into the systemic circulation after central venous catheter heparin lock. Nephrol Dial Transplant. 2005;20(6):1238–40.

Alexander H. Heparin versus normal saline as a flush solution. Int J Adv Sci Arts. 2010;1(1):63–75.

Anderson BJ, Mitchell MD, Williams K, Umscheid C. A comparison of heparin and saline flush to maintain patency in central venous catheters. Nurs Times. 2010;106(6):15–6.

Barbour MC, McGah PM, Ng CH, Clark AM, Gow KW, Aliseda A. Conective leakage makes heparin locking of central venous catheters ineffective within seconds: experimental measurements in a model superior vena cava. ASAIO J. 2015;61(6):701–9.

Baskin J, Pui C, Reiss U, Wilimas J, Metzger M, Ribeiro R, Howard S. Management of occlusion and thrombosis associated with long-term indwelling central venous catheters. Lancet. 2009;374(9684):159–69. https://doi.org/10.1016/s0140-6736(09)60220-8.

Baskin JL, Reiss U, Williams JA, Metzger ML, Ribeiro RC, Pui C-H, Howard SC. Thrombolytic therapy for central venous catheter occlusion. Haematologica. 2012;97(5):641–50.

Bishop L, Dougherty L, Bodenham A, et al. Guidelines on the insertion and management of central venous access devices in adults. Int J Lab Hematol. 2007;29(4):261–78.

Bodenham A, Babu S, Bennet J, et al. Safer vascular access. AAGBI Anaesth. 2016;71(5):573–85.

Breitling M. Malposition of a central venous catheter in the internal thoracic vein. Can J Anesth. 2010;57(S206):0832–610X.

Btaiche IF, Kovacevich DS, Khalidi N, Papke LF. The effects of needleless connectors on catheter-related thrombotic occlusions. J Inf Nurs. 2011;34(2):89–95.

Bunce M. Troubleshooting central lines. Mod Med Netw. 2003;66:28.

Carlo JT, Lamon JP, McCarthy TM, et al. A prospective randomised trial demonstrating valved implantable ports have complications and lower overall cost than nonvalved implantable ports. Am J Surg. 2004;188(6):722–7.

County Durham & Darlington NHS Foundation Trust. Reducing the occlusion rates of peripheral midlines, our 5-year experience using Bionector TKO needle free connectors. CDDFT IV Team; 2016.

Cummings-Winfield C, Mushani T. Restoring patency to central venous access devices. Oncology Commons. 2008;12(6):925–34.

Deitcher S, Fesen M, Kiproff P, Hill P, Li X, McCluskey E, Semba C. Safety and efficacy of alteplase for restoring function in occluded central venous catheters: results of the cardiovascular thrombolytic to open occluded lines trial. J Clin Oncol. 2002;20(1):317–24.

Dougherty L, Lister S. The Royal Marsden manual of clinical nursing procedures. 9th ed. Oxford: John Wiley & Sons; 2015.

Elli S, Abbruzzese C, Cannizzo L, Lucchini A. In vitro evaluation of fluid reflux after flushing different types of needleless connectors. J Vasc Access. 2016;17(5):429–34. https://doi.org/10.5301/jva.5000583.

Ferroni A, Gaudin F, Guiffant G, Flaud P, Durussel JJ, Descamps P, Berche P, Nassif X, Merckx J. Pulsative flushing as a strategy to prevent bacterial colonisation of vascular access devices. Med Devices (Auckl). 2014;7:379–83.

Field K, McFarlane C, Cheng AC, Hughes AJ. Incidence of catheter-related blood stream infection among patients with a needleless valve-based intravenous connector on an Austrailian Hematology-Oncology Unit. SHEA. 2007;28(5):610–3.

Gabriel J. Venous access devices part 2: Preventing and managing complications of CVADS. Nurs Times. 2013;109(40):20–3.

Goossens GA. Diagnostic accuracy of the Catheter Injection and Aspiration (CINAS) classification for assessing the function of totally implantable venous access devices. Support Care Cancer. 2016;24(2): 755–61.

Goossens GA. Flushing and locking of venous catheters: available evidence and evidence deficit. Nurs Res Pract. 2015;2015:985686.

Goossens GA, Jérôme M, Janssens C, Peetermans WE, Fieuws S, Moons P, Verschakelen J, Peerlinck K, Jacquemin M, Stas M. Comparing normal saline versus diluted heparin to lock non-valved totally implantable venous access devices in cancer patients: a randomised, non-inferiority, open trial. Ann Oncol. 2013;24(7):1892–9.

Gorji MAH, Rezaei F, Jafari H, Cherati JY. Comparison of the effects of heparin and 0.9% sodium chloride solutions in maintenance of patency of central venous catheters. Anaesth Pain Med. 2015; 5(2):e22595.

Gorski LA. Infusion therapy standards of practice. Home Healthcare Now. 2016;35(1):10–8.

Gorski L, Hadaway L, Hagle M, McGoldrick M, Orr M, Doellman D. Infusion therapy standards of practice. J Infus Ther. 2016;39:1S.

Guiffant G, Durussel JJ, Merckx J, Flaud P, Vigier JP, Mousset P. Flushing of intravascular access devices (IVADS)—efficacy of pulsed and continuous infusions. J Vasc Access. 2012;13(1):75–8.

Hackert T, Tjaden C, Kraft A, Sido B, Dienemann H, Buchler MW. Intrapulmonal dislocation of a totally implantable venous access device. World J Surg Oncol. 2005;3(1):19.

Hadaway L. Heparin locking for central venous catheters. J Assoc Vasc Access. 2006a;11:224–3.

Hadaway L. Technology of flushing vascular access devices. J Infus Nurs. 2006b;29(3):137–45.

Hadaway L. Flushing vascular access catheters: risks for infection transmission. Infect Control Res. 2009;4(2):1–7.

Hadaway L. Needleless connectors for IV catheters. How to avoid complications associated with various models and practices. Am J Nurs. 2012;112(11):32–44.

Hadaway L, Richardson D. Needleless connectors. A primer on terminiology. J of Inf Nurs. 2010;33(1):22–31.

Hanchet M. Needleless connectors and bacteremia: is there a relationship? Infect Control Today 2005:1–9.

Hoffer EK, Borsa J, Santulli P, et al. Prospective randomised comparison of valved versus nonvalved peripherally inserted central vein catheters. Am J Roentgenol. 1999;173:1393–8.

Hoffer EK, Bloch RD, Borsa JJ, Santulli P, Fontaine AB, Francoeur N. Peripherally inserted central catheters with distal versus proximal valves: prospective randomized trial. J Vasc Interv Radiol. 2001;12(10):1173–7.

Hull GJ, Moureau NL, Sengupta S. Quantitative assessment of reflux in commercially available needle-free IV connectors. J Vasc Access. 2018;19(1):12–22.

Jarvis WR. Choosing the Best Design for Intravenous Needleless Connectors to Prevent Bloodstream Infections. Infection Control Today. 2010;14(8).

Jarvis WR, Cathryn M, Hall KK, Fogle PJ, Karchmer TB, Harrington G, Salgado C, Giannetta ET, Cameron C, Sherertz RJ. Health care-associated bloodstream infections associated with negative or positive-pressure or displacement mechanical valve needleless connectors. Clin Infect Dis. 2009;49:1821–7.

Jasinsky LM, Wurster J. Occlusion reduction and heparin elimination trial using an antireflux device on peripheral and central venous catheters. J Infus Nurs. 2009;32(1):33–9.

Jonker MA, Osterby KR, Vermeulen LC. Does low dose heparin maintain central venous access device patency?: a comparison of heparin versus saline during a period of heparin shortage. JPEN. 2010;34(4):444–9.

Justo JA, Bookstaver PB. Antibiotic lock therapy: review of technique and logistical challenges. Infect Drug Resist. 2014;7:343–63.

Kelly LJ, Jones T, Kirkham S. Needle-free devices: keeping the system closed. Br J Nurs. 2017; 26(2):S14–9.

Keogh S, Flynn J, Marsh N, Higgins N, Davies K, Rickard CM. Nursing and midwifery practice for the maintenance of vascular access device patency. A cross-sectional survey. Int J Nurs Stud. 2015;52:1678–85.

Keogh S, Flynn J, Marsh N, Mihala G, Davies K, Rickard CM. Varied flushing frequency and volume to prevent peripheral intravenous catheter failure: a pilot, factorial randomised controlled trial in adult medical-surgical hospital patients. Biomed Central. 2016;17:348.

Klockgether-Radke AP, Gaus P. Malposition of a central venous catheter in a patient with severe chest trauma. Anasthesiol Intensivmed Notfallmed Schmerzther. 2004;39(5):292–6.

Krzywda EA, Andris DA. Twenty-five years of advances in vascular access: bridging research to clinical practice. SAGE J; 2005.

Lapalu J, Losser MR, Albert O, Levert H, Villiers S, Faure P, Douard MC. Totally implantable port management: impact of positive pressure during needle withdrawal on catheter tip occlusion (an experimental study). J Vasc Access. 2010;11:46–51.

Logan R. Neutral displacement intravenous connectors: evaluating new technology; 2013.

Lopez-Britz E. Garcia R, Cabello JB. Heparin versus 0.9% sodium chloride intermittent flushing for prevention of occlusion in central venous catheters in adults. Cochrane quality and production topics; 2014.

Losert H, Prokesch R, Grabenwoger M, et al. Inadvertent transpericardial insertion of a central venous line with cardiac tamponade failure of preventative practices. Intensive Care Med. 2000;26:1147–50.

Loveday HP, Wilson JA, Pratt RJ, Golsorkhi M, Tingle A, Bak A, Browne J, Prieto J, Wilcox M. EPIC3: national evidence-based guidelines for preventing healthcare-associated infections in NHS hospitals in England. J Hosp Infect. 2014;S86(1):S1–S70.

Lyons MG. An evidentiary review of flushing protocols in home care patients with peripherally inserted central catheters. Infusion. 2012;18:32–44.

Macklin D. The impact of IV connectors on clinical practice and patient outcomes. J Assoc Vasc Access. 2014;15(3):139. https://doi.org/10.2309/java.15-3-4.

Markota I, Markota D, Tomic M. Measuring of the heparin leakage into the circulation from central venous catheters- an *in vivo* study. Nephrol Dial Transplant. 2009;24:1550–3.

Marschall J, Mermel LA, Fakih M, Hadaway L, Kallen A, O'Grady N, Pettis A, Rupp ME, Sandora T, Maragakis LL, Yokoe D. Strategies to prevent central line-associated bloodstream infections in acute care hospitals: 2014 update. Infect Contr Hosp Epidemiol. 2014;35(7):753–71. http://digitalcommons.wustl.edu/open_access_pubs/3453

Mitchell MD, Anderson BJ, Williams K, Umscheid CA. Heparin flushing and other interventions to maintain patency of central venous catheters: a systematic review. J Adv Nurs. 2009;65(10):2007–21.

Miyagaki H, Nakajima K, Hara J, Yamasaki M, Kurokawa Y, Miyata H, Takiguchi S, Fujiwara Y, Mori M, Doki Y. Performance comparison of peripherally inserted central venous catheters in gastrointestinal surgery: a randomized controlled trial. Clin Nutr. 2012;31(1):48–52.

Moureau NL. Safe patient care when using vascular access devices. Br J Nurs. 2013;22(1):S14–21.

Moureau NL, Flynn J. Disinfection of needleless connector hubs: clinical evidence systematic review. Nurs Res Pract. 2015;2015:1–20.

Muslimani AA, Ricaurte B, Daw HA. Immune heparin-induced thrombocytopenia resulting from preceding exposure to heparin flushes. Am J Hematol. 2007;82(7):652–5.

National Institute for Health Care Excellence (NICE). Intravenous fluid therapy in adults in hospital. NICE CS174. 2017. https://www.nice.org.uk/guidance/cg174.

NICE. Clinical Guideline 139—Healthcare-associated infections: prevention and control in primary and community care. 2012. https://www.nice.org.uk/guidance/cg139/evidence/control-full-guideline-pdf-185186701. Accessed Sept 2017.

NICE. The 3M Tegaderm CHG IV securement dressing for central venous and arterial catheter insertion sites. 2015. https://www.nice.org.uk/guidance/mtg25. Accessed Sept 2017.

O'Grady N, Alexander M, Burns L, Dellinger E, Garland J, Heard S, et al. Centers for Disease Control Guidelines for the prevention of intravascular catheter-related infections. Clin Infect Dis. 2011;52(9):e162–93.

Ong CK, Venkatesh SK. Prospective randomised comparative evaluation of proximal valve polyurethane and distal valve silicone peripherally inserted central catheters. J Vasc Interv Radiol. 2010;21(8):1191–6.

Pereira S, et al. When one port does not return blood: two case reports of rare causes for misplaced central venous catheters. Soc Anaesthesiol. 2013;66(1):78–81.

Pikwer A, Baath L, et al. The incidence and risk of central venous catheter malpositioning: a prospective cohort study in 1619 patients. Anaeth Intensive Care. 2008;36(1):30–7.

Pittiruti M, Hamilton H, Biffi R, et al. ESPEN guidelines on parenteral nutrition: central venous catheters (access, care, diagnosis and therapy of complications). Clin Nutr. 2009;28:365–77.

Polaschegg H-D. Loss of catheter locking solution caused by fluid density. ASAIO J. 2005;51(3):230–5.

Polaschegg H-D, Shaht C. Overspill of catheter locking solution: safety and efficacy aspects. ASAIO J. 2003;49(6):713–5.

Ponec D, Irwin D, Haire W, Hill P, Li X, McCluskey E. Recombinant tissue plasminogen activator (Alteplase) for restoration of flow in occluded central venous access devices: a double-blind placebo-controlled trial—the cardiovascular thrombolytic to open occluded lines (COOL) efficacy trial. JVIR. 2001;12(8):951–5. https://doi.org/10.1016/S1051-0443(07)61575-9.

Randolph AD, Cook DJ, Gonzales CA, Andrew M. Benefit of heparin in peripheral venous and arterial catheters: systematic review and meta-analysis of randomised controlled trials. Br Med J. 1998;316(7136):969–75.

Rolden CJ, Paniagua L. Central venous catheter intravascular malpositioning: causes, prevention, diagnosis and correction. Weston J Emerg Med. 2015;16(5):658–64.

Royal College of Nursing. Standards for infusion nursing. 4th ed. London: Royal Collage of Nursing; 2016.

Royon L, Durussel JJ, Merckx J, et al. The fouling and cleaning of venous catheters: a possible optimisation of the process using intermittent flushing. Chem Eng Res Des. 2012;90(6):803–7.

Ryder M. Needlefree connectors. Canadian Vascular Access Association presentation. 2010. https://cvaa.info/en/news-events/conference-2011/speakers-presentations-2010/itemid/214. Accessed 4 Aug 2019.

Sauerland C, Engelking C, Wickham R, Corbi D. Vesicant extravasation part 1: mechanisms, pathogenisis and nursing care to reduce risk. Oncol Nurs Forum. 2005;33(6):1134–42.

Semba CP, Deitcher SR, Li X, Resnansky L, Tu T, McCluskey ER, Investigators C. Treatment of occluded central venous catheters with alteplase: results in 1,064 patients. J Vasc Interv Radiol. 2002;13(12):1199–205.

Shallom ME, Prentice D, Sona C. Heparin or 0.9% sodium chloride to maintain central venous catheter patency: a randomised trial. Crit Care Med. 2012;40(6):1820–6.

Sona C, Prentice D, Schallom L. National survey of central venous catheter flushing in the intensive care unit. Crit Care Nurse. 2012;32(1):e12–9.

Sungur M, Eryuksel E, Yavas S, et al. Exit of catheter lock solutions from double lumen acute haemodialysis catheters an in vitro study. Nephrol Dial Transplant. 2007;22:3533–7.

Vigier JP, Merckx J, Coquin JY. The use of a hydrodynamic bench for experimental simulation of flushing venous catheters: impact of the technique. ITBM-RBM. 2005;26(2):147–9.

Part VII

Right Evaluation

20

VHP Program: Implementation and Evaluation

Lisa A. Gorski

Abstract

A thorough and methodical evaluation of any program is imperative in determining its effectiveness. Prior to this chapter, a multitude of evidence-based practices and the importance of their application in promoting and ensuring vessel health and preservation have been described. The question is, how do we promote and ensure adherence to these sound practices and guidelines that when implemented will improve patient clinical outcomes and patient experience? How do we best implement these practice changes? And, what is the "right" way to evaluate components of a vessel health and preservation program? The objective of this chapter is to describe implementation strategies and to explore strategies for evaluation of a VHP program.

Keywords

Evaluation · Audit and feedback
Implementing change · Audit and feedback strategies

L. A. Gorski (✉)
Ascension At Home, 12403 N Hawks Glen Ct. Mequon, Milwaukee, WI 53097, USA

20.1 Introduction

The last quadrant of the VHP model includes processes to evaluate the success of your implementation, identify gaps and weaknesses, consider evaluation of new products to meet a need, and focus on patient and clinician satisfaction measurements. Improvement of care is impossible without an established process of evaluation. Right evaluation for VHP program application includes outcome measurement of complications, observation of policy performance, and plan to provide education for staff departments and units with negative outcomes or practice deficiencies. A multimodal quality program applies education of guidelines and recommendations ensuring that practices are consistent, and that staff is well informed. Adding new products should involve an established process for evaluation and trialing to ensure performance at the company stated levels. Integrated within a VHP program is the evaluation of products, supplies, and technology, both existing and considering new product trial testing. Each product should undergo periodic assessment to determine performance according to the facility needs and expected application. Each of these areas of evaluation requires measurement criteria, periodic checks for application, and compliance, all to ensure a successful and high-quality program.

According to the VHP model, the right evaluation must include audits and outcome monitoring which lead to identification of educational needs and use of products that can contribute to improved outcomes (Moureau and Carr 2018). Outcomes include complication rates, observation of compliance to organizational policies and procedures, and evaluation of clinician competencies. Examples of specific outcome measurements include catheter-related bloodstream infection rates, venous thrombosis rates in patients with PICCs, peripheral IV-related complications, and catheter occlusion rates. Process outcomes that might be evaluated in a VHP program include appropriate use of PICCs versus midline catheters, site care, and dressings performed in accordance with policy, intactness of VAD dressings, prompt removal of VADs when no longer necessary, and compliance with adhering to the components of the central line insertion checklist.

Outcomes are not just measured but are used to validate performance or to identify needed areas for quality improvement interventions. Audit and feedback are a widely used and recommended strategy in implementation and evaluation of practice changes. It is defined as a summary of clinical performance that may include recommendations for action; information is gathered over a specified period of time and used to increase group awareness of theirs and/or others' practice (RNAO 2012; Ivers et al. 2012). Audit and feedback are usually used in conjunction with other interventions, namely, educational strategies. As stated by Ray-Barruel (2017), ongoing audits are used to ensure compliance with care and will provide the evidence required to ensure that an organization is on track to excellence in VAD care. Clearly, without attention to program evaluation, deficiencies and patient outcomes would not be identified, and opportunities for performance improvement including necessary clinician education would not be identified.

20.2 Implementation and Quality Improvement Strategies

Both implementing and sustaining changes in practice are quite challenging. The Cochrane Effective Practice and Organization of Care (EPOC) group classifies quality improvement strategies used to change practice into four main categories (Flodgren et al. 2013). These strategies may be used either alone or in combination with improve adherence:

- **Organizational**: May include changes in professional roles or skill mix changes, for example, champion leaders or implementation of a specialty team.
- **Regulatory:** For example, government required healthcare initiatives.
  - **Example:** Requirements for infection or other outcome reporting.
- **Financial:** Constraints of reimbursement based on clinical outcomes or patient satisfaction. This is a strong motivator for implementing practice changes!
  - **Example**: In the United States, central line-associated bloodstream infection (CLABSI) rates in hospitals are publicly reported on the Medicare.gov website ("hospital compare"). Hospitals face penalties for high CLABSI rates, and *any* vascular access device-related BSI is considered a preventable event with treatment not reimbursable under medicare. The patient experience which includes satisfaction measures also factors into reimbursement.
- **Professional interventions:** The focus of this chapter may include educational strategies, the use of local opinion leaders, and the use of audit and feedback and reminders.

The Society for Healthcare Epidemiology/ Infectious Disease Society of America (SHEA/ IDSA) (Marschall et al. 2014) identifies an implementation strategy for CLABSI prevention that can also be applied to implementation of other evidence-based practices. It includes the following four steps:

- **Engage:** Includes multidisciplinary teams that include frontline and senior leadership in the process and outcome improvement plan, identification of local champions (e.g., vascular access/infusion clinicians), and focus on a culture of safety.
- **Educate:** The use of a variety of educational methods and strategies.
- **Execute**: Use quality improvement methodologies (e.g., plan-do-study-act) to structure prevention efforts, to standardize care processes (e.g. guidelines, bundles), and to create "redundancy" such as with visual reminders, checklists, posters, screen saver messages, etc.
- **Evaluate**: Include audits of both process (e.g. compliance with insertion bundle) and outcome (CLABSI rate) measures and link to initial and ongoing competency assessments and the critical step of providing feedback to all healthcare staff. Examples include compliance with insertion checklists with graphs showing cumulative compliance with process measures.

In the Infusion Therapy Standards of Practice, the Infusion Nurses Society addresses the importance of quality improvement programs including monitoring of adverse outcomes including infection rates, reporting such data regularly to both clinicians and leadership, and minimizing and eliminating barriers to change and improvement (Gorski et al. 2016). The Standards for Infusion Therapy from the Royal College of Nursing (2016) include similar recommendations and specifically address the need for auditing as an ongoing process in order to monitor, maintain, and improve clinical practice in infusion therapy and the need for timely dissemination of audit results to develop a culture of learning and quality improvement. The epic3 guidelines (Loveday et al. 2014) recommend the use of quality improvement interventions to support and manage VADs including the use of audit and feedback of compliance with practice guidelines.

The Registered Nurses' Association of Ontario (RNAO 2012) provides a "knowledge to action" framework. Prior to implementation of interventions, an important step is to recognize and understand barriers or roadblocks as well as "facilitators" to practice change. Facilitators are positive characteristics supporting practice change such as positive staff attitudes and beliefs, leadership support, organizational "champions," and interorganizational collaboration and networks (RNAO 2012). Examples of barriers to implementing practice changes include:

- Potentially negative attitudes by clinical staff, often related to organizational problems or issues such as inadequate staffing, high patient acuity levels, and organizational changes.
- Lack of interest or lack of knowledge which may also be impacted by many competing clinical priorities (e.g., reduce incidence of falls, pressure ulcers, nonvascular-associated infections).
- Guidelines or practice changes are not integrated or "hard-wired" into organization practices or policies/procedures (RNAO 2012).

It is important to acknowledge that the presence of policies does not result in adherence to best practices. In a survey of 975 US hospitals enrolled in the National Health and Safety Network, data were provided on the presence of policies in 1534 ICU units. There was a widespread presence of policies relative to CLABSI prevention (87–97%); however adherence to such policies ranged from 37 to 71% (Stone et al. 2014).

Another potential barrier to implementing evidence-based practices is how and in what way do key persons assess and champion the evidence. If the evidence is believed to be weak, implementation of a practice is not likely. The perceived strength of evidence relative to evidence-based infection prevention practices was studied in a survey of infection prevention personnel (Saint et al. 2013). Relative to CLABSI prevention, 90% or more survey respondents perceived the following evidence as strong: skin antisepsis with chlorhexidine, maximal sterile barrier precautions, and avoiding the femoral site. The researchers recommend that when translating evidence into practice, consideration should be given as to how key individuals assess the strength of evidence.

Conduction of an organizational survey may be a helpful strategy for identifying facilitators and barriers. Once understood, it is important to build upon identified facilitators and examine ways to tackle the barriers. Examples include addressing the educational needs and the level/type of education needed, providing adequate time for implementation, and exploring motivational strategies.

20.3 Exploration and Effective Use of Audit and Feedback Strategies

As stated earlier, audit and feedback are a widely used and recommended strategy in implementation of practice changes. A systematic review of literature was performed to explore features of educational interventions that led to competence in aseptic central line insertion and care in acute care settings (Cherry et al. 2010). Based upon a review of 47 studies that met the researchers' inclusion criteria, educational interventions were most effective and more likely to result in outcome improvement when used in conjunction with audit and feedback as well as availability of the clinical supplies consistent with the education. Education alone is not enough to improve outcomes and clinical practice!

In a Cochrane study including 140 randomized trials involving audit and feedback, the effect on professional behaviors and patient outcomes ranged from little/no effect to a substantial effect (Ivers et al. 2012). While most of the reviewed studies measured impact on physician practice, some involved nurses and pharmacists. Concluding that audit and feedback can lead to small but important improvements in practice, the researchers found audit and feedback strategies are most effective when:

- Baseline performance is low to begin with.
- It is provided more than once.
- It is provided by a supervisor or colleague.
- It is provided verbally as well as in writing.
- There are clear goals/targets and an action plan.

In a follow-up analysis to the Cochrane review, Ivers et al. (2014) state that audit and feedback are one of the most studied quality improvement interventions. While again asserting that audit and feedback lead to small but potentially important practice changes, they state that "the appropriate question is not: 'can audit and feedback improve professional practice?' but: 'how the effect of audit and feedback interventions can be optimized?'" (Ivers et al. 2014). Citing evidence that repeated feedback is more effective, the researchers opine that studies continue to evaluate interventions after only one cycle of feedback. There remains the need to identify the key, active ingredients of audit and feedback that will lead to a greater impact of interventions, and produce more generalizable outcomes.

Using a modified grounded theory approach involving 72 clinicians, including nurses, in ICU settings, the use of audit and feedback was perceived as fragmented and variable, not transparent, and provided information that was neither timely nor "actionable" (Sinuff et al. 2015). To improve the process, the researchers suggest the following: providing rationale for practice changes and for the audit process, incorporating feedback into daily activities such as rounds, developing audit and feedback criteria that are specific and transparent, and providing information that can be translated into specific actions. Furthermore, the feedback must be timely. For example, finding out that there were two-line infections in the previous month gives little information if the patient is not identified and what were potential breaches in expected practice. Participants in the study feedback should provide specific actions "which can be acted upon more immediately" (Sinuff et al. 2015: 396).

Another small qualitative study sought to describe the perception of nurses on the effectiveness of audit and feedback (Christina et al. 2016). Nursing practice relative to hand hygiene, the use of smart pumps, and intravenous site assessments was evaluated by a nurse manager or clinical nurse specialist who entered the patient's room with a checklist and documented the nurse's work weekly or biweekly. Feedback was provided to the nurse shortly after the audit. Three themes identified by the nurses included:

1. Relevance: The need to understand the purpose of audit and feedback and the link between the audit criteria and patient outcomes.
2. Timing and feedback: Some nurses felt that the audit process occurred too early during the shift, and they were not able to complete the expected work in such limited time.
3. Individual factors: A perception of criticism resulted in greater tendency to respond in a more negative manner.

Summarizing implications for nurse managers, the researchers suggest making the audit and feedback process relevant and transparent in its purpose, involving nurses in planning and developing the process and providing feedback with clearly evident goals and action plans to make feedback less personal (Christina et al. 2016).

Strategies for improving the audit and feedback process are summarized in Table 20.1.

Table 20.1 Strategies for improving the audit and feedback process

The audit process is transparent and relevant and includes:
• Rationale for practice changes
• Rationale for the audit process
• There is a link between audit criteria and patient outcomes
• Provide both written and verbal feedback
• Information obtained can be translated into clear goals and action plans
• Feedback is provided more than once

20.4 Examples: Successful Integration of Audit and Feedback into Practice

A quality improvement project implemented in a two-site hospital system involved the use of nurse-specific report cards providing feedback on central line management (Morrison et al. 2017). Using both visual and documentation audits, the authors sought to understand if known risk factors (e.g., maintaining dry intact dressing, maintaining IV set integrity) associated with central line-associated bloodstream infection (CLABSI) could be decreased. Using feedback intervention theory, information that is timely, detail focused, based on goals, and aimed at changing behavior and improving performance was provided. Nurses were provided a four-part computer-based educational module, and a trial of an alcohol disinfection cap was initiated before the audits. During the auditing period, additional interventions included house-wide implementation of the alcohol disinfection cap, updating of policies and procedures, and redesigned central line dressing/implanted port needle insertion trays. The weekly visual audit consisted of observation of dressings (e.g., dry and intact, chlorhexidine-impregnated dressings, dressings dated) and administration sets (e.g., labeling, use of disinfection caps, no looping) and also a documentation review (e.g., site assessment and care, catheter patency, dressing change date corresponds to date on dressing).

Over the 16-week period, 487 nurses received a "report card," which included 620 central lines; 113 failed the visual audit with 54% having at least one CLABSI contributing factor. Over time, there was a decrease in CLABSI contributing factors which the authors believed resulted from the personalized report cards. The nurses' responses to the report cards were briefly discussed and included justification of failures (not my fault), excuses (float nurse), and dismay. Outcome data included a decrease in CLABSIs; statistical significance of this outcome was not reported. Based upon the evaluation of this quality improvement study data, additional organizational changes were made including a face-to-face line care module for newly hired nurses, mandatory annual CLABSI prevention education, immediate intervention to correct failures at the time of the audit, and redesign of the electronic medical record IV documentation (Morrison et al. 2017).

In another example, a reduction in CLABSIs was reported over a 5-year period. Daily rounds of all central lines in an ICU setting revealed a substantial number of occluded lines as well as inadequate clinical practices including unlabeled dressings, improperly placed chlorhexidine foam dressings, and breaches in aseptic technique (Matocha 2013). Outcome data was used to support practice changes, product changes, and education and competency training.

In an emergency department, placement and care of peripheral IV catheters (PIV) was addressed using audit and feedback (Fakih et al. 2012). A quasi-experimental pre- and post-study methodology was used. Pre-study data included 10–20 observations of PIV placement per week, evaluation of documentation, and about 10 intravenous medication administrations observed per week. Steps observed include hand hygiene, skin antisepsis including air drying, maintaining aseptic technique during placement, and application of a sterile dressing. Implementation included education with a pre- and posttest as well as the same observations done pre-study. Two hundred twenty completed PIV placements were observed during the study period. Very poor compliance and lack of knowledge was evident relative to proper insertion technique pre-implementation (4.8%) and improved over time (30.9% during implementation, 31.7% post-implementation).

While the researchers found that audit and feedback were associated with a statistically significant improvement in documentation and compliance with PIV procedural steps, it is notable that overall compliance with the PIV insertion steps only improved to a little over 30%. When breaking down compliance into the five steps, hand hygiene prior to patient contact was about 20% pre-implementation and remained under 40% during implementation and post-implementation. Compliance was much greater, approaching or greater than 80% with the other PIV steps.

In a study of compliance with a transfusion bundle, monthly team audit and feedback were compared to monthly team audit and feedback *plus* individual feedback (Borgert et al. 2016). Compliance was significantly improved when the individual nurse was provided timely feedback in addition to the monthly team audit and feedback.

20.5 Summary

Implementing and sustaining evidence-based practice changes *is* challenging but is imperative in providing the best care and outcomes for the patients we serve. Increasingly, organizations are facing regulatory and reimbursement requirements and constraints that compel changes in clinical practice. Key interventions steps in implementation include involvement of a team that includes leadership, local champions, and clinical experts, an understanding of both positive characteristics of an organization that support practice change and barriers to change, and employment of sound quality improvement strategies. It is important to realize that education and well-written policies and procedures, while important and certainly needed as part of any implementation plan, are not enough.

Once implemented, there must be an ongoing evaluation of its effectiveness. The *right* evaluation of a vessel health and preservation program must include audit and feedback which is used in conjunction with other interventions including educational strategies. Audits will include clinician feedback, patient responses, process (e.g., the presence of inadequate dressings), and outcome (e.g., CLABSI, other complications) measures (Figs. 20.1 and 20.2).

Patient Name: ______________________ Date: ____ /_____ /_____ Clinician: ___________________
Day Month Year

Vessel Health and Preservation Evaluation Tool

This evaluation tool is a compliance tool to be used prior to patient being released from the hospital

(Key points reduces replacement of devices, reduces delays related to IV device and reduced cost with efficiency of IV device)

1. Was the right line protocol used to determine the best vascular access device. . for this patient? ☐ Yes ☐ No

2. Was the "right line" daily evaluation process completed throughout the stay?. . . ☐ Yes ☐ No

3. Was the vascular access device selected in the protocol placed within the first 24 hours of patient admittance?. . . . ☐ Yes ☐ No

4. Was the same vascular access device used during the entire hospital stay?. . . . ☐ Yes ☐ No

   If No, how many vascular access devices did the patient receive? _________

   What were the additional vascular access devices? ____________________

   Why were they necessary? ____________________________________

5. Were there any complications during the insertion procedure? . . . . ☐ Yes ☐ No

   If Yes, please explain: ____________________________________

   ____

6. Were there any complications throughout therapy? . . . . ☐ Yes ☐ No

   If Yes, please identify the complication and explain below:

   ☐ Phlebitis ☐ Infection

   ☐ Thrombosis ☐ Other: ______________________________

   Explanation: ____

   ____

7. What was the original vessel health assessment for this patient?

   ☐ Very Poor ☐ Good

   ☐ Poor ☐ Very Good

   ☐ Fair ☐ Excellent

8. What is the vessel health assessment at the time of discharge for this patient?

   ☐ Very Poor ☐ Good

   ☐ Poor ☐ Very Good

   ☐ Fair ☐ Excellent

Fig. 20.1 Clinician evaluation tool for VHP (used with permission of Teleflex)

Vessel Health and Preservation
Patient Satisfaction and Evaluation Tool

Patient Initials (if applicable): _______ **Date:** ___/___/___ (dd mm yyyy) **Pt Adm Date:** __/__/___ (dd mm yyyy)

Evaluator's Name: ____________________________ ☐ **RN** ☐ **MD** ☐ **PHARM D** ☐ **Other:** _______

Using the chart below, rate your satisfaction of your experience with your intravenous devices during your stay

Your Response	Very Satisfied	Satisfied	Neutral	Not Satisfied	Very Unsatisfied	Don't Know or Not Applicable
a. Were you satisfied with the intravenous (IV) device placed for your hospital treatment?	☐ 1	☐ 2	☐ 3	☐ 4	☐ 5	☐ N/A
b. Did you receive an adequate amount of information about your IV device, the purpose and need for the IV device?	☐ 1	☐ 2	☐ 3	☐ 4	☐ 5	☐ N/A
c. Were you satisfied with the choice of IV device and the reason for the device?	☐ 1	☐ 2	☐ 3	☐ 4	☐ 5	☐ N/A
d. Were you satisfied with the skill of the person placing the IV?	☐ 1	☐ 2	☐ 3	☐ 4	☐ 5	☐ N/A
e. Was the intravenous insertion procedure acceptable and relatively free from pain?	☐ 1	☐ 2	☐ 3	☐ 4	☐ 5	☐ N/A
f. Were you satisfied with the number of attempts necessary for the IV device?	☐ 1	☐ 2	☐ 3	☐ 4	☐ 5	☐ N/A
g. When your treatment was complete were you satisfied with how quickly your IV device was removed?	☐ 1	☐ 2	☐ 3	☐ 4	☐ 5	☐ N/A
h. Were you satisfied with the infection prevention education you received on how you can protect yourself??	☐ 1	☐ 2	☐ 3	☐ 4	☐ 5	☐ N/A
i. Were you satisfied with the attention to handwashing, scrubbing the hub and other infection prevention procedures practiced by the staff?	☐ 1	☐ 2	☐ 3	☐ 4	☐ 5	☐ N/A
j. Were you satisfied with your involvement as a participant in your treatment plan specific to IV devices and treatments?	☐ 1	☐ 2	☐ 3	☐ 4	☐ 5	☐ N/A
k. OVERALL your opinion of your IV therapy experience during your stay?	☐ 1	☐ 2	☐ 3	☐ 4	☐ 5	☐ N/A

1. What did you **NOT** LIKE about your IV experience?
2. What concerns, if any, about the staff or IV device?
3. What suggestions do you have for improvement?
4. Would you recommend this hospital to others?

☐ Yes ☐ No, because ____

Other commends? ____

Fig. 20.2 Patient evaluation tool for VHP (used with permission of Teleflex)

Audit and feedback are provided in a timely manner, provided more than once, provided by a supervisor or colleague both verbally and in writing, and should include clear goals/targets and an action plan. Furthermore, the audit and feedback process should be transparent to and understood by clinicians. Future research must focus on the key components of audit and feedback that will lead to greater impact of interventions.

Case Study

Most of the patients on the hospital's large surgical unit have peripheral IV catheters placed for routine fluid replacement and IV medication administration. During a team meeting, the nurses have expressed that they frequently remove and replace the catheters due to phlebitis. A review of medical records led by the unit's quality improvement team documented a high phlebitis rate of 30%. Additionally, based upon a 2-day point prevalence study of observed peripheral IV sites, the team noted that most of the catheters were placed in the hand/wrist area. A review of the clinical policy relative to peripheral IV catheter placement, care, and management was found to be outdated. A hospital-wide team was pulled together to revise the policy and update to current recommendations especially relative to site selection and catheter gauge size.

1. What next steps could be taken in promoting the updated peripheral IV catheter policy?
2. How might adherence to the new policy changes be measured?
3. How should the measurement process be presented to the staff nurses?
4. How might the changes be addressed in a daily practice?

Summary of Key Points

- When planning to implement changes in practice, put together a team that includes leadership, local champions, and clinical experts.
- Explore and understand organizational characteristics that will support practice changes as well as any barriers to change.
- Staff education and policies/procedures are necessary in implementation of practice changes, but they are not enough.
- The *right* evaluation of a vessel health and preservation program must include audit and feedback that includes both process and outcome measures.
- Audit and feedback must be provided in a timely manner, provided more than once, provided by a supervisor or colleague both verbally and in writing.
- Clear goals/targets and an action plan should be part of the audit and feedback process.
- The audit and feedback process should be transparent to and understood by clinicians.

References

Borgert M, Binnekade J, Paulus F, Goossens A, Vroom M, Dongelmans D. Timely individual audit and feedback significantly improves transfusion bundle compliance—a comparative study. Int J Qual Health Care. 2016;28(5):601–7.

Cherry MG, Brown JM, Neal T, Shaw NB. What features of educational interventions lead to competence in aseptic insertion and maintenance of CV catheters in acute care? BEME guide no. 15. Med Teach. 2010;32(3):198–218.

Christina V, Baldwin K, Biron A, Emed J, Lepage K. Factors influencing the effectiveness of audit and feedback: nurses' perceptions. J Nurs Manag. 2016;24:1080–7.

Fakih MG, Jones K, Rey JE, et al. Sustained improvements in peripheral venous catheter care in non-intensive care units: a quasiexperimental controlled study of education and feedback. Infect Control Hosp Epidemiol. 2012;33(5):449–55.

Flodgren G, Conterno LO, Mayhew A, Omar O, Pereira CR, Shepperd S. Interventions to improve professional adherence to guidelines for prevention of device-related infections. Cochrane Database Syst Rev. 2013;(3):CD006559. https://doi.org/10.1002/14651858.CD006559.pub2.

Gorski LA, Hadaway L, Hagle M, McGoldrick M, Orr M, Doellman D. 2016 infusion therapy standards of practice. J Infus Nurs. 2016;39(1S):S1–S159.

Ivers N, Jamtvedt G, Flottorp S, Young JM, Odgaard-Jensen J, French SD, O'Brien MA, Johansen M, Grimshaw J, Oxman AD. Audit and feedback: effects on professional practice and healthcare outcomes. Cochrane Database Syst Rev. 2012;(6):CD000259. https://doi.org/10.1002/14651858.CD000259.pub3.

Ivers NM, Grimshaw JM, Jamtvedt G, Flottorp S, O'Brien MA, French SD, Young J, Odgaard-Jensen J. Growing literature, stagnant science? Systematic review, meta-regression and cumulative analysis of audit and feedback interventions in health care. J Gen Intern Med. 2014;29(11):1534–41.

Loveday HP, Wilson JA, Pratt RJ, Golsorkhi M, Tingle A, Bak A, et al. J Hosp Infect. 2014;86(suppl 1):S1–S70.

Marschall J, Mermel LA, Fakih M, Hadaway L, Kallen A, O'Grady NP, et al. Strategies to prevent central line-associated bloodstream infections in acute care hospitals: 2014 update. Infect Control Hosp Epidemiol. 2014;35(7):753–71.

Matocha D. Achieving near-zero and zero: who said interventions and controls don't matter. JAVA. 2013;18(3):157–63.

Morrison T, Raffaele J, Brennaman L. Impact of personalized report cards on nurses managing central lines. Am J Infect Control. 2017;45:24–8.

Moureau NL, Carr PJ. Vessel health and preservation: a model and clinical pathway for using vascular access devices. Br J Nurs. 2018;27(8, suppl):S28–35.

Ray-Barruel G. Using audits as evidence. Br J Nurs. 2017;26(8):S3.

Registered Nurses of Ontario. Toolkit: implementation of best practice guidelines. 2nd ed. Toronto, ON: Registered Nurses of Ontario; 2012.

Royal College of Nursing. Standards for infusion therapy. 4th ed. London: Royal College of Nursing; 2016.

Saint S, Greene MT, Olmsted RN, Chopra V, Meddings J, Safdar N, Krein SL. Perceived strength of evidence supporting practices to prevent health care-associated infection: results from a national survey of infection prevention personnel. Am J Infect Control. 2013;41:100–6.

Sinuff T, Muscedere J, Rozmovitz L, Dale CM, Scales DC. A qualitative study of the variable effects of audit and feedback in the ICU. BMJ Qual Saf. 2015;24:393–9.

Stone PW, et al. State of infection prevention in US hospitals enrolled in the National Health and safety network. Am J Infect Control. 2014;42:94–9.

21

Competency Attainment and Evaluation among the Staff

Linda J. Kelly

Abstract

Effective teaching and subsequent evaluation of the competence of practitioners is crucial if patient safety is to be assured. Learning is a very complex process, and despite many years of research, it remains difficult to articulate how educational and training methods enable effective learning. We are, however, aware that the actions and attitudes of both the teacher and the learner affect the outcome of the teaching and learning experience. Unfortunately, many individuals teach others without the formal knowledge of how learners learn. Often the teacher lacks the concept to understand, explain and articulate a process during the learning process. This chapter intends to give a general overview of teaching and learning; it develops by exploring and discussing the issue of competency attainment and competency evaluation. Issues of continuous assessment will be considered as will the notion of lifelong learning.

Keywords

Competency · Competency assessment Education · Evaluation · Adherence to protocols

L. J. Kelly (✉)
Edinburgh Napier University,
School of Health and Social Care, Edinburgh, UK
e-mail: Linda.kelly@vygon.co.uk

21.1 Approaches to Teaching and Learning

The training and education of healthcare professionals have changed greatly in recent years. Gone are the days of 'learning on the job' or the 'see one, do one, teach one' method that had been the norm for so many a year. Historically, these were the traditional methods of teaching surgical procedures but raised concerns regarding patient safety. Although this method of teaching has since fallen out of favour, Kotsis and Chung (2013) argue that this method may still be valid if combined with a variety of other adult learning principles. Despite this claim, education and training are generally very structured processes, and academia is typically included. This approach allows the ability to clearly apply theory to practise.

To ensure that education is effective, it is important to have knowledge of some of the major views of learning. In psychology, there are several ideas about how learning occurs. In the twenty-first century, cognitive and social theories were most commonly used, with constructivism (how humans learn) as the most common approach to learning. The approach to teaching and learning clinical skills such as vascular access device insertion and care and maintenance should be underpinned by a constructivism or adult learning philosophical framework such as experiential learning. This is because higher-level skills such as those required for vascular access device insertion are generally mastered following repeated experiences of the task. According to Bradley (2006), learners construct their understanding through their interaction with it. A facilitator is required to help practitioners construct their knowledge and skills. Once the theory has been learned, skills are evaluated by the learner using a reflective process which is continuous. Thereafter, learning is constructed from the experience, and practice is improved as evaluation and reflection continue (Hulse 2013).

21.2 Experiential Learning (Learning by Doing)

Experiential learning is a model of learning where learning and meaning are derived from repeated patient care experiences. According to McLeod (2012), professional judgement and higher-level skills can be gained from repeated exposure to these experiences. Learning of this type takes place either within a clinical setting or a simulated environment. These learning experiences are designed and supported to ensure that a complete learning cycle is completed. This includes a concrete and tangible experience, observations and reflections, formation of abstract concepts and generalisations, followed by the testing of implications of concepts learned in new situations (Kolb 1983) (Fig. 21.1).

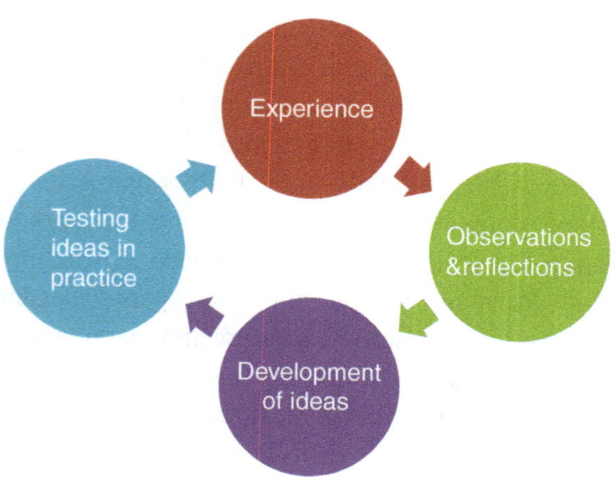
Experience
Observations &reflections
Development of ideas
Testing ideas in practice

Fig. 21.1 Model of experiential learning process (used with permission L. Kelly)

Theoretical perspective and empirical knowledge are gained from various disciplines including psychology, sociology, ethics, management, education and biological sciences.

The principle of experiential education is a methodology that involves educators or mentors engaging with learners in direct experience. This is followed by reflection which helps the learner to increase knowledge, further develop their skills and clarify values (Caldwell and Grobbel 2013). When applying experiential learning, account must be taken of the learner's previous experience, their knowledge base and their theoretical preparation. An example of this is when an individual has had previous experience of the procedure of peripherally inserted central venous catheter insertion. If service development takes place and this individual's role expands to insert tunnelled central venous catheter, their learning curve will be different to that of someone who had never inserted a central venous catheter. In other words, the learning needs and context of each learner will always vary. This teaching method takes this variation into account, and each educational intervention guides the learner from being dependent towards becoming a participant under supervision, before finally becoming an independent practitioner. This can also be described as the journey from novice to expert (Fig. 21.2) (Benner 1982).

21.3 Developing Competence: From Novice to Expert

21.3.1 Situated Learning

In contrast to the tradition classroom learning that involves abstract knowledge which is out of context, it is argued that learning should be 'situated' as learners acquire a greater learning experience when knowledge is presented in settings and situations that would normally involve that knowledge (Wacquant 1992). Social interaction and collaboration are important components of situated learning, and learners become involved in a 'community of practice'. As the novice learner moves from the fringes of a

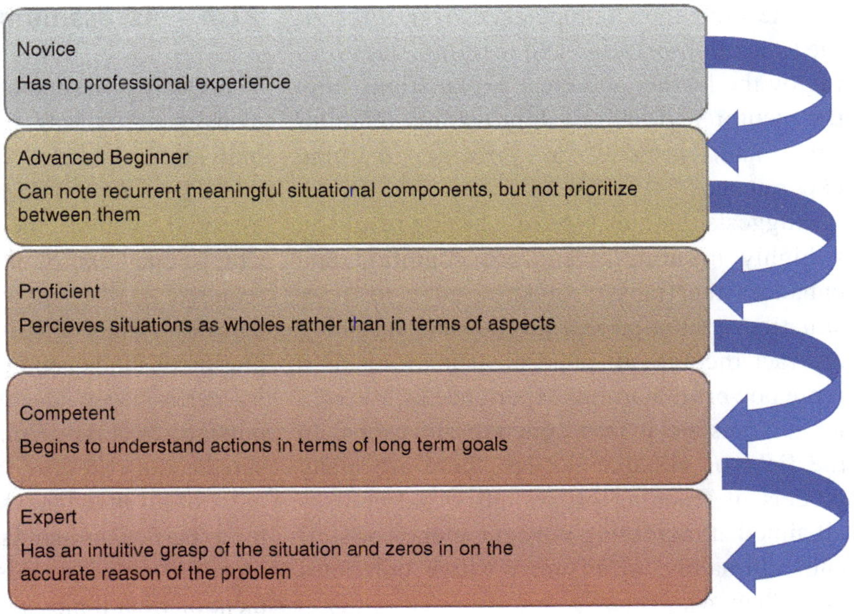

Fig. 21.2 Novice to expert modified

community to its centre, they become more actively engaged in the values and principles and eventually assumes the role of an expert (Collins and Greeno 2010). Within nurse education, simulated care environments are now commonly used to allow learners the opportunity to gain and practise skills in as close to clinical as possible (Onda 2012). Part-task simulation has been recognised as a positive learning tool within vascular access (Kelly et al. 2015). In this learning model, an experienced practitioner or mentor is the most valuable resource available to the learner. To ensure an effective partnership, it should be assured that the mentor - learner relationship is one that is dynamic and active. A positive learning environment is also one that will foster effective learning.

21.3.2 Situated Cognition and Cognitive Apprenticeship

The learning of vascular access skills in clinical practice can be characterised as situated learning. Usually, following a period of theory and learning the procedures of ultrasound guidance and device insertions on phantoms and models, nurses will then go into clinical practice to gain confidence and competence in the insertion procedure. Because these skills are being honed in the same or similar environment that the learner will be in once competence is achieve, this could be viewed as situated learning. Cognitive apprenticeship was introduced as an instructional model for situated learning and comprises of six teaching methods to support learning. These methods are:

- Modelling.
- Coaching.
- Scaffolding.
- Articulation.
- Reflection.
- Exploration.

The methods used in this model are very specific and designed to enhance learning in clinical practice. The cognitive processes of the experts play a critical role during complex task performance. They should aim to perform complex tasks in ways that simplifies it for the learner who is observing. This makes it easier for the learner to eventually reproduce the task on their own. Therefore, someone learning the skill of vascular access device insertion should work closely with a mentor and use observation of this competent person to learn skills and develop their competence over time. At the time of observation and learning, questioning by the learner and clear explanations from the mentor will help to improve this relationship and provide a positive learning experience.

Suggests that this type of learning results in a highly meaningful situated cognition and enhances the transfer of knowledge to other situations. Situated learning, unlike the more abstract theoretical, preclinical learning, is a more powerful learning experience as it is easier to translate it into concrete situations. In the field of vascular access, there are many models of teaching programmes and courses all aimed at increasing the competency of staff and, ultimately, to ensure positive outcomes (see Chap. 4).

Practitioners in vascular access roles are typically adult learners who are undertaking a programme of study that includes both didactic and practical hands-on practices of the procedure (Jamison et al. 2006). Practitioners in the learning stages should be able to recognise their learning needs, plan ways in which to address these needs and participate in information seeking. Once learning has been completed, it is vital to assess and evaluate this learning to ensure skills attainment, knowledge and understanding.

21.4 Assessment of Learning

The Quality Assurance Agency (QAA) defines assessment as 'any process that appraises an individual's knowledge, understanding, abilities or skills'. Assessment of clinical practice is essential within the healthcare profession. Competency can be defined as 'possessing the required skills, knowledge, qualifications or capacity', while defines competency as 'the integration of fundamental knowledge, clinical ability, performance, and attitude in the context of a nursing situation'. Competence is usually measured against set criteria and involves the assessment of an individual's performance in relation to a particular standard (Quinn 2000). With regard to vascular access, there is general agreement of what topics should be incorporated into an education and training package for device insertion and subsequent care and maintenance as noted in Chap. 4 (RCN 2016; Moureau et al. 2013).

Once a programme of training has been designed, it is important to ensure that the teaching and assessment are aligned constructively (Biggs 1999) (see Fig. 21.3). According to Biggs, teaching should be a balanced system in which all components support each other. This means that the learning outcomes and choice of assessment must match to allow competency to be

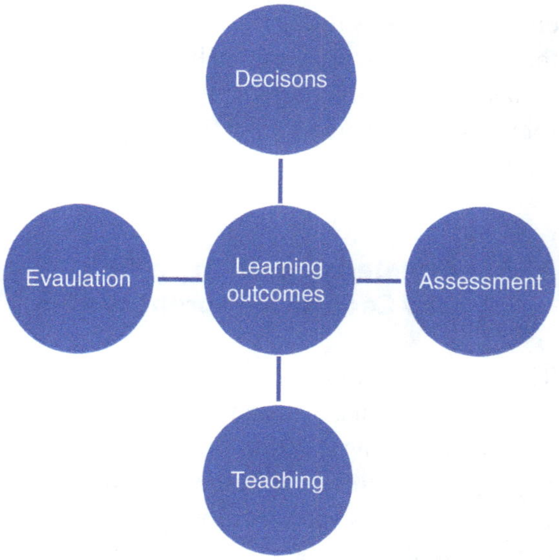

Fig. 21.3 Basic model of curriculum development (used with permission L. Kelly)

achieved. The teaching, learning and assessment strategies that we participate in must engage in a scholarly manner. To prevent surface teaching, ensure that:

- Learning outcomes are achievable.
- Levels and standards expected at various stages are clearly defined.
- Learning tasks and assessment are aligned.

21.5 Learning Outcomes/ Alignment to Assessment Methods

In terms of vascular access insertion education, examples of learning outcomes (LO) and how they can be aligned are provided below:

LO: *Demonstrate* knowledge of the physiology of blood flow and its importance in device and vein selection.

- Teaching centred on theory, self-directed study and practical sessions using ultrasound.
- Assess knowledge using a variety of methods, e.g. discussion with mentor, written work and diagrammatical explanation, during a patient assessment.

LO: *Critically discuss* the pathophysiology of thrombosis formation, Virchow's triad and how it is affected by vascular access device selection, insertion technique and location.

- Teaching would be didactic, self-directed study (reading) and practical teaching using ultrasound.
- Assess learning outcome by requiring a written piece of work. This allows student to formulate arguments and develop critical analysis skills.

LO: *Demonstrate* a skilful, successful ultrasound-guided vein puncture.

- Teaching would involve supervised practice, theory and practice in clinical practice or simulation using part-task phantoms and videos.
- As a practical skill, assess learning outcome using formal visual assessment by the mentor. This could either be done using part-task simulation or direct observation of an insertion procedure.

LO: *Identifies and explains* the signs and symptoms of arterial puncture and explains immediate interventions.

- Teaching would take place during didactic session, self-directed study (reading) and reflection.
- Assess learning outcome prior to hands-on practice. The assessment could involve discussions with the mentor and could also include some written work to allow for a complete assessment of knowledge and understanding.

21.6 Clinical Competence: Demonstration, Assessment and Evaluation

The validation of competency can have a direct impact on patient outcomes. In fact, in today's healthcare, patients expect competent care (Carney and Bistline 2008). Once competency has been acquired, assessment and evaluation of competency is necessary. There are a variety of ways in which clinical competency is demonstrated, assessed and evaluated. However, the most common method of assessing clinical competence is with competency assessment tools (Franklin and Melville 2015). Competency assessment tools have been in use for many years now, particularly within undergraduate programmes (Harris et al. 2010). To ensure that clinical assessments tools accurately measure the competence of learners, it is imperative that the tool be both reliable and valid:

- **Validity**—The degree to which a measure assesses what it was intended to measure.
- **Reliability**—The degree to which a score of other measure remains unchanged upon test and retest (when no change is expected).

The evaluation method must also be objective, observable and measurable. Therefore, it is imperative that those performing the evaluations be trained in using methods such as rater reliability studies that ensure consistency or test/retest which is a straightforward way of testing the stability or reliability of something. Global rating scales also allow for some degree of consistency in vascular access device insertion. The individual performing the evaluation has a vital role and must ensure the evaluation is performed the same way each time with no variation (Hyrkäs and Shoemaker 2007). It is suggested that standardised documentation for evaluation is useful to help increase compliance with guidelines. Competency should be measurable and evaluated regularly to ensure positive patient outcomes. Competency assessments should, whenever possible, reflect real-life situations such as that achieved in a simulation suite (Butler et al. 2011; Carney and Bistline 2008). It is usually recommended to use more than one assessment tool to produce as accurate an assessment as possible (Franklin and Melville 2015). The way in which competence can be evaluated is by direct observation either in the clinical setting or within simulated environments using part-task training arms.

One of the principal areas of concern regarding the use of clinical competency tools is that we often end up with a 'one-size-fits-all' document. Additionally, the documents produced are generally only able to measure the psychomotor aspects or the 'science' of a procedure but less able to assess the softer 'art' of nursing, such as intuition (Benner 1982). There are many considerations to consider when developing clinical assessment tools. The aim is to have a meaningful tool that is not just a tick box.

To gather this evidence of competence, Boritz and Carnaghan (2003) suggest that rather than a snap shot, the competency assessment be performed on multiple occasions, periodically and across a variety of contexts. The number of multi-faceted approaches to assessment is vast. Wilbeck in 2011 (Wilbeck et al. 2011) identified 11 methods of evaluating competency, namely:

- Benchmarking.
- Checklist evaluation.
- Global rating assessment.
- Simulation.
- Standardised patient.
- Observed Structured Clinical Examination (OSCE).
- Objective Structured Assessment of Technical Skills (OSATS).
- Peer review/rating.
- Portfolio.
- Procedure log.
- 360° evaluation.

21.7 Evaluating Staff Competence in Vascular Access Procedures

Following specific guidelines for vascular access, device insertion can reduce the risk of central line-associated bloodstream infections (Ciocson et al. 2014). Clinicians should adhere to standards and guidelines that have been proven to reduce and eliminate CLABSIs. According to the National Healthcare Safety Network, these standards include:

- Observation: Accountability to ensure inserter is following protocol.
- Experience and comfort of inserter: Inserter must have received special training to insert device.
- Reason for insertion: Is the access device necessary?
- Performance of hand hygiene prior to central line insertion: Basis for aseptic technique.
- Maximal sterile barrier precautions used: Keep sterile fields clear from contamination.
- Skin preparation: Kill bacteria prior to insertion to eliminate infection.
- Selection of insertion site: Healthy vasculature available to deliver therapy.
- Number of lumens: Use least number of lumens necessary to deliver therapy.

Insertion of a vascular access device is viewed as an evidence-based 'high-impact' intervention.

studied the effectiveness of the care bundle approach to reducing venous catheter-related complications in critical care. In this study, it was proven that adherence to the evidence-based recommendations from the Centre for Disease Control and Prevention (CDC) resulted in a significant decrease in catheter-related bloodstream infections. The low-level evidence base included the following interventions:

- Handwashing.
- Surgical-ANTT.
- Chlorhexidine skin prep.
- Minimise use of femoral approach.
- Remove device when no longer medically necessary.

These interventions led to a dramatic reduction in catheter-related bloodstream infections per 1000 days from 27 to 0 in 3 months. Following this study, a similar programme with an audit has since been rolled out internationally. Therefore, we know that the care bundle approach can be very effective, but compliance to the care bundle is required to ensure this outcome.

21.8 Evaluation of Competence: Focus on Vascular Access Care Bundles

Only after being deemed competent is a clinician allowed to perform device insertion without supervision. Often, a combination of methods is used to demonstrate competency. Many institutions continue to base competency on a required number of procedures performed. This approach has been challenged by ACGME, who suggests that it is not simply the number of procedures carried out that is important but that competency should be reviewed using a formal evaluation process. It has been suggested that competency be defined by the percentage of times in which successful independent skills performance is achieved and that an 80% to 90% success rate be required prior to independent device insertions.

Intermittent evaluation of the insertion procedure on a regular basis (e.g. annually) is required to ensure competency is maintained. In addition to device insertion, the day-to-day care and maintenance of the device should be carried out in a systematic and evidence-based fashion. Once again, evaluation of the care and maintenance on a regular basis is required to ensure all interventions are carried out.

Overall, competency in vascular access can be demonstrated by four competency assessment steps linking theory to practice:

1. Knowledge of the field of vascular access (devices, relevant anatomy and physiology, care and maintenance, prevention of complications, etc.)
2. Competence in techniques such as 'scrubbing the hub', effective flushing techniques.
3. Performance of skills such as ultrasound guidance, device insertion, etc.
4. Action (Ilic 2009).

In addition to knowledge, skills and attitudes, competence also includes the practitioner's problem-solving abilities, critical thinking skills, decision-making and reasoning skills, as well as excellent communication skills and the ability to work as an effective team member. All of these factors are taken into consideration when determining whether or not a clinician is competent to perform an insertion procedure alone.

Within vascular access, specific individual practices are known to improve care. When these practices are performed together as part of a care 'bundle', they produce a substantially greater improvement of care and reduction in infection rates than when performed indiscriminately. Following a group of practices such as an 'insertion bundle' or a 'care and maintenance' bundle ensures patient safety as well as successful implementation of the VHP framework.

A key principle of care bundles involves the level of adherence to the bundle; clinical variation should be avoided unless there is clinical indication for it, as the bundles have been established through evidence-based studies and are proven to reduce patient risks. Variation should never be the result of passive omission. Elements of the bundles should be implemented in every patient 100% of the time. Compliance of adherence to the bundle is of utmost importance. It must be assured that every step of the bundle is capable of being audited – it was completed, or it was not completed. Please note, the audit will only assess that the intervention was completed and not how well or poorly this was done. This information is often recorded in a simple tick box. If all aspects of the bundle are completed, it can be said that the care bundle has been completed. Occasionally, due to good reason such as patient allergy, aspects of a care bundle may be omitted. If there is not a good reason for omission of one or more steps in a care bundle, this can be seen as a failure of care.

21.9 How Can We Improve Compliance to Care Bundles?

- Validate evidence supporting bundle practices while making the information available to clinicians adopting the practices.
- Increase compliance with the introduction of care bundle checklists or end-of-bed charts.
- Make care bundle compliance part of a quality marker with the inclusion of a financial implication.

21.10 Lifelong Learning

In addition, as professionals we are responsible for continuously updating our practice and must now consider the notion of lifelong learning (Numminen et al. 2013). Adaptive practitioners should be committed to lifelong learning. Once a skill is acquired and competency met, there should be mechanisms put in place to ensure that competence is maintained, and the individual remains competent and therefore safe enough to continue to perform the procedure.

21.11 Summary

The right competency assessment ensures that practitioners are adequately prepared and safe to perform procedures or care for patients. Vascular access has changed vastly over the past two decades, and we are now aware of the many factors that ensure vessel health. The right approach to teaching and learning is the first step in this process. Following education, it is vital that the learning is assessed and that the right knowledge and skills have been gained. Competency is then achieved and validated using a recognised and effective method or tool. Finally, learning and competence should not be viewed as a one-off event; lifelong learning should become the norm.

Case Study

Jane French was delighted to be offered a staff nurse role within a busy vascular access service. One of the key roles would be to insert peripherally inserted central catheters (PICCs). Following her general orientation to the role, she began to focus on the procedure of device insertion.

Jane was given a competency document to guide her through the process. She was teamed up with a mentor, Oliver, who would act as her teacher and supervisor. She was instructed to approach any team member at any time with questions and queries if Oliver was unavailable.

Jane was supplied with an in-depth competency framework to guide her through her learning. This consisted of:

- Reading up on anatomy and physiology of arm veins as related to vascular access.
- Physiology of blood flow.
- Information on device selection.
- Patient assessment.
- Infection prevention and control.
- Ultrasound guidance.

- Device insertion techniques.
- ECG tip location device information and use.
- Complications (prevention, recognition and management).

Each of these sections contained reflective sections, further reading and questions to ensure learning had taken place.

In addition, Jane spent time in a simulation suite and put her learning into practice. With the use of part-task simulation, she gained practice and skills in:

- Ultrasound-guided venous access using phantoms.
- PICC insertion using a simulated model.
- Use of ECG tip location device.
- Dressing and flushing.

Once confident, she spent time working alongside Oliver, first, in an observational stance and then performing the procedure under supervision with Oliver scrubbed up with her. Jane reflected on each procedure performed and wrote this up in her competency document.

The number of supervised insertions was decided between Jane and Oliver, and this continued until Jane deemed herself competent and felt comfortable with the procedure and when Oliver agreed with her decision. The final competency sheet was signed by both parties to indicate competency had been attained.

Jane and Oliver continued to meet regularly and discuss her progress and to discuss any issues or concerns. Periodic competency assessment was integrated as part of the facility policies.

After 2 months, Jane was practising independently but continued to reflect and build her knowledge and skills in vascular access device insertion.

Summary of Key Points

1. Providing the right approach to teaching and learning is the first step in preparing competent practitioners.
2. Following education, it is vital that learning is assessed on a regular basis to ensure that the right knowledge and skills have been gained.
3. Competence assessment using a recognised and effective method or tool ensures that practitioners are adequately prepared to perform procedures or care for patients.
4. As professionals, we are responsible for continuously updating our practice. We therefore need to commit to lifelong learning. Learning and competence should not be viewed as a one-off event.

References

Benner P. From novice to expert. Am J Nurs. 1982;82:402–7. https://doi.org/10.1097/01.NUMA.0000313089.04519.f4.

Biggs J. Assessing for learning quality: II. Practice. In: Teaching for quality learning at University; 1999. p. 165–203. https://doi.org/10.1097/00005176-200304000-00028.

Boritz JE, Carnaghan CA. Competency-based education and assessment for the accounting profession: a critical review*. Can Account Perspect. 2003;2(1):7–42. https://doi.org/10.1506/5K7C-YT1H-0G32-90K0.

Bradley P. The history of simulation in medical education and possible future directions. Med Educ. 2006;40:254–62. https://doi.org/10.1111/j.1365-2929.2006.02394.x.

Butler MP, Cassidy I, Quillinan B, Fahy A, Bradshaw C, Tuohy D, O'Connor M, Mc Namara MC, Egan G, Tierney C. Competency assessment methods—tool and processes: a survey of nurse preceptors in Ireland. Nurse Educ Pract. 2011;11(5):298–303. https://doi.org/10.1016/j.nepr.2011.01.006.

Caldwell L, Grobbel C. The importance of reflective practice in nursing. Int J Caring Sci. 2013;6(3):319–26. International Journal of Caring Sciences September–December 2013; Vol 6 Issue 3.

Carney DM, Bistline B. Validating nursing competencies using a fair format. J Nurs Staff Dev.

2008;24(3):124–8. https://doi.org/10.1097/01.NND.0000300881.48802.b7.

Ciocson MAFR, Hernandez GM, Atallah M, Amer SY. Central vascular access device: an adapted evidence-based clinical practice guideline. J Assoc Vasc Access. 2014;19(4):221–37. https://doi.org/10.1016/j.java.2014.09.002.

Collins A, Greeno JG. Situated view of learning. In: International encyclopedia of education; 2010. p. 335–9. https://doi.org/10.1016/B978-0-08-044894-7.00504-2.

Denton A. Standards for infusion therapy. Royal College of Nursing; 2016. p. 41 t/m 42. Publication code: 005704.

Franklin N, Melville P. Competency assessment tools: an exploration of the pedagogical issues facing competency assessment for nurses in the clinical environment. Collegian. 2015;22(1):25–31. https://doi.org/10.1016/j.colegn.2013.10.005.

Harris P, Snell L, Talbot M, Harden RM. Competency-based medical education: implications for undergraduate programs. Med Teach. 2010;32(8):646–50. https://doi.org/10.3109/0142159X.2010.500703.

Hulse AL. Clinical competency assessment in intravenous therapy and vascular access: part 2. Br J Nurs. 2013;22(17):1008–13. https://doi.org/10.12968/bjon.2013.22.17.1008.

Hyrkäs K, Shoemaker M. Changes in the preceptor role: re-visiting preceptors' perceptions of benefits, rewards, support and commitment to the role. J Adv Nurs. 2007;60(5):513–24.

Ilic D. Assessing competency in evidence based practice: strengths and limitations of current tools in practice. BMC Med Educ. 2009;9(1):53. https://doi.org/10.1186/1472-6920-9-53.

Jamison RJ, Hovancsek MT, Clochesy JM. A pilot study assessing simulation using two simulation methods for teaching intravenous cannulation. Clin Simul Nurs. 2006;2(1):9–12. https://doi.org/10.1016/j.ecns.2009.05.007.

Kelly LJ, Green A, Hainey K. Implementing a new teaching and learning strategy for CVAD care. Br J Nurs. 2015;24(8):S4–8, S9, S12. https://doi.org/10.12968/bjon.2015.24.Sup8.S4.

Kolb D. David A. Kolb on experiential learning. 1983. www.infed.org/biblio/b-explrn.htm. https://doi.org/10.1177/0255761407088489.

Kotsis SV, Chung KC. Application of see one, do one, teach one concept in surgical training. Plast Reconstr Surg. 2013;131(5):1194–201. https://doi.org/10.1097/PRS.0b013e318287a0b3.

McLeod S. Bruner—learning theory in education | simply psychology. Simply Psychology. 2012. http://www.simplypsychology.org/bruner.html.

Moureau N, Lamperti M, Kelly LJ, Dawson R, Elbarbary M, Van Boxtel AJH, Pittiruti M. Evidence-based consensus on the insertion of central venous access devices: definition of minimal requirements for training. Br J Anaesth. 2013;110(3):347–56. https://doi.org/10.1093/bja/aes499.

Numminen O, Meretoja R, Isoaho H, Leino-Kilpi H. Professional competence of practising nurses. J Clin Nurs. 2013;22(9–10):1411–23. https://doi.org/10.1111/j.1365-2702.2012.04334.x.

Onda EL. Situated cognition: its relationship to simulation in nursing education. Clin Simul Nurs. 2012;8(7):e273–80. https://doi.org/10.1016/j.ecns.2010.11.004.

Quinn F. Curriculum theory and practice. In: Principles and practice of nurse education; 2000. p. 131–51. http://medcontent.metapress.com/index/A65RM03P4874243N.pdf%5Cn; http://books.google.com/books?hl=en&lr=&id=qILGb7xcXFIC&oi=fnd&pg=PP1&dq=Curriculum+theory+and+practice&ots=MuS4sZlKmu&sig=2-a0BmsV34nUfqpi4pFMsFxDSgU.

Wacquant L. Cognition in practice: mind, mathematics, and culture in everyday life. Actes de la recherche en sciences sociales. 1992; https://doi.org/10.2307/2073537.

Wilbeck J, Murphy M, Heath J, Thomson-Smith C. Evaluation methods for the assessment of acute care nurse practitioner inserted central lines: evidence-based strategies for practice. J Assoc Vasc Access. 2011;16(4):226–33. https://doi.org/10.2309/java.16-4-5.

22

Products, Equipment and Devices: A Study of Evaluation Processes

Linda J. Kelly

Abstract

The global medical device market is worth billions. In fact, a new report by the independent media company Visiongain predicts that the global medical devices market will reach $398 billion in 2017. In the field of infusion and vascular access, there is an enormous range of products, supplies, equipment and instruments available. The right evaluation of a product is necessary to test the clinical application, expected outcomes, performance, infection prevention, safety, efficacy, reliability and cost of these new products. Facts gained from product evaluations provide vital information that will either support the introduction of the product or provide reasons to reject it. Effective, well-informed product evaluation and purchasing can prove to ensure best patient outcomes, reduce rising costs or, in the best-case scenario, offer a balance of these two outcomes.

Keywords

Product evaluation · Purchasing decisions · Product evaluation form · Product evaluation process · Goals for product evaluation

L. J. Kelly (✉)
Edinburgh Napier University, School of Health and Social Care, Edinburgh, UK

22.1 Introduction

Product evaluation is a fundamental component in the promotion of patient safety requiring a structured, multidisciplinary approach to ensure effectiveness. It is important that clinical end users are involved in the evaluation of infusion and vascular access-related technologies as they are the best qualified to evaluate the performance, safety, effectiveness and efficiency of products used in their clinical area or healthcare setting (Philips 2017). A clinical evaluation should not be a discrete event, but rather, part of an ongoing process conducted throughout the life of a medical device, from initial product design and development, to regulatory review and approval, and finally, throughout product use once placed on the market.

This chapter provides general information about the evaluation of products, equipment and devices. It provides guidance for the evaluation process, discusses who should be involved in the evaluation, what to do with findings from the evaluation and the role of manufacturers in the evaluation process.

22.2 Product Evaluation

The reasons for introducing new products into the workplace are multiple and include replacing products no longer available, standardization across organizations, meeting the request or need of clinicians, cost-saving initiatives and attempts to improve patient and staff safety through improving patient outcomes. Emerging technologies have also led to the development of new products that require evaluation prior to adoption. In recent decades, there have been major advances in medical technologies. These advances have had a positive impact on patient outcomes by improving diagnoses and enabling more effective treatments (Burns et al. 2007). These advances do not come without a cost, and therefore we must be certain that decisions regarding the introduction of innovative technologies, devices, equipment and supplies are well evaluated.

In current times, a plethora of infusion and vascular access products are available, and there is a need to ensure that evidence is available to support the introduction or change of product. This is important due to the competition for limited finances, which is often fierce. Within the field of vascular access, we have seen such growth of new and innovative products. Many of these new products promise to improve patient outcomes by reducing infections or occlusions. There are also products, devices and equipment that claim to increase safety for both staff and patients and finally those that will improve the success of device insertion. As with any product, efforts should be made to validate claims within the specific facility and practice through product evaluation and trialling prior to final adoption. Even after adoption, a plan to follow-up by checking compliance and performance is needed to prove continued value and need for a product. The following section will provide an overview of some of these innovative products.

22.3 Emerging Technologies in Intravenous Therapy and Vascular Access

As we are aware, vascular access devices are utilized for most types of intravenous therapy and provide reliable access in most healthcare settings. With the development of healthcare technology, easier and safer insertion techniques and a greater selection of devices to choose from, the number of vascular access devices on the market continues to grow. Apart from the obvious groups of devices (peripheral venous cannula, extended dwell cannula, midline and peripherally inserted central catheter, tunnelled central venous catheter and totally implanted port), each of these devices can be further categorized as they are designed in numerous ways and with varying designs:

- Materials such as polyurethane or silicone.
- Can have valves incorporated or remain open ended (tapered or non-tapered).
- Can be impregnated with silver, antibiotics, etc.
- Introduction of safety devices.

Because of the range of devices available, there is often a selection of similar devices with differing design and materials available in a single organization. To improve patient safety and to reduce any potential risk, the decision is often made to standardize products.

22.3.1 Dressings

Once a vascular access device is inserted, the aim is for it to remain in situ for the treatment period. The consequences of a failed or dislodged catheter include interruption of medical treatment and the need for a replacement vascular access device which comes with potential insertion complications and possible negative patient experience (Robinson-Reilly et al. 2016). The purpose of a dressing is to:

- Protect the site from microbial contamination from the surrounding skin and environment.
- Prevent dislodgement.
- Prevent micromotion within the vein which increases the risk of phlebitis (Ullman et al. 2016).

The range and design of dressings has and continues to increase and now includes:

- Chlorhexidine-impregnated dressing.
- Sutureless securement devices (SSDs).

- Integrated securement devices (ISDs).
- Tissue adhesives, a medical grade super glue.

22.3.2 Needle-Free Connectors

Since their introduction, the range of needle-free connectors (NFCs) has exploded, and there is now a vast array of NFCs with various characteristics available. These numerous branded products also vary in their design and function (Kelly et al. 2017). The differences include:

- Visual appearance: Colour, shape, etc.
- Differences in internal mechanisms which are responsible for how the device functions.
- Presence of an integrated and extension line (single or multiple).
- Incorporation of valves and filters.
- Inclusion of occlusion management systems.

22.3.3 Port Cleaning Caps

Port cleaning or disinfecting caps are devices that offer an engineered solution to hub disinfection. Their use is aimed at reducing compliance of needle-free connector disinfection (Moureau and Flynn 2015; Cameron-Watson 2016). These caps are impregnated with a disinfection solution. The cap is placed on the hub of a needless connector and remains in place until the device is next accessed, allowing for standardization and compliance. Following use, the cap is discarded and a new one is then attached. The caps are available with various antimicrobial solutions including 70% alcohol, iodinated alcohol, povidone-iodine gauze and chlorhexidine/alcohol (Moureau and Flynn 2015).

22.3.4 Vein Visualization Technology

Ultrasound technology has been found to be invaluable in vascular access procedures, particularly for deep veins (Lamperti et al. 2012; Simon and Saad 2012). However, there is now a range of near-infrared devices available that are useful for peripheral cannulation of the more superficial veins (Kelly 2013; Lamperti and Pittiruti 2013). This technology is still relatively new, and although there have been some evaluations, to properly understand the potential benefits of this technology, further evaluations are necessary (Phipps et al. 2012).

22.3.5 Tip Location Devices

Historically, the tip of a PICC position was estimated by external landmarking and confirmed using a chest X-ray. The success rate of this technique remains variable between practitioners (Roldan and Paniagua 2015). Chest X-ray tip confirmation has also raised controversy in the literature (Plkwer 2008). Technologies to assist in tip guidance and location continue to evolve, and there are a wide range of such technologies now available. They rely on electrocardiology tracings, but once again, these products vary in design and function, and differences in products include:

- Inclusion of magnetics—external systems for locating tip position.
- ECG only technology without magnets.
- Doppler technology.

22.4 How Do We Decide Which Is the Right Product?

The selection and adoption of the right products involves a lot of effort, and decisions made must be fully justified. When faced with such a wide-range and diverse number of products, decision-making must be evidence-based, and product evaluation helps to provide practical evidence of the product in clinical situations. To be effective, product evaluations must be systematic and well planned. One way to ensure this is to set early goals and aims of what is expected from the evaluation. Examples of product goals include:

- To reduce the rate of occlusions.
- To reduce the rate of infections.
- To increase compliance.
- To save nursing hours.

Setting goals allows you to pinpoint and focus on the expected outcomes of the product introduction or change. Once the decision is made to introduce a new product, a structured approach should be taken to ensure that the process runs smoothly. This first step is to produce a written proposal of intent and to begin to explore the options that are available on the market.

22.5 Discovering New Products

Part of the role of practitioners in infusion and vascular access specialties is to be aware of the market and any new or innovative technologies emerging. There are a few ways in which we become aware of emerging technologies, and to do so effectively requires a thorough exploration of the market. Information can be obtained from an independent review of literature. Journal articles focusing on product evaluations and research papers provide invaluable information giving details of the outcomes of product use in practice (Jeanes and Bitmead 2015; Ventura et al. 2016; Barton et al. 2017). Conferences, study days and trade shows are also a fantastic arena for companies to display and demonstrate products. Detailed product brochures are often available and can be taken away for future perusal. A trade show or conference that is clinically focused and aimed at specific specialties such as intravenous access provides an ideal environment for the exploration of available products. In these settings, the ability to question the manufacturers and get hands-on demonstrations helps to narrow the field in the preliminary stages of product evaluation. Visits to other hospital sites currently using the product provides another way to gain information and to visualize the product in use. This sharing of experience and outcomes generally proves to be one of the most valuable evaluation stages.

22.6 The Right Evaluation Form

The use of an evaluation tool is vital to help standardize the evaluation. This tool should glean the following information:

- Does the product meet the objective?
- Does the product meet the need of the patient?
- Does the product solve a problem?
- Does the product prove cost-effective?
- Does the product improve patient care?
- Does the product compare with others?

The use of an evaluation tool encourages objective ratings in addition to make comparisons of comparable products. Again, the information gained from this stage of evaluation will narrow the field of suitable products and guide you toward the products that will eventually be included in the 'hands-on' evaluation. The general information detailed on the evaluation form includes:

- Name of product.
- Manufacturer.
- Name of evaluator.
- Date of evaluation.

The evaluation tool should subsequently focus on the product and gain more specific information. An example of an evaluation tool for a midline device is shown below.

22.7 Midline Catheter Evaluation

Product name:
Manufacturer:
Name of person completing evaluation: Designation:
Date of evaluation:

Features	Consideration	Comments
Packaging	Size: will the storage and discarding of the packaging be an issue? Is the product package easy to open? Can sterility be maintained easily during opening?	
Length	Are all necessary device lengths available?	
Lumen	Are all necessary Fr sizes available? Is it available in millilumen options?	

Material	Is the device radiopaque? Is the device power injectable? Is the device flexible on insertion? Does the device maintain its shape?	
Ease of insertion	Is the needle sharp? Does it have sharp safe features? Is the wire of an adequate length? Does the device advance smoothly? Is device securement easy to obtain?	
Product information	Is the information contained in the package clear and detailed?	

22.8 Who Is Involved in a Product Evaluation?

Evaluation is often performed on an 'ad hoc' basis without clear goals and objectives (Keselman et al. 2004). A team is created through the coordination of experts from various departments dependent on the device being evaluated. The process varies between hospitals and departments. Because the decision-making process for medical devices is very complex and subject to numerous constraints such as individual practitioner's choice, time and cost, the process of evaluation can be difficult at times. In addition to the functional aspects of devices, there exists another form of functionality referred to as 'soft functionality' (McDonagh et al. 2002). Soft functionality includes the emotional and other intangible, qualitative needs that affect the relationship of the user with the product. Soft functionality is a principal factor in the development of products and can have a bearing on the evaluation processes undertaken. Manufacturers are becoming keener to distinguishing their products from others and continue to explore innovative approaches to improve the symbolic dimensions of their products. One should be aware of their own emotions around products and how they 'feel' about them, as often the emotional needs of users are considered and exploited during the design of products (McDonagh et al. 2002). Group decision-making is imperative, and all stakeholders should have an input into product evaluation. This approach achieves goals that are beyond the range of one independent individual, as it is unlikely that one individual possesses the full skill set to allow a robust decision to be made. The evaluation team should be multidisciplinary and interdepartmental. Suggested members of this team include:

- End users.
- Infusion nurses.
- Nursing staff in areas that the products will be used.
- Medical staff.
- Infection control department.
- Pharmacy.
- Materials management.
- Purchasing/procurement department.
- Radiology physicians.
- Anaesthetic physicians.
- Biomedical department.
- Microbiology.
- Manufacturer.

Each of these committee members comes with a different agenda, be it costs, infection prevention or patients' safety. The purpose of this committee is to review all information gained from the preliminary evaluation using the evaluation tool. The committee acts as an end reviewer for product decisions, considers the qualities of each of the products and assesses the range available. Finally, the committee is responsible to either endorse or deny product selection, introduction or replacement.

22.9 Working with Manufacturers During Evaluation

The support of manufacturers during evaluations is invaluable. If any issues occur during evaluation of a product, the manufacturer should be responsive and offer help, advice and support. Many manufacturers now offer 'added-value' services. This means that rather than a focus only on product sales, clinical support by specialist clinicians is part of the service offered. This approach gives companies a competitive advantage (Trombetta 2010) as advice and support is delivered on site and helps to ensure correct use of products during the evaluation process. Many hospitals now see this added value as essential and recognize a level of dependence on them during evaluation processes.

22.10 Right Evaluation Process

Establish a clear timeframe during which an evaluation will take place; the length of time should be confirmed and agreed upon in advance. Decide as to where the evaluation will take place. Will this be in one department or clinical setting or across several settings? Introduce the evaluation tool to the evaluators, and explain the importance of detailed completion of the forms to all involved. Evaluation should provide feedback from all stakeholders and members of a team that will be using it. Additionally, ensure that individuals of the evaluation team have effective training regarding the use of the product to ensure correct use of the product or device and a more robust and meaningful evaluation. Ideally, the training is provided by the manufactures who are familiar with the products and take place as close to the evaluation commencement date as possible. Following the evaluation process, the results are collated, and findings are disseminated to the committee. Details of the chosen product should be communicated to all necessary individuals. Following introduction of the product, provide training to all practitioners who will be involved with its use. Thereafter, continuous evaluation of the product is imperative.

22.11 Conclusion

The number and range of products available within the field of vascular access continues to expand. New and innovative products that aim to reduce infections, prevent occlusions and improve patient safety are plentiful. To ensure the most suitable products are on our shelves, we must ascertain that the right evaluation of products is undertaken. The aim of product evaluation is multifaceted and includes identifying products and devices that meet specific performance outcomes, are safe for both patients and staff, ensure positive patient outcomes and are cost-effective for all stakeholders (Ventola 2008).

Case Study

Staff nurse Ricky Goldsworth attended a local Vascular Access Conference. One of the presentations involved a nurse practitioner discussing the introduction of a new vascular access device into her department. The presenter explained that, due to the design of the product, it was successfully dwelling for longer periods of time than traditional peripheral cannulas. She presented impressive audit results that demonstrated cost savings and, more importantly, an improved patient experience. This was the first time that Ricky had heard about such a device but was impressed with the results that had been presented. Ricky approached the presenter during the tea break and spoke a bit more about the devices. He found out that some of the companies that made the devices were exhibiting at the conference. He visited the appropriate stands and discussed the products with the company sales executives. He also picked up information on the product that he could take with him and read at his own convenience.

Once back at work, Ricky sat down with his manager and told her about the device. She asked him to write a proposal detailing how introducing the device might improve practice and patient care. She advised him to conduct an audit to determine what the situation was at present. This would give them a baseline to work from and evidence to show that change was required. She also gave him support to go and visit the nurse who had presented at the conference. This would give him a better insight into the product in practice.

Ricky wrote his proposal, provided published evidence and argued that introducing the devices could:

- Save money.
- Save time.
- Improve the patient experience.
- Potentially reduce infectious complications.

After the proposal was submitted, a multidisciplinary group was set up to commence an evaluation. An evaluation tool was developed to cover all required key points.

Devices from two companies that fit the criteria were included in the evaluation. A timeframe of 1 month was set for the evaluation. The evaluation took place in one ward area only. Full training was provided to key members of staff prior to the evaluation date.

Following the evaluation period, results were collated and discussed by the committee. The evaluation was successful and very positive. One product scored more highly than the others, and this device was selected as the most appropriate to purchase.

Subsequent training was rolled out ward by ward and department by department. Audit was continued and will continue to ensure the product remains effective and complication free.

Summary of Key Points

1. Clinical end users should be involved in the evaluation of infusion and vascular access-related technologies as they are the best qualified to evaluate the performance, safety, effectiveness and efficiency of products used in their clinical area or healthcare setting.
2. When possible, published evidence on performance of a product should be included in the product evaluation.
3. To ensure a successful product evaluation, before commencement, ensure there are clear goals and objectives set and that there is a multidisciplinary/interdepartmental evaluation team in place.
4. Effective, well-informed product evaluation and purchasing can prove to ensure best patient outcomes.

References

Barton A, Ventura R, Vavrik B. Peripheral intravenous cannulation: protecting patients and nurses. Br J Nurs. 2017;26(8):S28–33. https://doi.org/10.12968/bjon.2017.26.8.S28.

Burns LR, Bradlow ET, Lee JA, Antonacci A. No title. Int J Technol Assess Healthc. 2007;23(4):445–63.

Cameron-Watson C. Port protectors in clinical practice: an audit. Br J Nurs. 2016;25(8):S25–31. https://doi.org/10.12968/bjon.2016.25.8.S25.

Jeanes A, Bitmead J. Reducing bloodstream infection with a chlorhexidine gel IV dressing. Br J Nurs. 2015;24(19):S14–9. https://doi.org/10.12968/bjon.2015.24.Sup19.S14.

Kelly LJ. Vascular access: viewing the vein. Br J Nurs. 2013;22(19 Suppl):S16–8. https://doi.org/10.12968/bjon.2013.22.Sup19.S16.

Kelly LJ, Jones T, Kirkham S. Keeping the system closed. Br J Nurs. 2017;26(2):S14–9. IV Therapy Supplement.

Keselman A, Tang X, Patel VL, Johnson TR, Zhang J. Institutional decision-making for medical device purchasing: evaluating patient safety. Stud Health Technol Inform. 2004;107(Pt 2):1357–61. D040004983 [pii].

Lamperti M, Pittiruti M. II. Difficult peripheral veins: turn on the lights. Br J Anaesth. 2013;110(6):888–91. https://doi.org/10.1093/bja/aet078.

Lamperti M, Bodenham AR, Pittiruti M, Blaivas M, Augoustides JG, Elbarbary M, Pirotte T, Karakitsos D, Ledonne J, Doniger S, Scoppettuolo G, Feller-Kopman D, Schummer W, Biffi R, Desruennes E, Melniker LA, Verghese ST. International evidence-based recommendations on ultrasound-guided vascular access. Intens Care Med. 2012;38:1105–17. https://doi.org/10.1007/s00134-012-2597-x.

McDonagh D, Bruseberg A, Haslam C. Visual product evaluation: exploring users' emotional relationships with products. Appl Ergon. 2002;33(3):231–40. https://doi.org/10.1016/S0003-6870(02)00008-X.

Moureau NL, Flynn J. Disinfection of needleless connector hubs: clinical evidence systematic review. Nurs Res Pract. 2015;2015:796762. https://doi.org/10.1155/2015/796762.

Philips N. Berry & Kohn's operating room technique. 12th ed. Ohio: Elsevier; 2017.

Phipps K, Modic A, O'Riordan MA, Walsh M. A randomized trial of the vein viewer versus standard technique for placement of peripherally inserted central catheters (PICCs) in neonates. J Perinatol. 2012;32:498–501. https://doi.org/10.1038/jp.2011.129.

Plkwer A. Does the position of the central venous catheter tip matter? Int J Intens Care. 2008;15(4):120–3. http://www.embase.com/search/results?subaction=viewrecord&from=export&id=L354396138

Robinson-Reilly M, Paliadelis P, Cruickshank M. Venous access: the patient experience. Support Care Cancer. 2016;24(3):1181–7. https://doi.org/10.1007/s00520-015-2900-9.

Roldan CJ, Paniagua L. Central venous catheter intravascular malpositioning: causes, prevention, diagnosis, and correction. West J Emerg Med. 2015;16(5):658–64. https://doi.org/10.5811/westjem.2015.7.26248.

Simon PO, Saad WE. Ultrasound-guided vascular access. Ultrasound Clin. 2012;7(3):283–97. https://doi.org/10.1016/j.cult.2012.04.001.

Trombetta B. Category captain management: an idea whose time has come in the pharmaceutical industry? Int J Pharmaceut Healthc Market. 2010;4(2):157–74. https://doi.org/10.1108/17506121011059768.

Ullman AJ, Kleidon T, Gibson V, Long DA, Williams T, McBride CA, Hallahan A, Mihala G, Cooke M, Rickard CM. Central venous access device SeCurement and Dressing Effectiveness (CASCADE) in paediatrics: protocol for pilot randomised controlled trials. BMJ Open. 2016;6(6):1–9. https://doi.org/10.1136/bmjopen-2016-011197.

Ventola CL. Challenges in evaluating and standardizing medical devices in health care facilities. P & T. 2008;33(6):348–59.

Ventura R, O'Loughlin C, Vavrik B. Clinical evaluation of a securement device used on midline catheters. Br J Nurs. 2016;25(14):S16–22. https://doi.org/10.12968/bjon.2016.25.14.S16.

Appendix

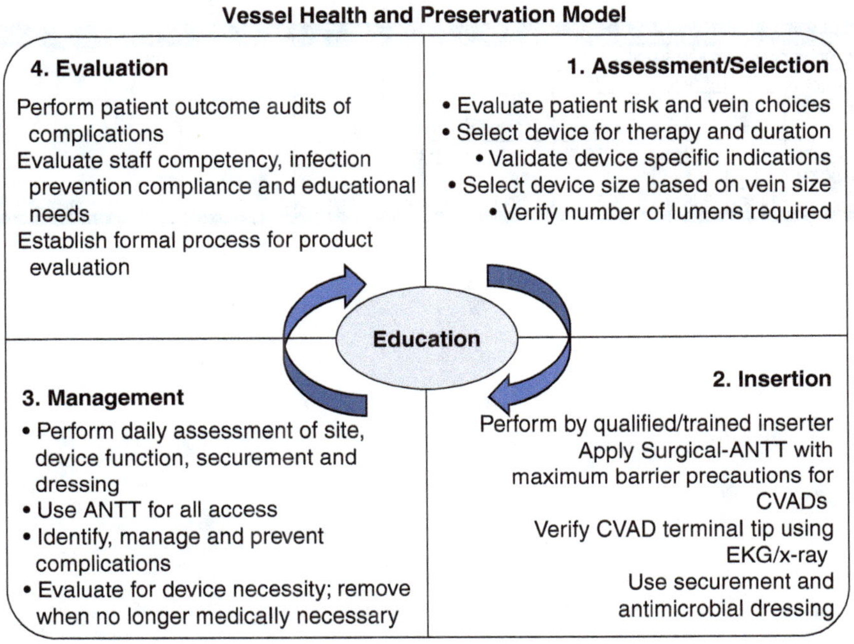

Fig. A.1 Vessel health and preservation: four quadrants of care (used with permission from N. Moureau (PICC Excellence)

CATHETER/VEIN SCALE

Chart for determining catheter size/length versus appropriate vein diameter and depth from ultrasound assessment

Peripheral vascular access devices

PICC Excellence, Inc.

FRENCH SIZE	2	2.5	3	3.5	4	4.5	5	5.5	6	7	8
CATHETER GAUGE SIZE	24	22	20	19	18	17	16	15	14		12
CATHETER MEASUREMENT mm	0.55	0.75	0.9	1.06	1.27	1.47	1.65	1.8	2.1	2.3	2.7
INCHES	0.022	0.026	0.0355	0.042	0.05	0.058	0.065	0.072	0.083	0.092	0.105
VESSEL SIZE needed 1/3 vs 2/3 catheter to blood flow. French size is desired vein size	2mm	2.5mm	3mm	3.5mm	4mm	4.5mm	5mm	5.5mm	6mm	7mm	8mm

INS RECOMMENDATION for 2/3 catheter in vein

DEPTH using 45 degrees	0.25	0.5	.75	1.0	1.25	1.5
CATHETER LENGTH needed	1.2cm	2cm	3.2cm	4.25cm	5.25	6.4cm
DEPTH using 30 degrees	0.25	0.5	.75	1.0	1.25	1.5
CATHETER LENGTH needed	1.5cm	3cm	4.5cm	6cm	7.5cm	8cm

www.piccexcellence.com

Vessel Health and Preservation Protocol
Right Patient Tool – Risk Factors

Directions: Check all that apply.
These risk factors may require a referral or a consult for a vascular access specialist to place indicated device.

Stage 1:

Patient conditions require clinician to use care with skin access, vein selection, and catheter size determination.

- ❑ Elderly skin/loss of elasticity
- ❑ Abrasions
- ❑ Psoriasis, skin breakdown
- ❑ Rash or allergies
- ❑ Long-term steroid use
- ❑ Small peripheral veins accommodating 22g or smaller while still allowing 50% space around catheter
- ❑ Diabetes
- ❑ History of cancer treatment to peripheral veins
- ❑ Dehydration or fluid restrictions
- ❑ Malnutrition

These conditions are known to commonly require multiple restarts. Any patient requiring 2 or more restarts within 24 hours should automatically be referred to Stage 2 and a vascular access consultation.

Stage 2:

Patient conditions require extra care and referral to Vascular Access Specialist for consultation.

- ❑ High volume fluid needs: blood or blood by-products, intravenous medications, antibiotics, pain meds, TPN/PPN, chemotherapy, inotropes, other types (list not inclusive)
- ❑ Limited peripheral access due to single side mastectomy, chest or neck surgery, amputation of arms, infection, cellulitis, fistula, trauma or Injury, burns, hematomas, obesity >250lbs
- ❑ Circulatory status: Stroke, hemiparesis, thrombosis to upper extremity, sign of illegal drug use, elevated INR, fistulas or shunts, severe dehydration or edema/fluid overload, DVT
- ❑ Previous complications: presence of CVC, frequent IV restarts, history of poor access, hourly blood draws, required central line access in past
- ❑ Critical factors: Acuity, life sustaining infusions, inotropes, unstable cardiac status, confirmed MI, arrhythmia, respiratory compromise
- ❑ Pediatric patient: less than 8 years old, child with high activity level (Pediatric specialist)
- ❑ Creatinine levels >2.0. Requiring nephrologist OK prior to PICC line placement.

Do not attempt to place device yourself. Refer to Vascular Access Specialist for consultation and placement.

Stage 3:

Patient conditions require clinician to refer patient to Interventional Radiology or Surgeon for placement of any vascular access device.

- ❑ History of radiology access placement
- ❑ Renal failure requiring Dialysis catheter
- ❑ Upper extremity DVT

Do not attempt to place device yourself. Refer to Interventional Radiology or Surgeon for placement.

Vessel Health and Preservation Protocol Right Line Contraindication Tool

Place patient label here

Use this tool to determine any risk factors or contraindications that may prevent use of the "right line" as determined by **PAGE 1** of the Right Line Tool.

PIV INDICATED UNLESS:	Choose this device instead
❑ Infection, injury or surgery that interferes with access	Internal Jugular or CVC
❑ Meds/fluids that are known irritants	PICC
❑ Continuous infusion of vesicant meds	PICC
❑ Meds as chemotherapeutic agents	PICC
❑ Thrombosis/Clots	CVC
❑ Mastectomy (same side)	CVC
❑ Peripheral neuropathy	Internal Jugular

PIV INDICATED UNLESS:	Choose this device instead
❑ Therapy required for > 4 weeks	PICC
❑ Irritating or vesicant medications	PICC
❑ Fluids that exceed 900mOsm	PICC
❑ Vancomycin is considered an irritant	PICC
❑ Thrombosis/Clots	CVC

PIV INDICATED UNLESS:	Choose this device instead
❑ Thrombosis, peripheral neuropathy, circulatory impairment	CVC
❑ Cellulitis, injury to one or both arms	CVC
❑ History of CVA, mastectomy, upper extremity fistulas	CVC
❑ Fistula; Renal Failtue or Creatinine >2.0	Internal Jugular

PIV INDICATED UNLESS:	Choose this device instead
❑ Elevated INR	Reconsider PICC or PIV
❑ Central or deep vein thrombosis (DVT)	Reconsider PICC or PIV
❑ Low platelet level (<50,000)	Reconsider PICC or PIV
❑ Critical status of patient exceeds risk	Reconsider PICC or PIV
❑ Ventilator	Reconsider PICC or PIV
❑ Tracheotomy	Reconsider PICC or PIV
❑ Existing Dialysis Catheter	PIV hand vein or Internal Jugular
❑ Elevated Creatinine >2.0	Internal Jugular

TIPS

- **Always use the smallest device that will administer treatment.**
- **Use the least number of lumens, single when possible.**
- **Consider vein size and catheter size to fit without tourniquet.**
- **Total size of the catheter lumen should not exceed 50% of the vein size.**
- **Each morning complete Daily Assessment for VHP to determine IV device necessity.**
- **Remove IV devices as soon as possible (ASAP).**
- **During ANTT cleanse hubs with frictional scrub before each access to prevent contamination.**
- **When any cap is removed from a catheter or intravenous tubing always apply a sterile cap, never reuse same cap.**
- **Flush all intravenous devices well (10-20ml) after any blood draws.**

❑ No Contraindications present ❑ Device Contraindicated ❑ Device Contraindicated ____________________

Person determining contraindication of device: ______________________________

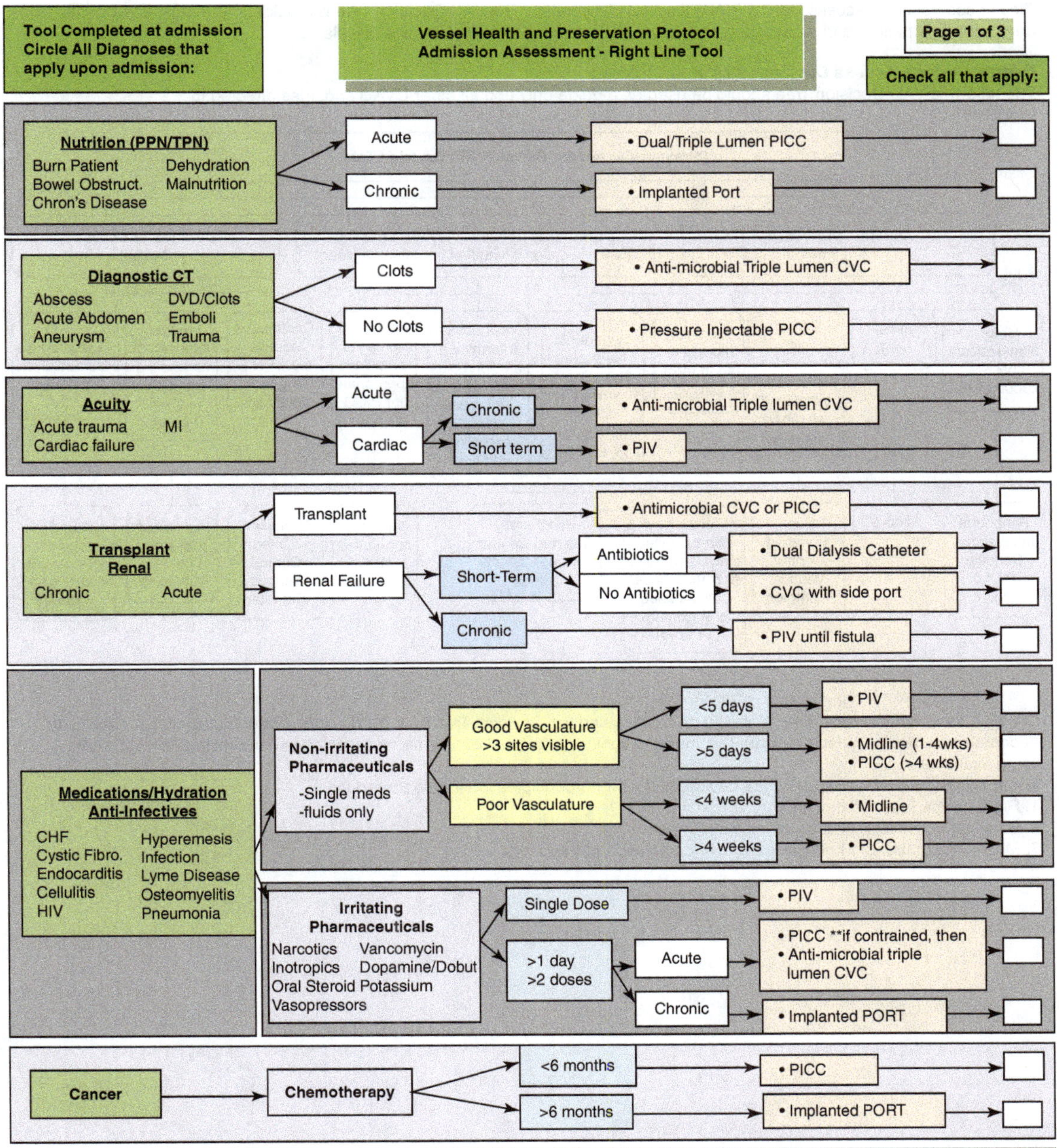

Circle device indicated. ***If more than one box checked, choose the device that most safely delivers **ALL** required infusions with lowest risk. Device indicated should be placed within 24 hours of admission.

****Refer to contraindications tool (page2) to confirm device****

Vascular Access Device indicated according to protocol: ______________________________

Name of Clinician performing assessment: ______________________________ Date: ____________

Scope of protocol: this order set pertains to patients admitted at any portal of hospital entry for purposes of initiating venous access and management for the duration of the hospitalization.

****** See Page 2 Right Line Contraindication Tool to confirm device******

Please see Vascular Access Device (VAD) Decision Tree below. The VAD Decision Tree is a guide to the most appropriate device for your patient and should guide device selection when VAMS NP is not available.

Central Venous Access Devices (CVAD) in Children

The following VAD Decision Tree should be used as a guide only and all other CVAD enquiries directed to VAMS NP

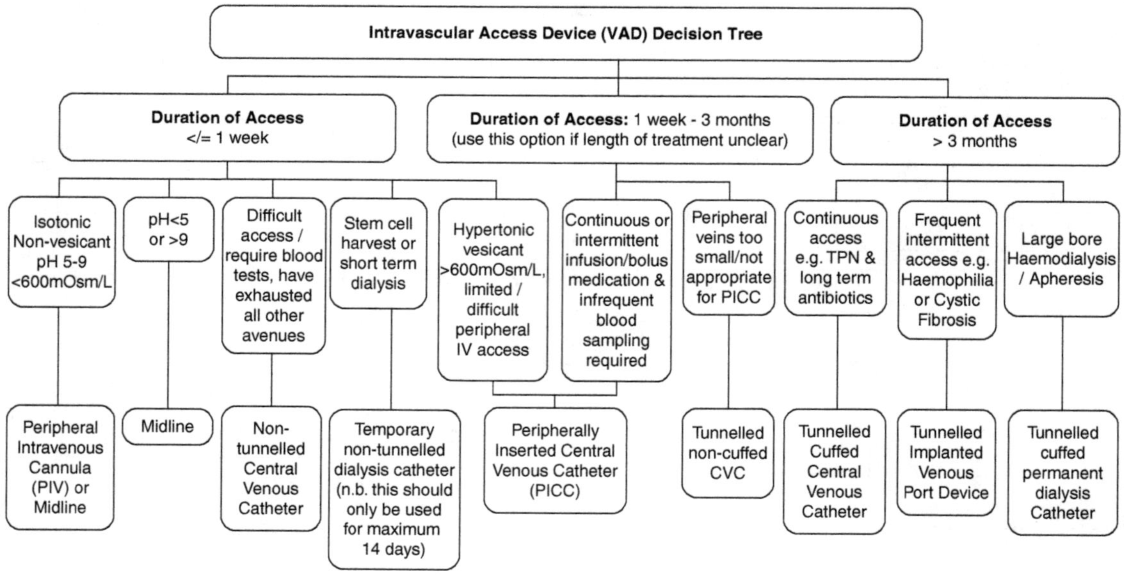

Decision for venous access device should be made using the Decision Tree as a **guide only**. For complex cases, especially neonatal lines, device selection should be made in conjuction with all clinical teams involved in care, including VAMS NP when available.

When choosing the most appropriate device the following principles must be adhered to:

1. Right device inserted first time
2. Smallest possible device for completion of treatment
3. Minimum number of lumens required for completion of treatment

Daily Vessel Health Assessment Tool

Patient Medical ID #: ______________________ **Date:** ____ / ____ / ______
dd mm yyyy

Nursing Information

1. How comfortable is the patient with their vascular access device? (ask the patient)
   - ☐ 5 - Extremely comfortable ☐ 2 - Somewhat uncomfortable
   - ☐ 4 - Somewhat comfortable ☐ 1 - Very uncomfortable
   - ☐ 3 - Comfortable ☐ N/A due to confusion /sedation or other ______________

   If #2 or #1 checked, please explain the reason for discomfort: ______________

2. What is the current device(s)? (check all that apply)

Type:	☐ PIV	☐ Midline	☐ PICC	☐ CVC	☐ Port	☐ Dialysis	
Number of Lumens		☐ 1	☐ 2	☐ 3	Which Device?	☐ PICC	☐ CVC
No. of Lumens in Use		☐ 1	☐ 2	☐ 3	Which Device?	☐ PICC	☐ CVC

3. What complications, if any occurred within the last 24 hours (PIV)? (check all that apply)
   - ☐ Infiltration ☐ Multiple restarts in 24 hrs
   - ☐ Phlebitis/thrombophlebitis ☐ Infection ☐ Other ______________

4. Did any complications occur within the last 24 hours with Central Venous Access Device(s)? ☐ Yes ☐ No
   If Yes, check all that apply. Which Device? ☐ PIV ☐ Midline ☐ PICC ☐ CVC ☐ Port ☐ Dialysis
   - ☐ Infection ☐ Phlebitis ☐ Occlusion
   - ☐ Partial Withdrawal Occlusion ☐ Thrombosis ☐ Other

5. Is this patient having any difficulty with eating and drinking? ☐ Yes ☐ No
6. Are there IV medications ordered other than PRN? ☐ Yes ☐ No
7. Is the VAD absolutely necessary for blood draws with this patient? ☐ Yes ☐ No

Nursing Recommendation: **Print Name:** ______________ RN/NP/PA/IVRN (circle)

8. Referring to the VHP Right Line Tool is the venous access device(s) most appropriate for the current treatment plan? ☐ Yes ☐ No

   If No, What device would apply based on Right Line Tool Selection? ______________

9. Is there any reason to maintain the current device(s)? ☐ Yes ☐ No
   If Yes, (other than the above reason) Why? ______________

RECOMMENDATIONS:
- ☐ Discontinue device(s) ☐ Maintain device(s)
- ☐ Consider new device(s) from VHP Assessment Trifold Recommended new device(s) ______________

Physician/Pharmacist Info: **Print Name:** ______________ MD/PharmD (circle)
(Information can be obtained by interview or by phone)

10. Would switch to all oral medications be contraindicated at this time for this patient? ☐ Yes ☐ No
11. Is there an active blood stream infection? ☐ Yes ☐ No
12. Will access be required once the patient is released? ☐ Yes ☐ No
13. What is the current discharge plan? # of days left
14. Is the current IV device still necessary for this treatment plan and this patient? ☐ Yes ☐ No
    If Yes, please explain:
    - ☐ IV needed additional days Number of additional day(s) ______________
    - ☐ Critical condition ☐ Other ______________

MD Action Plan:
See nursing recommendation(s). If two or more NO answers, consider discontinuation of all IV devices to reduce risk to patient.

FINALACTION:
☐ Discontinue device(s) ☐ Maintain device(s) ______________ # day(s)

For internal review: ☐ 25% ☐ 50% ☐ 75% ☐ 100%

Fig. A.2 Daily Assessment Tool (used with permission of Teleflex)

SAMPLE DAILY MONITORING TOOL

Clinical assessment due between 7A and 7p shift each day for each patient

Patient Name and Room Number: Date:

Clinician Name:

Please notify PICC/VAS Team if advanced assessment of device is needed.

Daily Assessment for Site Necessity:

Current Intravenous Devices (list all with quantity):

PIV **#1** Location: R / L; describe location size length of time in place (hrs/days)

Describe usage:

PIV **#2** Location: R / L; describe location size length of time in place (hrs/days)

Describe usage:

PICC Location: R / L; describe location size lumens **Describe usage:**

CVC Location (Chest /Neck): R / L; describe location lumens **Describe usage:**

Port Location: R / L; describe location **Describe usage:**

Current Infusions:

☐ Fluid Infusion - Type ☐ Intravenous Medications Check all that apply: ☐ Antibiotics ☐ Pain Meds ☐ TPN/PPN ☐ Chemotherapy ☐ Inotropes ☐ Other types

☐ Blood Draws from CVC, frequency _____

Venous Access Requirements:

☐ Peripheral sites adequate for prescribed therapy currently

☐ Peripheral vein sites available (prescriptive medications include known vein irritants)

Consider: ☐ Temporary Antimicrobial CVC ☐ PICC ☐ Tunneled CVC ☐ Port

☐ Limited peripheral sites – Central Venous Catheter needed

Consider: ☐ Temporary Antimicrobial CVC ☐ PICC ☐ Tunneled CVC ☐ Port

☐ Refer to Advanced Inserter under Vein Sparing Protocol -assessment related to patient diagnosis, complications as an inpatient and infusion history

https://www.ncbi.nlm.nih.gov/pmc/articles/PMC5417573/pdf/wocn-44-211.pdf

CVAD-Associated Skin Impairment (CASI) Algorithm

EXIT SITE INFECTION
Redness, induration (hard), and/or tenderness within 2 cm of the catheter exit site; possibly with other signs and symptoms of infection, such as fever or purulent drainage at exit site, concomitant bloodstream infections

If Exit Site Infection is Suspected:
- Culture site and draw blood cultures
- Collaborate with practitioner; may need to remove catheter
- Topical antimicrobial agent† (based on culture results) or consider non-CHG antimicrobial dressing
- If there is no resolution with topical therapy or it is accompanied by purulent drainage, start systemic antibiotics
- Consider cauterizing exuberant granulation tissue at site of long-term CVAD

†Confirm compatibility with dressing and catheter

SKIN INJURY
- Stripping: Shallow irregular lesions; shiny skin
- Tears: Partial or full thickness
- Tension blisters

- Consider non-alcohol antiseptic agent
- If skin flap present, approximate viable skin flap edges prior to dressing application

SKIN IRRITATION/CONTACT DERMATITIS
Skin color change (red, dark, shiny, dull) persisting 30 min. after dressing change (often mimics shape of dressing) and/or burning, itchy skin and/or lesions (macules, papules, vesicles, bullae)

- Rule out infiltration/extravasation, thrombophlebitis and other skin conditions (e.g., eczema, impetigo)
- Identify and avoid suspected irritant:
  - Change type/concentration of cleansing solution (**see Fig. 1**)
  - Ensure solution and barrier film are allowed to dry fully before dressing application
  - If no resolution, change brand/type of dressing
  - Consider open application test of dressing/antiseptic solution on unaffected skin (**see Fig. 2**)

WEEPING/OOZING
(Non-infectious)
Assess color, consistency, odor, amount and location of exudate

- Control bleeding: pressure at site, alginate and/or hemostatic agent under dressing
- Apply non-alcohol barrier film and absorbent dressing

- Apply alcohol-free barrier film and appropriate dressing
- Consider anti-inflammatory, anti-pruritic agents and/or analgesics; cool compresses (applied on top of dressing)
- Assess irritated skin every 24 hrs; monitor for signs and symptoms of infection
  - If no improvement to sites with suspected contact dermatitis, consider short-term use of topical corticosteroid (do not apply directly on exit site
- If no improvement within 3–7 days, consult wound/skin specialist

- Educate staff and/or patients/caregivers on proper dressing selection, atraumatic application/removal, site care
- Identify patients at risk and take precautions with site care (e.g., malnutrition, dehydration, elderly/neonates, dermatologic conditions, low/high humidity, radiation therapy, medications [chemotherapy, anti-inflammatories, including long-term corticosteroid use, anticoagulants])

Fig. 1–Reaction to CHG w/ Alcohol

Try CHG w/o alcohol
No improvement?
Try Povidone Iodine
No improvement?
Try sterile normal saline

Fig. 2–Open Application Test
1. Apply product to forearm
2. Monitor for 30–60 min.
3. Reassess in 3–4 days for signs of dermatitis

Dressing Usage Guide for CVAD Skin Impairment Management

Dressing*	Skin Injury (e.g., tear/blister)	Skin Irritation	Drainage Low	Drainage Med	Drainage High	Able to see site
Non-adherent non-woven gauze** (if skin intact or topical agent applied)		•	•			
Transparent film		•				Yes
Absorbent clear acrylic	•	•	•	•	•	Yes
Hydrocolloid (do not apply directly on CVAD exit site)		•	•	•		
Foam (silicone or low-tack)	•	•	•	•	•	
Alginate (also has hemostatic properties)	•			•	•	
Skin glue (2-octylcyanoacrylate alcohol-free topical bandage) + Cover Dressing	if skin flap can be approximated					Yes
Antimicrobial dressing***			•	•	•	

- Apply sterile alcohol-free skin barrier film prior to dressing (let dry before applying dressing)
- If skin damage/drainage is away from the exit site, isolate wound and exudate from exit site: apply absorbent dressing over area of injury and transparent dressing over exit site and prepped skin.
- If exudate leakage, use a different dressing with higher fluid handling capacity

*Stabilize catheter with securement device/dressing
**Does not provide a microbial barrier
***Assess manufacturer's contraindications. Recommend consult wound/skin specialist and/or physician.

Vessel Health and Preservation
Patient Satisfaction and Evaluation Tool

Patient Initials (if applicable): _________ Date: ___/___/____ Pt Adm Date: __/__/___
dd mm yyyy dd mm yyyy

Evaluator's Name: ______________________________ ☐ RN ☐ MD ☐ PHARM D ☐ Other: _______

Using the chart below, rate your satisfaction of your experience with your intravenous devices during your stay

Your Response	Very Satisfied	Satisfied	Neutral	Not Satisfied	Very Unsatisfied	Don't Know or Not Applicable
a. Were you satisfied with the intravenous (IV) device placed for your hospital treatment?	☐ 1	☐ 2	☐ 3	☐ 4	☐ 5	☐ N/A
b. Did you receive an adequate amount of information about your IV device, the purpose and need for the IV device?	☐ 1	☐ 2	☐ 3	☐ 4	☐ 5	☐ N/A
c. Were you satisfied with the choice of IV device and the reason for the device?	☐ 1	☐ 2	☐ 3	☐ 4	☐ 5	☐ N/A
d. Were you satisfied with the skill of the person placing the IV?	☐ 1	☐ 2	☐ 3	☐ 4	☐ 5	☐ N/A
e. Was the intravenous insertion procedure acceptable and relatively free from pain?	☐ 1	☐ 2	☐ 3	☐ 4	☐ 5	☐ N/A
f. Were you satisfied with the number of attempts necessary for the IV device?	☐ 1	☐ 2	☐ 3	☐ 4	☐ 5	☐ N/A
g. When your treatment was complete were you satisfied with how quickly your IV device was removed?	☐ 1	☐ 2	☐ 3	☐ 4	☐ 5	☐ N/A
h. Were you satisfied with the infection prevention education you received on how you can protect yourself?	☐ 1	☐ 2	☐ 3	☐ 4	☐ 5	☐ N/A
i. Were you satisfied with the attention to handwashing, scrubbing the hub and other infection prevention procedures practiced by the staff?	☐ 1	☐ 2	☐ 3	☐ 4	☐ 5	☐ N/A
j. Were you satisfied with your involvement as a participant in your treatment plan specific to IV devices and treatments?	☐ 1	☐ 2	☐ 3	☐ 4	☐ 5	☐ N/A
k. OVERALL your opinion of your IV therapy experience during your stay?	☐ 1	☐ 2	☐ 3	☐ 4	☐ 5	☐ N/A

1. What did you **NOT** LIKE about your IV experience?
2. What concerns, if any, about the staff or IV device?
3. What suggestions do you have for improvement?
4. Would you recommend this hospital to others?

☐ Yes ☐ No, because ____

Other commends? ____

Patient Name:____________________ **Date:** ____ / ____ / ____ **Clinician:**__________________

Day Month Year

Vessel Health and Preservation Evaluation Tool

This evaluation tool is a compliance tool to be used prior to patient being released from the hospital

(Key points reduces replacement of devices, reduces delays related to IV device and reduced cost with efficiency of IV device)

1. Was the right line protocol used to determine the best vascular access device. . for this patient? ☐ Yes ☐ No

2. Was the "right line" daily evaluation process completed throughout the stay?. . . ☐ Yes ☐ No

3. Was the vascular access device selected in the protocol placed within the first 24 hours of patient admittance?. . . . ☐ Yes ☐ No

4. Was the same vascular access device used during the entire hospital stay?. . . . ☐ Yes ☐ No

   If No, how many vascular access devices did the patient receive? ________

   What were the additional vascular access devices? __________________

   Why were they necessary? __________________________________

5. Were there any complications during the insertion procedure? . . . . ☐ Yes ☐ No

   If Yes, please explain: __________________________________

   ____

6. Were there any complications throughout therapy? . . . . ☐ Yes ☐ No

   If Yes, please identify the complication and expain below:

   ☐ Phlebitis ☐ Infection

   ☐ Thrombosis ☐ Other: ________________________________

   Explanation: ____

   ____

7. What was the original vessel health assessment for this patient?

   ☐ Very Poor ☐ Good

   ☐ Poor ☐ Very Good

   ☐ Fair ☐ Excellent

8. What is the vessel health assessment at the time of discharge for this patient?

   ☐ Very Poor ☐ Good

   ☐ Poor ☐ Very Good

   ☐ Fair ☐ Excellent

Permissions

All chapters in this book were first published by Springer; hereby published with permission under the Creative Commons Attribution License or equivalent. Every chapter published in this book has been scrutinized by our experts. Their significance has been extensively debated. The topics covered herein carry significant information for a comprehensive understanding. They may even be implemented as practical applications or may be referred to as a beginning point for further studies.

The contributors of this book come from diverse backgrounds, making this book a truly international effort. We would like to thank all the contributing authors for lending their expertise to make the book truly unique. They have played a crucial role in the development of this book. Without their invaluable contributions this book wouldn't have been possible. They have made vital efforts to compile up to date information on the varied aspects of this subject to make this book a valuable addition to the collection of many professionals and students.

This book was conceptualized with the vision of imparting up-to-date and integrated information in this field. To ensure the same, a matchless editorial board was set up. Every individual on the board went through rigorous rounds of assessment to prove their worth. After which they invested a large part of their time researching and compiling the most relevant data for our readers.

The editorial board has been involved in producing this book since its inception. They have spent rigorous hours researching and exploring the diverse topics which have resulted in the successful publishing of this book. They have passed on their knowledge of decades through this book. To expedite this challenging task, the publisher supported the team at every step. A small team of assistant editors was also appointed to further simplify the editing procedure and attain best results for the readers.

Apart from the editorial board, the designing team has also invested a significant amount of their time in understanding the subject and creating the most relevant covers. They scrutinized every image to scout for the most suitable representation of the subject and create an appropriate cover for the book.

The publishing team has been an ardent support to the editorial, designing and production team. Their endless efforts to recruit the best for this project, has resulted in the accomplishment of this book. They are a veteran in the field of academics and their pool of knowledge is as vast as their experience in printing. Their expertise and guidance has proved useful at every step. Their uncompromising quality standards have made this book an exceptional effort. Their encouragement from time to time has been an inspiration for everyone.

The publisher and the editorial board hope that this book will prove to be a valuable piece of knowledge for students, practitioners and scholars across the globe.

Index

M

N

P

Q

R

S

T

V

Printed in the USA
CPSIA information can be obtained
at www.ICGtesting.com
LVHW080034211023
761596LV00010BA/1759

9 781646 465866